Management of Chronic
Pelvic Pain

Management of Chronic Pelvic Pain

A Practical Manual

Edited by

Michael Hibner
Arizona Center for Chronic Pelvic Pain, Scottsdale, Arizona

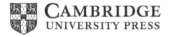

CAMBRIDGE
UNIVERSITY PRESS

University Printing House, Cambridge CB2 8BS, United Kingdom

One Liberty Plaza, 20th Floor, New York, NY 10006, USA

477 Williamstown Road, Port Melbourne, VIC 3207, Australia

314–321, 3rd Floor, Plot 3, Splendor Forum, Jasola District Centre,
New Delhi – 110025, India

103 Penang Road, #05–06/07, Visioncrest Commercial, Singapore 238467

Cambridge University Press is part of the University of Cambridge.

It furthers the University's mission by disseminating knowledge in the pursuit of
education, learning, and research at the highest international levels of excellence.

www.cambridge.org
Information on this title: www.cambridge.org/9781108819886
DOI: 10.1017/9781108877084

First published 2021
Reprinted 2022

Printed in Great Britain by Ashford Colour Press Ltd.

A catalogue record for this publication is available from the British Library.

Library of Congress Cataloging-in-Publication Data
Names: Hibner, Michael, editor.
Title: Management of chronic pelvic pain : a practical manual / edited by Michael Hibner, St Joseph's
Hospital & Medical Center, Phoenix, AZ.
Description: Cambridge, United Kingdom ; New York, NY : Cambridge University
Press, 2020. | Includes bibliographical references and index.
Identifiers: LCCN 2020019042 (print) | LCCN 2020019043 (ebook) | ISBN 9781108819886 (paperback) |
ISBN 9781108877084 (ebook)
Subjects: LCSH: Pelvic pain – Treatment. | Chronic pain – Treatment.
Classification: LCC RG483.P44 M36 2020 (print) | LCC RG483.P44 (ebook) | DDC 616/.0472–dc23
LC record available at https://lccn.loc.gov/2020019042
LC ebook record available at https://lccn.loc.gov/2020019043

ISBN 978-1-108-81988-6 Paperback

Every effort has been made in preparing this book to provide accurate and up-to-date information that is in accord with accepted
standards and practice at the time of publication. Although case histories are drawn from actual cases, every effort has been made to
disguise the identities of the individuals involved. Nevertheless, the authors, editors, and publishers can make no warranties that the
information contained herein is totally free from error, not least because clinical standards are constantly changing through research
and regulation. The authors, editors, and publishers therefore disclaim all liability for direct or consequential damages resulting from
the use of material contained in this book. Readers are strongly advised to pay careful attention to information provided by the
manufacturer of any drugs or equipment that they plan to use.

Contents

Contributors

Nicole Afuape, MD
Division of Surgery and Pelvic Pain,
St. Joseph's Hospital and Medical Center,
Creighton University School of Medicine,
Phoenix, AZ, USA

Diana T. Atashroo, MD
Division of Minimally Invasive Gynecologic Surgery
Stanford University
Palo Alto, California, USA

Elizabeth Banks, MD
Department of Obstetrics & Gynecology, University
of Pennsylvania, PA, USA

Bolesław Bendek, MD
Phoenix, AZ, USA

Karen Brandon, DPT
School of Allied Health Professionals,
Loma Linda University, Loma Linda, CA,
USA

Charles Butrick, MD, FPMRS
The Urogynecology Center, Overland Park, KS,
USA

Jorge Carrillo, MD
Gynecology Section, Division of Surgery, Orlando
VA Medical Center, Orlando, FL; and University of
Central Florida College of Medicine, Orlando, FL,
USA

Mario E. Castellanos, MD
Division of Surgery and Pelvic Pain, St. Joseph's
Hospital and Medical Center, Creighton University
School of Medicine, Phoenix, AZ, USA

Richard Cockrum, MD
Division of Minimally Invasive Gynecologic Surgery
NorthShore University Health System
Evanston, IL, USA

Mark Dassel, MD
Center for Endometriosis and Chronic Pelvic Pain,
Cleveland Clinic; and Case Western Reserve
University, Cleveland, OH, USA

Nita Desai, MD
Division of Surgery and Pelvic Pain, St. Joseph's
Hospital and Medical Center, Creighton University
School of Medicine, Phoenix, AZ, USA

Katherine de Souza, MD
Division of Minimally Invasive Gynecologic
Surgery, Penn State Health Milton S. Hershey Medical
Center, Penn State College of Medicine, Hershey, PA,
USA

Katherine M. Fretz, MSc
Pain Research Lab, Department of Psychology,
Queen's University, Kingston, ONT, Canada

Sheena Galhotra, MD
Division of Minimally Invasive Gynecologic Surgery
University of Arizona Medical Center
Phoenix, Arizona

Ashley L Gubbels, MD
University of Rochester Medical School, Rochester,
NY, USA

Alyssa Herrmann, MD
Cleveland Clinic, Cleveland, OH, USA

Michael Hibner, MD, PhD
Arizona Center for Chronic Pelvic Pain, Scottsdale,
AZ, USA; and University of Arizona College of
Medicine, Phoenix, AZ, USA

Lauren Hill, PT, DPT, WCS
Division of Surgery and Pelvic Pain, St. Joseph's
Hospital and Medical Center, Creighton University
School of Medicine, Phoenix, AZ, USA

Mohammad R. Islam, MD
Division of Minimally Invasive Gynecologic Surgery University of Arizona Medical Center Phoenix, Arizona, USA

Maryam R. Kashi, DO
Endoscopy Unit, Central Florida Gastroenterology & Hepatology, AdventHealth Medical Group, Orlando, FL, USA

Seetha Lakshmanan, MD
Department of Internal Medicine, Roger Williams Medical Center, Providence, RI, USA

Georgine Lamvu, MD, MPH
Division of Surgery, Gynecology Section, Orlando VA Medical Center; and University of Central Florida College of Medicine, Orlando, FL, USA

Javier F. Magrina, MD
Division of Gynecology, Mayo Clinic, Phoenix, AZ, USA

Joseph M. Maurice, MD, MS, FACOG
Department of Obstetrics and Gynecology,

Carle Illinois College of Medicine
Urbana, IL, USA

J. Curtis Nickel, MD, FRCSC
Department of Urology, Queen's University, Kingston, ONT, Canada

Anna Reinert, MD
Division of Obstetrics, Gynecology, and Gynecologic Sub-Specialties, Department of Obstetrics and Gynecology, Keck School of Medicine, University of Southern California, Los Angeles, CA, USA

Dean A. Tripp, PhD
Departments of Psychology, Anesthesia & Urology, Queen's University, Kingston, ONT, Canada

Debra Wickman, MS, MD, FACOG, CSE
Sexual Medicine, Banner – University Medicine Women's Institute, Phoenix, AZ; and Department of Obstetrics and Gynecology, University of Arizona College of Medicine, Tucson, AZ, USA

Foreword

Fred M. Howard, MS, MD

I am excited that Dr. Hibner has edited this comprehensive textbook on chronic pelvic pain. Such a broad-based book is needed to educate those new to the management of chronic pelvic pain and as a reference for those actively providing care to patients with chronic pelvic pain. Dr. Hibner has chosen authors with special expertise in pelvic pain, including several who have done post-residency fellowships in the discipline.

It is particularly moving to me to see such growth of interest in improving the care of women with chronic pelvic pain. In the 1980s, when I chose to dedicate much of my career to the care of women with chronic pelvic pain and to the education of healthcare providers about the affliction, there was very little interest in either. I was in private practice in Greenville, South Carolina, and kept seeing patients with chronic pelvic pain and realized I was not prepared to manage their conditions well. I started educating myself as best I could, but at that time there were few sources of good information. But fortunately, there were two physicians, Dr. John Steege and Dr. John Slocumb, who had strong interests in pelvic pain and were mentors from whom I learned much. When I left private practice to return to academic medicine in 1991, there was still little interest by most physicians in the care of women with chronic pelvic pain. My first publication as an academic physician was a long treatise on the role of laparoscopy in chronic pelvic pain. At that time, laparoscopy was viewed by gynecologists as essential to evaluation of pelvic pain and by many was thought to be the ultimate and definitive diagnostic test. In the 1990s it still was common practice after a negative laparoscopy to tell a patient one or more of the following:

1. Nothing is wrong.
2. The pain is in your head ("supratentorial" was a derogatory way we sometimes stated this to colleagues) and you need to see a psychiatrist for psychiatric problems.
3. You need a nerve-cutting procedure, such as a uterine nerve transection or presacral neurectomy.
4. The only thing left to do is a hysterectomy.
5. Nothing can be done and you must learn to live with the pain.

We have learned much in the 30 years since and now it would be rare for a gynecologist to counsel a patient with any of those five recommendations.

We now know laparoscopy has a limited role in diagnosing causes of pelvic pain. For example, in this textbook there are chapters on pelvic pain arising from endometriosis and pelvic pain arising from adhesive disease. These are disorders in which laparoscopy may have a diagnostic role. In contrast to these two chapters, there are eight chapters on disorders in which laparoscopy has no diagnostic role: pelvic pain arising from interstitial cystitis, pelvic pain arising from pelvic congestion syndrome, pelvic pain arising from irritable bowel syndrome, vulvodynia, pelvic pain arising from ovarian remnant syndrome, pudendal neuralgia, pain arising from mesh implants, and myofascial pain and pelvic floor muscle spasm.

This book will add significantly to the quality of care that women with chronic pelvic pain receive. My hope is that it will be widely read and its messages will be incorporated into the practice of all healthcare providers caring for women with pelvic pain. I commend Dr. Hibner and his colleagues on this work.

Introduction to Chronic Pelvic Pain

Michael Hibner, Nicole Afuape, and Bolesław Bendek

Editor's Introduction

Pelvic pain is a condition which is much more common than perceived by the medical and general community. Because it affects the most private aspects of human life such as sexuality and reproduction, patients are not willing to discuss it with their families, friends, and loved ones. Medical providers are also very likely to dismiss the symptoms and blame it on a psychological or psychiatric conditions. Chronic pelvic pain is real, it is common, and it is almost always due to some identifiable disease or injury. Patients with pelvic pain need to be heard and treated with dignity and respect, and the majority of them can be helped.

In at the conquer'd doors they crowd! I am possess'd!
Embody all presences outlaw'd or suffering,
See myself in prison shaped like another man,
And feel the dull unintermitted pain.
Walt Whitman, *Song of Myself*

Pain is one of the most feared and dreaded human sensations. It is derived from the Latin *poena* – punishment. Pain, thirst, and hunger responses are considered to be the most primordial of human emotions [1]. Unlike higher emotions such as love, hate, and anger, these primordial sensations involve lower brain regions such as the medulla, midbrain, and hypothalamus. Pain may occur as an acute event or as a persistent, long-term symptom. While acute pain or nociception serves as an alert of trauma and impending damage, chronic pain is a disease and can easily become one of the most debilitating conditions that one can endure.

In 1979 the International Association for the Study of Pain (IASP) defined pain as "an unpleasant sensory and emotional experience associated with actual or potential tissue damage, or described in terms of such damage" [2]. This definition is incomplete because it excludes the clinically significant social and cognitive components of pain. Also, describing pain merely as an unpleasant sensation minimizes patient suffering and may influence bias in the approach of practitioners.

Over the years our understanding of pain has changed dramatically. The pain experience is characterized by tremendous interindividual variability. By definition, pain is a subjective and personal experience, inherently making clinical practice and research challenging. A multitude of biological and psychological factors contribute to these differences: genetic, psychosocial, and demographic processes inherently influence each other, contributing to the overall pain experience. Historically, pain researchers have focused intellectual pursuits on legitimizing these differences.

Nociceptive pain originates in damaged tissues, usually secondary to a noxious stimulus, and neuropathic pain is caused by a disease of the nervous system. Superficial nociceptive pain originates in the pain receptors (nociceptors) located in the skin. Deep nociceptive pain may be either somatic or visceral. Deep somatic nociceptors located in the muscles, tendons, ligaments, bones, and blood vessels usually produce dull and poorly localized pain. Deep visceral nociceptive pain originates in the visceral receptors and may be well localized; however, this localization rarely corresponds with the area of injury because of pain referral patterns. This phenomenon is commonly seen in conditions such as painful bladder syndrome, in which presenting symptoms may include back or vulvar pain. Neuropathic pain may originate in the peripheral or central nervous system, as a result of disease or intrinsic malfunction. Peripheral neuropathic pain is more common, producing sensations of burning, tingling, electrical shocks, or pins and needles. Table 1.1 outlines common terms used in clinical descriptions of abnormal pain function.

Acute pain is an essential evolutionary sensation that prompts a change in position or behavior, usually in response to some noxious stimulus, with the

Table 1.1 Common terms used in pain conditions

Allodynia	Pain in response to the stimulus that is normally non painful
Hyperalgesia	Exaggerated response to a stimulus that is normally painful
Central sensitization	Up-regulation of central nervous system, causing the sensation of higher intensity pain with less provocation. Allodynia and hyperalgesia are signs of central sensitization
Analgesia	Absence of pain in response to painful stimulus
Dysesthesia	An unpleasant abnormal sensation. May be spontaneous or evoked
Paresthesia	An abnormal sensation. Unlike dysesthesia it does not need to be unpleasant
Hyperesthesia	Increased sensitivity to stimulation
Allotriesthesia	Pain caused by the sensation of a foreign body in the absence of a foreign body
Neuralgia	Pain in the distribution of the nerve. By definition it does not require nerve injury
Neuritis	Pain caused by inflammation of the nerve
Neuropathy	A disturbance of function or pathological change in a nerve
Noxious stimulus	A stimulus that is strong enough to damage normal tissues, usually prompting a reactive pain response
Peripheral sensitization	Increased sensitivity to an afferent nerve stimulus. Occurs after injury to the area, which results in the flare-up response
Nociceptive pain	Pain originating in the pain receptors in the skin (superficial), muscles, tendons, blood vessels (deep), or visceral organs, usually secondary to a noxious stimulus
Neuropathic pain	Pain originating in the peripheral or central nervous system, resulting from disease or intrinsic malfunction
Wind-up phenomenon	Perceived increase in pain intensity due to repetitive painful stimulus. Caused by activation of normally dormant receptors
Viscerosomatic convergence	Noxious stimulus to the viscera triggers pain referred to somatic sites
Viscerovisceral convergence	Noxious stimulus to the viscera triggers pain referred to other visceral sites
Functional somatic syndrome	Physical symptoms that are poorly explained. Encompasses conditions like chronic fatigue, fibromyalgia, irritable bowel syndrome, tension headache, and others
Somatization	Manifestation of mental phenomena as physical symptoms
Conversion disorder	Neurological symptoms such as numbness, blindness, or paralysis in the absence of organic cause and traced back to a psychological trigger

goal of preventing any further damage to tissues. Pain has been studied in numerous animal species, including fish and invertebrates such as the fruit fly. Across species, it has been demonstrated that acute pain serves not only as a warning of external trauma, but also as a symptom of numerous internal disease processes. In humans, acute pain may serve as a lifesaving symptom of medical emergencies such as myocardial infarction. Chronic pain, on the other hand, does not always serve a clear essential purpose and can actually become a disease of its own. The general mechanism of chronic pain has clear differences from that of acute pain. The majority of patients who experience tissue trauma with acute

pain will heal without any sequelae. After physical healing is complete, a small percentage of these patients will continue to experience pain. Chronic pain may result from a number of other mechanisms including degenerative disease resulting from aging or overuse, and abnormal or insufficient healing following acute physical trauma. Chronic pain may also present as a primary condition, lacking any identifiable cause. It is theorized that in some instances, the central nervous system may produce independent pain input without an external or internal pain stimulus. Regardless of origin, the mechanism of chronic pain generally has some relation to musculoskeletal or nervous system function.

Maladaptive plasticity changes in the nervous system that lead to a disruption in function, producing a disease state, have been described in a large number of clinical trials and animal studies. Additionally, these changes may also occur in sensory conduction pathways between the peripheral and central nervous system, resulting in the development and maintenance of chronic pain. Central sensitization represents the manner in which pain is uncoupled from the clear noxious stimulus that defines acute nociceptive pain. Instead, the features of pain are reflective of the functional state of the central nervous system, the memory of persistent pain, and the associated sensory conduction pathways. Central sensitization results in an alteration of the induction, spatial extent, intensity, and duration of pain [3].

A key difference between an acute episode of pain and chronic pain is that the persistence of this sensation can lead to a number of adverse sequelae including physical suffering, sleep disorders, fatigue, and substance abuse. Because chronic pain and mood control share the same neurotransmitters, these patients often suffer from mood disorders such as depression, bipolar disease, obsessive–compulsive disorder, and posttraumatic stress disorder. Persistent pain can also lead to significant social concerns including difficulty with intimacy, strain on personal relationships, and poor professional performance. Decline in physical activity in patients with chronic pain often causes weight gain, deconditioning, and other secondary morbidities.

Prevalence and Impact of Chronic Pain

The prevalence of chronic pain is difficult to estimate. In the industrialized world anywhere from 20% to 50% of people suffer from pain for more than 6 months during some point in their lifetime. In the United States the prevalence of chronic pain is approximately 30.7%, translating to an estimate of 90 million people living in pain. Chronic pelvic pain affects 5.7%–26.6% of reproductive-age women, with variation in these numbers influenced by population characteristics [4]. It is estimated that one in seven women meet clinical criteria of chronic pelvic pain at some point in their lives. In women the prevalence of chronic pelvic pain is higher than that of asthma, diabetes, and coronary artery disease and almost as high as that of back pain [5].

This vast number of affected individuals has led to significant social and economic sequelae. The total annual cost associated with pain in the United States has been estimated to be between 560 and 635 billion dollars, which is higher than the combined annual cost associated with heart disease and cancer. Other studies estimate the economic impact of chronic pain to be 3% of GDP.

Between 1999 and 2016, more than 630,000 people died from a drug overdose in the United States. In 2016, an estimated 48.5 million persons in the United States reported use of illicit drugs or misuse of prescription drugs in the past year, of which 4.3% were prescription pain relievers; this translates to 2 million individuals [6]. In 2017 healthcare providers wrote on average 58.5 prescriptions per 100 persons. Even though opioid prescribing continued to decrease through 2017, more efforts are needed to help healthcare providers adopt and maintain safe prescribing habits.

The Diagnostic Challenges of Chronic Pelvic Pain

Chronic pelvic pain is a common and often underdiagnosed condition occurring in both women and men. Although this book specifically focuses on chronic pelvic pain in women, chronic pain in men is equally frequent and devastating, with similar challenges in diagnosis and management.

The International Pelvic Pain Society defines chronic pelvic pain as pain located in the pelvis, persisting for 6 months or longer, with or without association with menstrual cycles and severe enough to cause functional disability [7]. Up to one in seven women meet this clinical criterion over the span of their lifetime. Despite this high prevalence, the condition remains relatively underdiagnosed and untreated. This is at least in part due to the suboptimal education of clinicians on the subject of female chronic pelvic pain. In the United States, most medical school curricula lack even a single lecture dedicated to chronic pelvic pain in women, and postgraduate obstetrics and gynecology training tends to limit this training to endometriosis and painful bladder syndrome. This approach produces clinicians who are ill prepared for the diagnosis and management of the wide range of gynecological and nongynecological conditions that can lead to chronic pelvic pain.

Most women with pelvic pain have more than one condition contributing to their pain, further complicating diagnostic workup. This is commonly true in the case of endometriosis. Dr. Fred Howard, a pioneer in the area of chronic female pelvic pain in the United States, made an observation in his practice that more than three-quarters of patients with endometriosis and pelvic pain have another etiology contributing to their pain, in addition to their endometriosis. This means that if the only intervention offered to these women is treatment of endometriotic lesions, more than half will likely not experience adequate improvement in their chronic pain.

The diagnosis of pelvic pain is further challenged by the fact that many patients with chronic pelvic pain do not have easily identifiable pathology. The American College of Obstetricians and Gynecologists (ACOG) highlights bloodwork, ultrasonography, cystoscopy, sigmoidoscopy, colonoscopy, and laparoscopy as potential workup modalities that may be helpful in working toward a diagnosis in patients with chronic pelvic pain, based on presenting symptoms [8]. It has been reported that up to 30% of women with pelvic pain have completely normal findings on laparoscopy [9]. In the remaining 70% of patients the most common surgical findings were lesions consistent with endometriosis and adhesions. The severity of endometriosis and adhesions tends to be only marginally correlated with the severity of chronic pelvic pain [10]. Only deep infiltrating endometriosis has been shown to be associated with more pain [11]. In light of the inconsistent findings in the clinical workup of patients with chronic pelvic pain, ACOG has previously concluded that "few, if any of the diseases thought to cause chronic pelvic pain meet traditional epidemiological criteria of causality"[12].

A final key point is that more than 70% of the causes of chronic pelvic pain may be nongynecological, further contributing to diagnostic challenges. Musculoskeletal causes of pain are often overlooked in the evaluation and workup of chronic pelvic pain, and data regarding the true prevalence are limited. Based on a retrospective, cross-sectional study conducted using a population in a single chronic pelvic pain specialty clinic, Tu et al. estimated that the prevalence of pelvic floor musculoskeletal disorders in their patients was 14%–22% [13]. Based on our practice experience, which is approaching two decades of work, this is a gross underestimation. Up to 74% of patients with chronic pelvic pain will have an identifiable abdominal wall trigger point with proper clinical evaluation, and 71% have focal areas of pain along the pelvic floor muscles (ie. levator ani, obturator interni) and piriformis muscles on vaginal exam [14]. The

most common musculoskeletal contributor to chronic pelvic pain is spasm of the pelvic floor muscles. This spasm may be primary or secondary. Causes of primary spasm are unknown but it may be due to genetic abnormalities or inherent diseases of the muscles that make them more prone to spasm. Secondary spastic pelvic floor may result from irritation of pelvic viscera, physical pelvic trauma, or psychological insult. Irritation of the pelvic viscera may be associated with endometriosis or pelvic inflammatory disease (PID). Accidents, athletic activity, or simply overworking pelvic and lower extremity muscles can lead to pelvic trauma. Pelvic surgery and childbirth with seemingly uncomplicated clinical course may provoke pelvic floor muscle spasms. Psychological insult may include psychological trauma and sexual violence. Musculoskeletal causes of pain will be discussed in detail in Chapter 20.

Another common cause of chronic pelvic pain is painful bladder syndrome. It will be discussed in detail in Chapter 9. Painful bladder syndrome is also often referred to as interstitial cystitis or bladder pain syndrome. This syndrome often coexists with other pelvic pain disorders. Painful bladder syndrome is not simply a disease of the bladder; it is a condition mediated by the intricate connection between the viscera, muscles, and central nervous system. Table 1.2 lists a number of other gynecological and nongynecological conditions that may manifest as chronic pelvic pain.

Table 1.2 Causes of chronic pelvic pain

Gynecological
Endometriosis
Adenomyosis
Primary dysmenorrhea
Pelvic congestion
Pelvic masses
Ovarian entrapment/remnant
Pelvic infections/pelvic inflammatory disease
Surgical
Adhesions
Urological
Interstitial cystitis/bladder pain syndrome
Urethritis
Urolithiasis
Gastroenterological
Irritable bowel syndrome

Table 1.2 (cont.)

Diverticulitis

Ileitis

Chronic appendicitis

Neurological

Nerve entrapment

Complex regional pain syndrome

Musculoskeletal

Spastic pelvic floor syndrome

Sacroiliac joint instability

Psychosomatic

Physical and/or sexual abuse

Depression

Anxiety

Personality disorder

We hope that this text will serve as a primary resource for addressing the challenges that clinicians face in caring for chronic pelvic pain patients. The following chapters will assist in defining the theories and components of chronic pelvic pain development. They will also provide diagnosis and management algorithms that can be used to optimize the care for these patients.

Five Things You Need to Know

- Chronic pelvic pain is defined as pain located in the pelvis, persisting for 6 months or longer, with or without association with menstrual cycles and severe enough to cause functional disability.
- In the industrialized world anywhere from 20% to 50% of people suffer from pain for more than 6 months during some point in their lifetime.
- Up to 70% of patients with chronic pelvic pain have a nongynecological cause of their pain.
- More than 60% of patients with chronic pelvic pain treated in general obstetrics/gynecology practice do not have a proper diagnosis.
- Most patients with chronic pelvic pain have multiple reasons for pain: endometriosis, interstitial cystitis, and irritable bowel syndrome coexist in many of these patients.

References

1. Denton D. *The Primordial Emotions: The Dawning of Consciousness.* Oxford: Oxford University Press; 2012. DOI: 10.1093/acprof:oso/9780199203147.001.0001.

2. Williams A, Craig K. Updating the definition of pain. *Pain.* 2016;**11**(1):2420–3.

3. Woolf CJ. Central sensitization: implications for the diagnosis and treatment of pain. *Pain.* 2011;**152** (3 Suppl):S2–15. DOI: 10.1016/j.pain.2010.09.030.

4. Ahangari A. Prevalence of chronic pelvic pain among women: an updated review. *Pain Physician.* 2014;**17** (2):E141.

5. Zondervan K, Barlow DH. Epidemiology of chronic pelvic pain. *Best Pract Res Clin Obstet Gynaecol.* 2000;**14**(3):403–14. DOI: 10.1053/beog.1999.0083.

6. CDC National Center for Injury Prevention and Control. 2018 Annual surveillance report of drug-related risks and outcomes.

7. Howard FM. The role of laparoscopy in chronic pelvic pain: promise and pitfalls. *Obstet Gynecol Surv.* 1993;**48**(6):357–87.

8. ACOG. *Chronic Pelvic Pain.* 2014

9. Howard FM. The role of laparoscopy in chronic pelvic pain: promise and pitfalls. *Obstet Gynecol Surv.* 1993;**48**(6):357–87. DOI: 10.1097/00006254-199306000-00001.

10. Vercellini P, Fedele L, Aimi G, Pietropaolo G, Consonni D, Crosignani PG, et al. Association between endometriosis stage, lesion type, patient characteristics and severity of pelvic pain symptoms: a multivariate analysis of over 1000 patients. *Hum Reprod.* 2007;**22** (1):266–71. DOI: 10.1093/humrep/del339.

11. Fauconnier A, Chapron C, Dubuisson JB, Vieira M, Dousset B, Bréart G. Relation between pain symptoms and the anatomic location of deep infiltrating endometriosis. *Fertil Steril.* 2002;**78**:719–26. DOI: 10.1016/S0015-0282(02)03331-9.

12. ACOG Committee on Practice Bulletins. Practice Bulletin No. 51. Chronic pelvic pain. *Obstet Gynecol.* 2004**103**(3):589–605 (out of print).

13. Tu FF, Sanie SA, Steege JF. Prevalence of pelvic musculoskeletal disorders in a female chronic pelvic pain clinic. *J Reprod Med.* 2006;**51**(3):185–9.

14. Slocumb JC. Neurological factors in chronic pelvic pain: trigger points and the abdominal pelvic pain syndrome. *Am J Obstet Gynecol.* 1984;**149** (5):536–43.

Neurobiological Basis of Pelvic Pain

Ashley L. Gubbels

Editor's Introduction

Nerve pain is more often than not a cause of pelvic pain. This is particularly true in patients in whom pain started after pelvic trauma, surgery, or vaginal delivery. Unfortunately, most of gynecologists who are often physicians of primary contact for pelvic pain patients are not trained in recognizing and treating patients with nerve injury pain. Patients with nerve injury pain can almost always pinpoint the moment when the pain started. It is often unilateral and neuropathic in nature. Patients have a burning, tingling sensation often associated with increased sensitivity to stimuli analogous to skin pain after sunburn. Pain is often exacerbated by body movements and certain body positions. It is very important for the first provider who sees patients with pelvic pain that pain may be related to nerve injury because expeditious treatment increases the chances of recovery. It is also important to instruct patients to avoid activity that started the pain in the first place and minimize activity that exacerbates the pain. Trial of muscle relaxants, gabapentin, or pregabalin may be appropriate first treatment; however, prompt referral to physical therapy, neurology, or a specialized pelvic pain center is often necessary.

Introduction

Chronic pain is defined by the International Academy for the Study of Pain as "pain without apparent biological value that has persisted beyond the normal tissue healing time (usually taken to be 3 months)" [1]. It has been estimated that more than 30% of Americans suffer from chronic pain. According to the 2011 Institute of Medicine Report "Relieving Pain in America: A Blueprint for Transforming Prevention, Care, Education, and Research," pain is a significant problem costing US society at least $560 to $635 billion annually [2]. Although repeat estimates have not been published, the rates of chronic pain and accompanying opioid abuse have only been increasing. The understanding of the pathophysiology of pain is constantly evolving and this chapter attempts to summarize our current knowledge.

Pertinent Anatomy

Abdominal and pelvic pain can originate from the gynecological, urological, gastrointestinal, neurological, or musculoskeletal systems. Often pain may stem from multiple systems simultaneously. To understand the complex interplay between these systems and structures, one must understand the neuroanatomy involved. Abdominal and pelvic pain can stem from the somatic system (T12–S5) or the visceral system (T10–S5). Somatic pain arises from skin, muscles, joints, and the pleural and peritoneal lining. Visceral pain arises from the hollow organs of the abdominopelvic cavity including the bladder, bowel, uterus, and fallopian tubes. The complexity of pelvic pain is in part related to the interactions between these two systems. Of importance, the visceral nerves converge on the same somatic levels in the thoracic, lumbar, and sacral spinal cord. This is termed viscerosomatic convergence and can result in visceral pain being perceived in somatic regions. With time, muscles innervated by the stimulated somatic nerves can develop trigger points leading to worsening somatic pain. Viscerovisceral convergence can also occur, leading to referred symptoms in other organs. This neural convergence can also be useful therapeutically to treat pain.

Somatic Pain

Peripheral neuropathic pain typically has a very specific localization along nerve distributions. Nerve injury can occur through a variety of mechanisms such as trauma, stretch, compression, fibrosis, or entrapment. Understanding neuroanatomical relationships, especially within the pelvis, is vital to both diagnosis and treatment.

The abdominal wall is innervated by the thoracoabdominal intercostal nerves (T6–T12) along with the iliohypogastric and ilioinguinal nerves. The intercostal nerves travel between the transversus abdominis and internal oblique muscles within the transversus abdominis plane (TAP). At the midaxillary line, perforating branches diverge to innervate the lateral abdominal wall. The segmental nerves of T6–T9 perforate the abdominal wall along the path of the anterior costal margin. The remaining intercostal nerves perforate the rectus abdominis sheath, providing sensation to the anterior abdominal wall. Near the anterior superior iliac spine (ASIS) the ilioinguinal and iliohypogastric nerves, which previously ran within the TAP, transition to travel between the internal and external oblique muscles.

The iliohypogastric nerve arises from the T12–L1 spinal segments. It travels through the psoas and transversus abdominis muscle, coursing medially below the internal oblique. It splits into two branches, with the anterior branch piercing the external oblique muscle at the level of the ASIS to provide cutaneous sensation to the mons pubis and the lateral branch to the posterolateral gluteal region. This nerve converges on the dorsal horn structures shared by the distal fallopian tube and ovary.

The ilioinguinal nerve arises from L1–L2 spinal segments. It follows a course similar to that of the iliohypogastric nerve but enters the inguinal canal 2 cm medial to the ASIS. It exits the superficial inguinal ring to provide sensation to the groin, labia majora, and the medial aspect of the thigh. It converges with the neurons of the proximal fallopian tube and uterine fundus.

The genitofemoral nerve also arises from the L1–L2 spinal segments and converges with neurons from the proximal fallopian tube and uterine fundus. It courses through the psoas muscle, exiting along its medial border at the L4 vertebral level, where it divides into a genital and femoral branch. The genital branch supplies the mons pubis and labia majora while the femoral branch supplies the skin of the femoral triangle. It can commonly be injured as a result of post-appendectomy fibrosis or hernia repair.

The obturator nerve arises from L2–L4 spinal segments and travels along the pelvic sidewall, exiting the pelvis through a tunnel in the pubic ramus, and then divides into two branches. The anterior branch sends motor fibers to the adductor longus, adductor brevis, and gracilis and sensory fibers to the distal medial two thirds of the thigh. The posterior branch sends motor fibers to the adductor magnus and sensory fibers to the knee joint.

The lateral femoral cutaneous nerve arises from L2–L3. It courses over the iliacus muscle, passing under the inguinal ligament to provide sensory fibers to the upper outer thigh. Although it does not innervate any structures in the pelvis, it converges with neurons from the uterus in the dorsal horn.

The pudendal nerve arises from S2–S4. It carries motor, sensory, and autonomic fibers. The sensory component of the nerve innervates the clitoris, labia, distal one third of the vagina, perineum, and rectum. The motor component innervates the external urethral sphincter, perineal muscles, and external anal sphincter. After exiting the sacrum, it travels inferiorly and laterally on the anterior surface of the piriformis muscle. Once it enters the gluteal region it joins the pudendal artery and vein, which accompany the nerve through its course. It briefly exits the pelvis through the greater sciatic foramen and reenters through the lesser sciatic foramen, where it passes between the sacrospinous and sacrotuberous ligaments approximately 1 cm medial to the ischial spine. In this location the nerve is the most dorsal structure. It then travels through the aponeurosis of the obturator internus muscle, an area referred to as Alcock's canal. On exiting the canal, it divides into the inferior rectal nerve, the perineal nerve, and the dorsal clitoral (penile) nerve. The pudendal nerve converges in the dorsal horn on neurons from the cervix, uterosacral ligaments, and vulvovaginal region. Reference Chapter 15 for further detailed information about the pudendal nerve and its involvement in chronic pelvic pain.

The nerve to the levator ani is separate from the pudendal nerve. This nerve arises from S3–S5 and travels along the superior surface of the coccygeal muscle and innervates the coccygeus, iliococcygeus, pubococcygeus, and puborectalis [3]. The nerves to the levator ani and the pudendal nerve run approximately 5–6 mm from one another at the level of the ischial spine; therefore, a pudendal nerve block often results in a block of both.

7

Visceral Pain

Visceral pain is mediated through the autonomic nervous system via the sympathetic and parasympathetic divisions. The autonomic innervation of the pelvis is via the superior and inferior hypogastric plexi. The superior hypogastric plexus overlies the L4–S1 vertebrae along the sacral promontory. It contains sympathetic fibers from the lumbar sympathetic chains and the aortic plexus. The inferior hypogastric plexus is formed by the hypogastric nerves carrying sympathetic fibers from the superior hypogastric plexus and parasympathetic fibers from the pelvic splanchnic nerves. Sympathetic fibers inhibit peristalsis of organs and stimulate muscle contraction during orgasm. Parasympathetic fibers stimulate peristalsis of the bladder and rectum to facilitate urination and defecation as well as erectile function.

The ganglion impar is a singular structure located retroperitoneally at the level of the sacrococcygeal junction. It is the terminal fusion of the two sacral sympathetic chains, and it provides nociceptive and sympathetic input to the perineum, distal rectum, urethra, and vagina. Blocks of the ganglion impar are used to treat intractable perineal pain, poorly localized visceral pelvic pain, and coccydynia.

Acute Pain Processing

To understand chronic pain, it is first important to understand the physiology of acute, nociceptive pain processing. Pain processing involves multiple steps: transduction, transmission, perception, and modulation. Any insult or injury to tissue activates nociceptors. These are free nerve endings that serve as sensory receptors to detect damage or threat of damage to tissue. The ability to sense pain is a protective biological mechanism. Nociceptors are found in the dermis, muscles, connective tissues, synovia, parietal pleura, and peritoneal membranes. Nociceptive activation occurs from stimulation of either visceral or somatic structures. Different classes of nociceptors respond to different stimuli such as mechanical, thermal, or inflammatory trauma. Aδ fibers are small myelinated fibers that sense temperature and sharp pain and conduct at a rate of 5–30 m/s [4]. Aβ fibers sense nonpainful touch. C-fibers are small-diameter unmyelinated axons that respond to multiple types of stimuli such as dull pain, temperature, and itch. They conduct signals at a rate of 0.4–1.4 m/s and represent about 70% of all nociceptive fibers in the body.

Somatosensory nociceptors have a single process emanating from the cell body in the dorsal root ganglion (DRG) that bifurcates, sending one axon to the peripheral tissue and another to synapses on second-order neurons within the dorsal horn of the spinal cord [5]. This functions to reduce the risk of conduction failure.

Initial injury leads to localized tissue damage that produces neurogenic inflammation and release of histamine, prostaglandins, bradykinin, and substance P at the site of injury. These peptides are sensed at the free nerve ending and transduced into an electrical signal that is then transmitted to the dorsal horn. Nociceptors are excitatory neurons and release glutamate as a primary neurotransmitter along with other peptides such as substance P, calcitonin gene-related peptide (CGRP), and somatostatin [5]. The second-order neuron in the spinal cord is then activated within the anterolateral system. The anterolateral system has both a direct pathway, in which Aδ fibers run within the spinothalamic tract, and an indirect pathway, in which C-fibers run within the spinoreticular tract [6]. The Aδ fiber second-order neurons cross over to the contralateral spinothalamic tract and transmit the information to the thalamus, where pain is perceived. They then synapse onto a third-order neuron that relays the signal to the somatosensory cortex for localization. The C-fiber first-order neurons first synapse onto interneurons. These interneurons then synapse on second-order neurons within the ipsilateral and contralateral spinoreticular tracts that convey information into the reticular formation in the brainstem. Impulses from the reticular formation are then relayed bilaterally to the thalamus, where they are perceived as well as relayed to the primary somatosensory cortex, hypothalamus, and limbic system.

Noxious stimuli or injury to tissue induces physiological processes meant to signal a problem and protect us from further injury. Following tissue damage, locally noxious substances are released leading to a decrease in the threshold of C-fibers for activation and pain perception. This is termed primary hyperalgesia. This process occurs by upregulation of existing receptors that results in an increased response to the same concentration of neurotransmitters or mechanical stimulus. There is also an increase in the number of receptors in response to nerve growth factor. This combination results in primary hyperalgesia of the injured area. The area surrounding the injury is termed the "zone of flare," which becomes increasingly sensitive to mechanical stimuli (secondary hyperalgesia) as well as exhibiting pain in response to innocuous stimuli (allodynia) [7]. This process is termed peripheral sensitization and evolutionarily served as a protective process to allow us to heal. For example, if you burn your hand, the injured tissue releases various noxious chemicals, which leads to neurogenic inflammation and a primary zone of injury. Surrounding uninjured tissue becomes further sensitized as a protective mechanism to keep you from grabbing things with your hand and potentially injuring it further. This eventually resolves because of plasticity in the nervous system. Once healing takes place, the system can and typically does revert back to its preinjured state.

The experience of pain is much more than the detection of noxious stimuli. Emotions have a significant effect on our experience of pain. According to the International Association for the Study of Pain (IASP), pain is defined as an unpleasant sensory and emotional experience associated with actual or potential tissue damage [8]. The perception of pain is influenced by mood, past experiences, and expectations and in short, it is the affective component that makes pain painful. While the somatosensory cortex determines characteristics such as location and duration, the anterior cingulate cortex (ACC) and insula, part of the limbic system, are responsible for the emotional aspects of pain perception. Our understanding of this aspect of pain sensation is more limited. A number of studies have found that even observing another individual in pain can activate some of these same areas of the brain in the observer. This can result in "priming" of the brain and effect the subject's subsequent experience of the same noxious stimulus [9].

Lastly, pain can undergo modulation by descending inhibitory pathways. Pain modulation involves several regions of the central nervous system (CNS), including the prefrontal cortex, ACC, insula, and periaqueductal gray (PAG). These regions modulate pain by either inhibiting or facilitating transmission of nociceptive input at the synapse of the first- and second-order neurons within the dorsal horn [10]. Serotonin, norepinephrine, and dopamine are the primary neurotransmitters involved in this inhibition. Modulation can be disrupted with the development of chronic pain.

Chronic Pain Processing

Chronic pain is defined as pain lasting more than 3 months. The development of chronic pain results from maladaptation of the aforementioned system whereby pain itself modifies the function of the nervous system. In the early phase, this sensitization is a normal protective response, but chronically it serves no physiological purpose. Chronic pain results from the initial nociceptive response followed by the acute phase described earlier, but chronic pain is not simply long-lasting acute pain. There are two characteristics of chronic pain that differ from acute pain: (1) the pain lasts longer than 3 months and (2) the pain occurs in addition to the pain from the original condition. In fact, the original condition may have healed but the pain persists as its own problem, independent of it.

Central sensitization is defined by the International Association for the Study of Pain as an increased responsiveness of nociceptive neurons in the CNS to their normal or subthreshold afferent input. It is a process by which CNS becomes more reactive to stimuli until it can begin to generate the sensation of pain itself without external stimulation. There are three phases of central sensitization: acute, late, and the disinhibition phase. The acute phase consists of two processes termed wind-up and long-term potentiation. Wind-up is a process of increasing response. The repetitive activation of C-fibers leads to progressive increases in the magnitude of the response evoked in dorsal horn neurons due to the action of glutamate at N-methyl-D-aspartate (NMDA) receptors. Normally a magnesium ion blocks the NMDA receptor but with repetitive stimulation the magnesium block is removed and the response of the second-order neuron becomes amplified. Activation of this receptor is an essential step in initiating and maintaining sensitization. This explains why NMDA antagonists such as ketamine can be utilized to attenuate or block the process of wind-up. Wind-up is a reversible and short-term form of sensitization. Long-term potentiation is a simultaneous process in which there is long-standing strengthening between synapses. Long-term potentiation consists of two phases. The early phase is independent of new protein synthesis and lasts up to 3 hours. This phase is reversible if the input ceases. The late phase can last for the lifetime of the individual. It involves protein synthesis and structural changes within the synapse, making the connection between neurons stronger. It has also been shown that a phenotypic switch occurs in the dorsal root ganglion, where large Aβ neurons, typically responsive to touch, begin to function like C-fibers and transmit pain [11]. This clinically manifests as allodynia. Phenotypic changes also occur in glial cells such as astrocytes and microglia, which can increase neuronal hypersensitivity.

In the late phase of central sensitization, the prolonged stimulus or reduced activation threshold leads to more semipermanent changes within the system. This phase is characterized by increased reactivity of the second-order neuron along with altered transcription of receptors in the dorsal horn. Neurons now become able to generate signals in response to inputs that would normally have been subthreshold and innocuous in nature.

Finally, in the disinhibition phase, there is both reduced activity and complete loss of inhibitory neurotransmitters and interneurons. Descending modulation from the brain is also altered. This can lead to persistent enhancement of pain sensitivity. Once these changes occur we lose the ability to place a "brake" on pain and the sensation becomes more permanent. It is thought that most of these changes occur in the dorsal horn but there is likely some component occurring in higher centers in the brainstem and cerebral cortex.

Many chronic pain conditions have been shown to be associated with changes in brain volume in specific regions involved in pain processing. Some areas demonstrate reduction in volume. Many theories exist to explain this volumetric reduction: direct neurotoxic effect from repetitive episodes of pain, effect of altered metabolic activity, neurodegeneration secondary to pain-related inactivity, and effect related to psychological changes from anxiety or depression [12]. Volume reductions are commonly found in the thalamus, ACC, and insula. While some areas shrink, others expand. A study by As-Sanie et al. in 2012 evaluated the changes in the brains of women with chronic pelvic pain. Interestingly, women with endometriosis but no pain had a volume increase in the PAG (an area important in descending pain inhibition) [13] and those with larger PAGs were able to tolerate increased pressure before reporting pain. It has been noted that these volumetric changes correlate with the duration of pain, suggesting that these changes are a consequence of pain.

Chronic pain is a potent stressor and affects the hypothalamic–pituitary–adrenal (HPA) axis. Cortisol is released in times of stress and has been shown to be central to stress-induced analgesia. This phenomenon can be seen when the flight or fight response has been activated and injured individuals are able to perform feats they would otherwise be unable to (i.e., lifting a car to save another). Chronic stress, however, leads to decreased cortisol levels and the reduction in cortisol may lead to exacerbations in pain. Abnormally low cortisol levels have been found in chronic pelvic pain conditions similar to other chronic pain conditions [14]. Studies have suggested that HPA axis dysfunction is a consequence of pain rather than a cause.

Changes in the enteric nervous system (ENS) have also been found in patients with chronic visceral pain. The intestinal wall contains a dense neuronal network including sensory, motor, and interneurons grouped into the nerve bundles of the myenteric (Auerbach's) and submucosal (Meissner's) plexi. This system controls motility, secretion, absorption, and immune function in the gut. Information from the ENS and CNS travels in a bidirectional manner and links the cognitive, emotional, and autonomic centers in the brain. The release of neuropeptides such as substance P and serotonin from intrinsic enteric afferents can initiate and intensify neurogenic inflammation, leading to sensitization of nearby extrinsic visceral nerves [14]. The gastrointestinal (GI) tract has dual extrinsic innervation through the splanchnic sympathetic and the vagal/pelvic parasympathetic systems. Visceral input to the spinal cord enters at multiple segments and is communicated to the brain via a three-neuron chain. This is one reason why pain experienced from the viscera is difficult to localize.

Visceral hypersensitivity occurs when there is an increased perception of the stimuli arising from the visceral organs, which typically are nearly insensate. This is commonly experienced in irritable bowel syndrome (IBS) and irritable bowel diseases such as Crohn's and ulcerative colitis. It is thought that immune cells within the gut may trigger peripheral sensitization through inflammation. Signals from the GI tract are modulated through the spinal cord and higher brain centers. A common finding in visceral pain disorders is overlap with other visceral systems (e.g., IBS and painful bladder syndrome). It is suspected that this is related to cross-sensitization between somatic structures and visceral organs, termed viscerosomatic and viscerovisceral cross-sensitization. In viscerosomatic cross-sensitization, primary afferents from viscera converge on the same second-order neurons in which somatic structures synapse. This overlap can lead to pain sensation in somatic structures correlating to the level of spinal input. In the pelvis, the most common example of this is spastic pelvic floor syndrome, in which the muscles of the pelvic floor become sensitized due to pain input from, for example, endometriosis. In visceroviseral cross-sensitization, primary afferents from multiple organs synapse onto the same second-order neuron [15]. The bladder is a frequent target of visceroviseral cross-sensitization. Colon to bladder sensitization is a common finding in patients with IBS, who often also exhibit bladder sensitivity and symptoms of nocturia, frequency, and urgency. Bladder to colon sensitization can also occur but seems to be less frequent. Patients with interstitial cystitis/bladder pain syndrome (IC/BPS) have been shown to have an increased association with IBS when compared to the baseline population.

Impact of Psychosocial Attributes

Patients' experience of pain is dependent on many psychosocial factors including personality style, cognitive appraisal, and coping ability. These have been extensively studied. Patient beliefs regarding pain impact their experience of it. Beliefs about acute pain are often applied to chronic pain and can end up becoming maladaptive. For example, while decreased activity can be beneficial following an acute injury, this similar decrease in activity in chronic pain can actually contribute to increased pain and debilitation [16]. Pain frequently leads to emotional distress, and patients with chronic pain are more vulnerable to the effects of this distress.

Catastrophizing is a common finding in patients who have more distress from pain. Catastrophizing is a process in which one assumes the worst and it negatively impacts memories and experiences. It is a strong predictor of pain-related disability and has been shown to lead to attenuation of centrally mediated diffuse noxious inhibitory control mechanisms [17]. Fear and anxiety are almost twice as common, and panic disorder and posttraumatic stress disorder (PTSD) are three times as common in patients with chronic pain as in the general population [18]. Depression is also a common comorbid condition with chronic pain and has been found to be present in more than 50% of patients in a specialized pain clinic [19]. The feeling of self-control or helplessness has been found to be linearly related to functionality in patients with chronic pain. Patients who lack a sense of control have greater pain and decreased ability to physically and psychologically cope. The perception of control can physiologically alter neuronal activity in the anterior cingulate cortex and insula, both of which are involved in emotional responses [20]. Coping skills also play an important role in the experience of pain. Patients with higher coping skills are typically better able to adapt to pain; however, it is important to point out that coping ability is variable over time and within specific situations. As coping is not a personality trait, it is modifiable with counseling and practice.

Conclusion

Chronic pain is a complex entity involving the interplay of multiple systems and neurologic pathways. Our understanding is constantly evolving as our knowledge of the neurobiological and psychosocial aspects of pain expands. The more we can understand the transition from acute to chronic pain and the associated modulating factors, the more we will be able to make an earlier clinical impact for our patients.

> **Five Things You Need to Know**
> - Knowledge of anatomical and physiological neural pathways is important in understanding chronic pain conditions.
> - Chronic pain is the result of maladaptive changes within the CNS and is not just a continuation of acute pain.
> - The CNS undergoes functional anatomical changes in the chronic pain states that perpetuate the ongoing nature of pain.
> - Viscerosomatic and visceroviseral convergence are key processes in overlapping pain conditions, especially within the abdomen and pelvis.
> - The psychosocial aspects of the experience of pain, such as beliefs, catastrophizing, lack of control, and coping skills, contribute significantly to the patient's perception and ability to manage chronic pain.

References

1. Harstall C, Ospina M. How prevalent is chronic pain? *Pain*. 2003;11(2):1–4.

2. Institute of Medicine Report from the Committee on Advancing Pain Research, Care, and Education. *Relieving*

Pain in America: A Blueprint for Transforming Prevention, Care, Education and Research. Washington, DC: National Academies Press; 2011.

3. Barber MD, Bremer RE, Thor KB, Dolber PC, Kuehl TJ, Coates KW. Innervation of the female levator ani muscles. *Am J Obstet Gynecol.* 2002;**187**(1):64–71.

4. Djouhri L, Lawson SN. Abeta-fiber nociceptive primary afferent neurons: a review of incidence and properties in relation to other afferent A-fiber neurons in mammals. *Brain Res Rev.* 2004;**46**(2):131–45.

5. Basbaum AI, Bautista DM, Scherrer G, Julius D. Cellular and molecular mechanisms of pain. *Cell.* 2009;**139**(2):267–84. DOI: 10.1016/j.cell.2009.09.028.

6. Raja SN, Meyer RA. Peripheral mechanisms of somatic pain. *Campbell JN Anesthesiology.* 1988;**68**(4):571–90.

7. Dubin AE, Patapoutian A. Nociceptors: the sensors of the pain pathway. *J Clin Invest.* 2010;**120**(11):3760–72.

8. IASP Task Force on Taxonomy. Part III: Pain terms: A current list with definitions and notes on usage. In Merskey H, Bogduk N. (eds), *Classification of Chronic Pain*, 2nd ed. Seattle: IASP Press; 1994, 209–14.

9. Bushnell, MC, Ceko M, Low LA. Cognitive and emotional control of pain and its disruption in chronic pain. *Nat Rev Neurosci.* 2013;**14**(7):502–11.

10. Kwon M, Altin M, Duenas H, Alev L. The role of descending inhibitory pathways on chronic pain modulation and clinical implications. *Pain Pract.* 2014;**14**(7);656–67.

11. Mifflin KA, Kerr BJ. The transition from acute to chronic pain: understanding how different biological systems interact. *J Anesth.* 2014;**61**:112–22.

12. Brawn J, Morotti M, Zondervan KT, Becker CM, Vincent K. Central changes associated with chronic pelvic pain and endometriosis. *Hum Reprod Update.* 2014;**20**(5):737–47.

13. As-Sani S, Harris RE, Napadow V, Kim J, et al. Changes in regional gray matter volume in women with chronic pelvic pain: a voxel-based morphometry study. *Pain.* 2012;**153**:1006–14.

14. Vermeulen W, DeMan JG, Pelckmans, PA, DeWinter BY. Neuroanatomy of lower gastrointestinal pain disorders. *World J Gastroenterol.* 2014;**20**(4):1005–20.

15. Brumovsky PR, Gebhart GF. Visceral organ cross-sensitization: an integrated perspective. *Auton Neurosci.* 2010;**153**(1–2):106.

16. Crofford LJ. Chronic pain: where the body meets the brain. *Trans Am Clin Climatol Assoc.* 2015;**126**:167–83.

17. Turk DC, Fillingim RB, Ohrback R, Patel KV. Assessment of psychosocial and functional impact of chronic pain. *Pain.* 2016;**17**(9):21–49.

18. McCracken LM, Zayfer C, Gross RT. The Pain Anxiety Symptoms Scale: development ad validation of a scale to measure fear of pain. *Pain.* 1992;**50**:67–73.

19. Bair MJ, Robinson RL, Katon W, Kroenke K. Depression and pain comorbidity: a literature review. *Arch Intern Med.* 2003;**163**:2433–45.

20. Salomons TV, Johnstone T, Backonja MM, Davidson DJ. Perceived controllability modulates the neural response to pain. *J Neurosci.* 2004;**24**:7199–203.

Chapter 3

History and Evaluation of Patients with Chronic Pelvic Pain

Nita Desai and Mario Castellanos

Patient Evaluation

A detailed history and physical examination are the most important first steps in evaluating a patient with chronic pelvic pain. The goal is to dissect the signs and symptoms that often represent multiple overlapping conditions. Adequate time should be reserved for the initial patient encounter to give the patient a chance to express her complex symptoms and to explore her concerns and treatment goals. Developing a good rapport is essential to gain trust and to reduce anxiety, especially in preparation for the physical examination. As well, healing begins with careful listening, acknowledgment of her pain and suffering, and with the offer of help.

History

Taking a history from patients with chronic pelvic pain may be overwhelming, as many will present with multiple symptoms across different organ systems. Therefore, using the approach for the evaluation of symptoms (quality, severity, location, radiation, aggravating/alleviating factors, and associated symptoms), although important, may not produce sufficient information to tease out all the associated anatomical structures contributing to the chronic pain. Proceeding in a stepwise and concentrated fashion is important [1].

Step 1: Allow the Patient to Tell Her Story

The initial question should be open ended: "How can I help you today?" "Tell me about your concerns." Allow the patient to express her symptoms and to tell you the story of her pain. It is important to take note of her concerns and chief symptoms so that you can address all issues by the end of the visit. For instance, the patient may present complaining of LLQ abdominal pain, but her main concern is that it prevents her from enjoying intercourse. Once you have a list of her concerns, and understand her situation, you can begin questioning to explore each of her problems. The patient will feel that she is being heard and will make the rest of her visit more productive.

Step 2: Develop a Timeline

Understanding how the pain started or with what event the patient associates the start of her pain can lead to identifying the root cause and help formulate a pertinent differential diagnosis. Instead of asking "How long have you had your pain?" you can ask "How did your pain start?" or "Can you associate anything with the start of your pain?" These questions may reveal underlying conditions and the cause of her pain. For example, a patient who presents with generalized pelvic pain and dyspareunia notes that the pain first started after a cesarean section 3 years ago and that her pain is mostly on the right aspect of her prior Pfannenstiel incision. This may suggest that the patient has an ilioinguinal nerve entrapment or adhesions from her Pfannenstiel scar. Operative reports are useful for investigating pain that started after a surgery, paying close attention to procedure details, positioning, and complications. Another example is a patient who presents with pelvic pain and sensation of pelvic/vaginal pressure that started after a pregnancy. Understanding that pregnancies place patients at risk of developing pelvic congestion syndrome would lead clinicians to consider this diagnosis. Specific events are not pathognomonic for a condition, but they can help focus or rule out pertinent differential diagnoses (Table 3.1).

Another approach is asking "When did you first start experiencing pain?" Obtaining a history in a timeline/chronological fashion may reveal a sequence of events and evolution of symptoms that may help identify the components of her pain. For example, a patient with generalized pelvic pain notes that she has always had painful periods (endometriosis) and that she later developed urinary frequency and suprapubic pain (bladder pain syndrome). She now has pain with sitting and painful intercourse and bowel movements (hypertonic pelvic floor disorder). When symptoms are broken down into a timeline, it is easier to address and explore her symptomatology (Figure 3.1).

Step 3: Map Out the Pain

Localization of pain using a pain map can elicit important diagnostic clues to identify anatomical sources of pain and to differentiate visceral, somatic, and

Table 3.1 Inciting events and associated chronic pelvic pain conditions

Event	Etiology
Hysterectomy	Pelvic adhesions, vaginal apex neuroma, peripheral nerve injury, pelvic floor tension myalgia, bladder pain syndrome
Vaginal delivery	Pelvic congestion syndrome, sacroiliac joint dysfunction, pubalgia, obturator and/or pudendal neuralgia
Cesarean section	incisional neuroma, ilioinguinal nerve entrapment, abdominal wall endometrioma, pelvic adhesions
Midurethral slings/ vaginal mesh	Pudendal neuralgia, pelvic floor tension myalgia, mesh erosion, obturator nerve injury
Falls/trauma	Pelvic floor tension myalgia, nerve injury
Stress, psychological event	Pelvic floor tension myalgia, bladder pain syndrome
Strenuous physical activity	Muscle spasms (obturator internus, levator ani, psoas), pudendal neuralgia
Urinary tract infections	Bladder pain syndrome, pelvic floor tension myalgia
Uterine ablation	Adenomyosis, post ablation tubal ligation syndrome
Pelvic inflammatory disease	Chronic endometritis, pelvic adhesions, hydrosalpinx

neuropathic origins. It may be difficult for patients to describe their pain and express the location of their pain using anatomical terms. Many patients may simple state "It hurts down there" or "I am having female pain." A pain map is useful in helping patients point out the location of their pain. Have the patient draw out or shade in the areas where she is experiencing pain on a pain map (Figure 3.2). Encourage the patient to write out descriptors or color code if she is experiencing multiple different pains. The pain map is a helpful tool to focus the patient during the encounter. This map should be completed prior to the patient visit.

Pain maps may reveal a pain pattern that is well localized, a viscerotome, a dermatome, or a combination of each. Well localized pain can be drawn as a dot or x to suggest a somatic source of pain. Shaded areas of the lower abdomen and umbilicus may correspond to referred pain from viscera. An outline may follow a specific dermatome, suggesting neuropathic pain. Usually, pain maps are not as

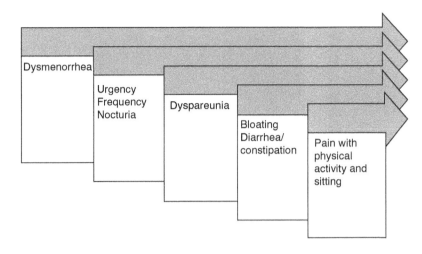

Figure 3.1 Pelvic pain timeline of a patient with endometriosis affecting multiple organ systems.

Dysmenorrhea

Urgency
Frequency
Nocturia

Dyspareunia

Bloating
Diarrhea/
constipation

Pain with
physical
activity and
sitting

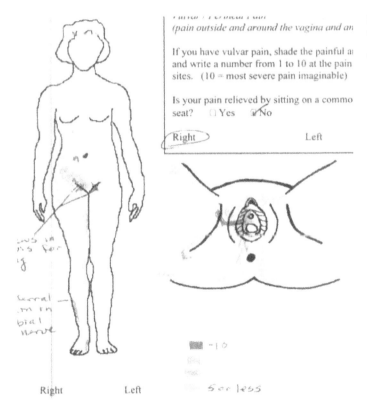

Figure 3.2 Pain map demonstrating a patient experiencing pudendal neuralgia on the left and ilioinguinal neuralgia on the right. Color-coding can help differentiated different pains based on quality or intensity.

straightforward because pelvic pain usually presents with many overlapping conditions. Nevertheless, a detailed pain map as in Figure 3.2 can be further explored with the patient to determine causes of pain.

Step 4: Know Your Triggers

Pelvic pain can occur in specific settings. These settings or triggers of the pain can help build a differential diagnosis. Patients whose pain is not constant should be evaluated for triggers by simply asking "When do you feel your pain?" The patient may reveal that her pain is felt when she sits, performs a specific physical activity, drinks coffee, or with intercourse. Pain with sitting that is relieved by standing is the hallmark symptom for pudendal neuralgia (Chapter 15). Stress is a very common trigger that usually indicates a pelvic floor disorder, bladder pain syndrome, or musculoskeletal pain. Dyspareunia is discussed separately in the text that follows.

Step 5: Factor It Out

Pelvic pain conditions may have corresponding alleviating and aggravating factors based on the type of pain the patient is experiencing. For instance, somatic pain, or musculoskeletal pain, is usually improved with rest and application of heat, while physical activity that utilizes the involved muscles worsens the pain. When pain is worsened by a physical activity, the muscles involved in that activity should be assessed. Neuropathic pain from peripheral nerve injuries often improves with cold and may be positional. In contrast, neuropathic pain is worsened by touch and the patient may avoid tight clothing or belts. Visceral pain may be aggravated by different foods (irritable bowel syndrome [IBS], interstitial cystitis/bladder pain syndrome [IC/BPS]) or menses (adenomyosis) and alleviated after completion of visceral function such as bladder emptying (IC/BPS) and bowel movement (IBS) (Table 3.2). One possible exception is pelvic congestion syndrome, which involves visceral pain that is positional. Patients with pelvic congestion syndrome have deep throbbing pain and a sensation of heaviness with standing that is alleviated with lying flat. This is thought to be from stasis of blood in incompetent dilated pelvic and gonadal veins (Chapter 10).

Associated symptoms can help determine contributing anatomy. Urinary frequency, urgency, and nocturia can help differentiate the urological origin of pain, while urinary hesitancy, the inability to void spontaneously, is associated with hypertonic pelvic floor disorders (Table 3.3).

Step 6: Does the Pain Cycle?

The menstrual cycle is often used to describe the timing of chronic pelvic pain. Cyclical pain can suggest gynecological conditions such as adenomyosis or endometriosis, especially if it is associated with heavy menstrual bleeding. However, during menses, pain

Table 3.2 Factors that can modify pelvic pain symptoms

Alleviating Factors	Etiology
Massage	Musculoskeletal
Bowel movement	IBS
Ice	Neuralgias
Voiding	IC/BPS
Lying down	Pelvic congestion syndrome, musculoskeletal
Heating pad/hot bath/rest	Musculoskeletal

Aggravating Factors	Etiology
Bowel movement	Pelvic floor tension myalgia, rectal endometriosis, IBS
Orgasm	Pelvic floor tension myalgia, pudendal neuralgia
Exercise, walking	Pelvic floor tension myalgia
Full bladder	IC/BPS, pelvic adhesions
Sitting	Pudendal neuralgia
Contact with clothing	Neuralgias
Certain foods	IC/BPS, IBS
Stress	Pelvic floor tension myalgia, IC/BPS, pelvic floor tension myalgia
Standing	Pelvic congestion syndrome, pelvic floor tension myalgia

IBS, irritable bowel syndrome; IC/BPS, interstitial cystitis/bladder pain syndrome.

may be secondary to musculoskeletal causes. In fact, "menstrual cramps" may be associated with spasms of the abdominal wall and pelvic floor muscles. This pain is usually felt across the pelvis and lower back, acting like a tight belt or vise. Uterine pain, on the other hand, is mostly throbbing midline pelvic pain or low back pain. Cyclical pain can be tracked with a calendar, thereby identifying pain with menses, before/after menses, and ovulation. For instance, pelvic congestion syndrome may present with worsening pain prior to menses that improves during menses. Nevertheless, it is important to note that a cyclical pattern of pain may be secondary to increased sensitivity to pain from sex steroids and not related to either endometriosis or adenomyosis. Women in the ovulatory phase demonstrate higher pain sensitivity than at other

Table 3.3 Symptoms associated with pelvic pain conditions

Associated Symptoms	Possible Etiology
Dysmenorrhea/ menorrhagia	Adenomyosis, endometriosis
Urinary hesitancy	Pelvic floor tension myalgia, interstitial cystitis
Vaginal/rectal pain with sitting with foreign body sensation	Pudendal neuralgia
Urinary frequency, urgency	Bladder pain syndrome
Constipation/diarrhea	Functional bowel disorders, pelvic floor tension myalgia

Table 3.4 Differential diagnosis of dyspareunia by pain occurrence

Pain Type	Differential Diagnosis
Touch/foreplay	Vestibulitis, vulvodynia, dermatoses, chronic vaginitis, clitorodynia
Initial penetration	Vestibulitis, vulvodynia, dermatoses, chronic vaginitis, hypertonic pelvic floor disorder
Deep penetration	Adenomyosis, endometriosis, pelvic floor tension myalgia
Orgasm	Pudendal neuralgia Pelvic congestion
Postcoital	Pelvic floor tension myalgia, fissures, atrophic vaginitis, dermatoses
Positional	Bladder pain syndrome, uterine/ adnexal pathology

times during their cycle. Estrogenic cycles may play a role in the development of chronic pelvic pain [2]. Thus, urological and gastrointestinal sources of pain may also follow a cyclical pattern. For example, bladder pain syndrome can present as suprapubic pain that becomes worse during menses and thus may be mistaken for dysmenorrhea of uterine origin.

Step 7: Address Sexual Pain

Although a common complaint, dyspareunia can result from multiple etiologies corresponding to external genitalia, vaginal epithelium, pelvic floor disorders, uterine and adnexal conditions, bladder pain syndrome, and gastrointestinal disorders. When a patient identifies she is having pain with intercourse, it is important to clarify which intercourse she is referring. Pain may be from penetrative intercourse (vaginal and/or anal), external genital stimulation, use of accessories, post activity pain, or orgasm. In addition, establishing what type of pain she is having is important for formulating a differential diagnosis (Table 3.4). Answering questions about one's sexual practices may be embarrassing and therefore clinicians should work toward developing a good rapport throughout the patient evaluation before asking these questions.

"When does it hurt with sex?" may be a good opening question to start a dialogue. Differentiating internal and external pain can help build a differential diagnosis and guide the physical examination. For instance, pain experienced with initial penetration or genital stimulation may suggest a vulvar dermatosis, vulvodynia, neuralgia, hypertonic pelvic floor disorders or urethral disorders. Deep pelvic pain with vaginal or rectal intercourse may suggest a visceral pathology such as adenomyosis, endometriosis, or bladder pain syndrome. Many of these patients are able to have intercourse as long as they control the depth of penetration. Vaginal or anal intercourse may be positional. Pain with vaginal intercourse in the quadrapedic (rear entry) position suggests the diagnosis of bladder pain syndrome, since intercourse in this position is more likely to affect the anterior vaginal wall and bladder. Patients who present with pain after a hysterectomy should be assessed for vaginal apex pain and pelvic adhesions. Lastly, pain with orgasm, postcoital pain, or vaginal throbbing may indicate a hypertonic pelvic floor disorder.

In patients with external pain, the location of pain should be explored. A pain map is very useful in these cases to help the patient describe the location. Unilateral pain, such as pain described as affecting one labium minus, should prompt exploration of organic pathology on physical examination or suspicion of a nerve injury or entrapment.

Step 8: Look to the Past

Patients with chronic pelvic pain have often seen multiple clinicians, obtained numerous tests, and undergone numerous treatments. If available, reviewing the medical records will allow the clinician to develop a timeline treatments and diagnostic procedures. The patient may have had some relief with some treatments or may have had worsening pain or a change in her pain after others. This can help the clinician not duplicate failed treatment options and medical testing.

Step 9: Establish Safety

As with all patients, patient with chronic pelvic pain should be screened for sexual abuse, depression, and intimate partner violence. Although sexual abuse has been associated with chronic pelvic pain, causality should not be assumed and careful assessment for etiologies of pain should take place regardless of sexual abuse history.

There are many screening questionnaires that can be used to help identify patients who may be experiencing intimate partner violence. We recommend using the form that can be best incorporated into the clinician's practice to ensure that all patients are screened. All patients should be asked "Do you feel safe at home?" There should also be leaflets and pamphlets in the office and in the restrooms that can direct patients to call a hotline and seek help.

The American College of Obstetricians and Gynecologists released a committee opinion and recommended the following screening questions [3]. Patients who answer a question positively should be referred for additional help.

1. Do you have someone special in your life? Someone you're going out with?
2. Are you now – or have you been – sexually active?
3. Think about your earliest sexual experience. Did you want this experience?
4. Has a friend, a date, or an acquaintance ever pressured or forced you into sexual activities when you did not want them? Touched you in a way that made you uncomfortable? Anyone at home? Anyone at school? Any other adult?
5. Although women are never responsible for rape, there are things they can do that may reduce their risk of sexual assault. Do you know how to reduce your risk of sexual assault?

Physical Examination

The objective of the physical examination is to identify all possible anatomical sources of pain (Table 3.5). This goal can be achieved by employing a systematic and methodical approach to the exam, with the goal of duplicating pain through palpation or positioning. This process can be quite anxiety provoking for patients; therefore proper consent should be obtained. Further, it may be reasonable to postpone a physical examination, to a later time and date, should the patient prefer. These authors suggest verbalizing all aspects of the exam to the

Table 3.5 Common signs and symptoms and their associated chronic pelvic pain condition

Symptom	Sign	Syndrome
Abdominal wall pain	Carnett's sign	Abdominal wall muscle spasm, nerve entrapment, hematoma
Painful urination or urethral discharge	Urethral mass	Urethral diverticulum
Bladder frequency	Suprapubic or bladder tenderness	IC/BPS
Bladder urgency	Muscle tenderness	IC/BPS +/– SPFS
Bladder pressure, pain, discomfort	Suprapubic or bladder tenderness +/– muscle tenderness	IC/BPS +/– SPFS
Bladder hesitancy or incomplete emptying	Muscle tenderness	SPFS
Pain with external vaginal touch	Vulvar tenderness	Vulvodynia or vulvar vestibulitis
Pain with intercourse: initial penetration, pain during arousal, and/or residual vaginal soreness (after intercourse or orgasm)	Muscle tenderness	SPFS
Pain with intercourse: deep penetration	Muscle tenderness +/– cervical or uterine pain	SPFS +/– female pelvic organ pain
Pain with defecatory urge	Muscle tenderness without pain on DRE	SPFS
Pain during defecation	Muscle tenderness with pain on DRE	SPFS, rectal sphincter
Perineal/vaginal/ rectal burning +/– foreign body sensation	Pain or discomfort throughout palpation, without specificity	Pudendal neuralgia

DRE, digital rectal exam; IC/BPS, interstitial cystitis/painful bowel syndrome; SPFS, spastic pelvic floor syndrome.

patient, during the process of the examination, and informing patients of both internal and external aspects of the examination, to alleviate these stressors and help build trust. The goal of the examination is not to reproduce pain in its most extreme state, but rather to identify dermatomes, tissues, nerves, muscles, and organs that reproduce pain, so as to define underlying causes and develop subsequent individualized treatment options.

General

General evaluation of the patient should be performed. This includes a review of vital signs and general assessment of the patient's overall health status. Patients presenting with unstable vital signs and/or acute abdominal/pelvic pain, in which life-threatening pathology such as ectopic pregnancy, appendicitis, or bowel perforation is suspected, emergent evaluation and intervention should be undertaken. Additionally, patients presenting with other acute etiologies of pain, such as ovarian torsion or pelvic inflammatory disease should also be expeditiously evaluated and treated. Once the vital signs and overall patient status are assessed and deemed stable, verbal consent is obtained. As gaining trust with these patients is important, it is reasonable to assess at this juncture whether the examination can be performed on the same day or should be postponed to a later date. Patient comfort is key in obtaining a thorough evaluation.

The initial physical assessment then begins with observation of a patient's gait and posture, in both sitting and standing positions. Patients with musculoskeletal sources of pain may present with antalgic or uneven gait, restricted range of motion, leaning to one side to avoid sitting on the painful side, or frequent adjustments in position [1]. At this point the patient is asked to sit on the examination table. Once the patient is seated, these same observations can be made in regard to posture, leaning, and difficulty sitting. These symptoms can suggest muscle floor spasm and/or pelvic neuropathies (see Chapter 20).

Back

The patient should be asked to localize areas of tenderness, if present, on the back. Any areas of scarring and associated pain should be noted. Care should be taken at this point to gently palpate the lumbar and sacral aspects of the spine, as well as the pelvic joints, including the hips and anterior superior iliac spine

(ASIS), sacroiliac (SI) joints, and the pubic symphysis. Pain in these areas is suggestive of intrinsic injury to the joint(s) as well as muscular dysfunction. Pain that originates during palpation of the SI joint in the posterior pelvis can radiate to the pelvis or lower extremities and may be found in nearly 50% of patients with musculoskeletal diagnoses [2]. Tenderness in the area of palpation as well as referral or radiation to the back and/or abdominal wall suggests a musculoskeletal cause of pain. Spinal curvature, abnormal posture, or asymmetry of the pelvic girdle or gait also suggests a musculoskeletal component to pain [3]. Pain at the pubic symphysis can indicate issues such as musculoskeletal inflammation. Based on the clinical history, it may be feasible to have the patient undergo evaluation by orthopedic or physical medicine and rehabilitation specialists, at a future date, should severe joint pain and/or ambulatory dysfunction be noted. Additionally, any pain or trigger points over the buttocks should be assessed and noted, as these can be present in patients with pelvic floor muscle spasm as well as pelvic neuropathies. Once evaluation of the back is complete, abdominal examination can begin.

Abdomen

The majority of the abdominal examination should take place with the patient in the supine position, knees bent. Initially, the patient should specify where on the abdomen her pain is located, as well as demonstrate how much pressure is required to elicit her pain. Care should be taken to notate areas of scarring and if there is associated pain. In particular, scars should be assessed for not only incisional hernias, but inguinal and Spigelian as well. Inguinal hernias are best evaluated in the standing position, where masses above and below the inguinal ligament crease may be more easily visible. If a hernia is suspected, with the fingers placed over the femoral region, the external inguinal ring, and the internal ring, have the patient cough. A palpable bulge or impulse located in any one of these areas may indicate a hernia [4]. Palpation for Spigelian hernias should be done just lateral to the lateral margin of the rectus sheath. Spigelian hernias are small, spontaneous, lateral ventral hernias that protrude through the transversus abdominis aponeurosis lateral to the edge of the rectus muscle, but medial to the "Spigelian line," which is the point of transition of the transversus abdominis muscle to its aponeurotic tendon. Spigelian hernias are most likely just below the level of the umbilicus, but they are difficult to palpate [3].

Once this is complete, palpation across the pubic symphysis should be performed to assess for pain, which can be indicative of issues specific to the symphysis, such as separation or osteitis, as well as muscular pain from the rectus sheath insertion site. We now evaluate the abdomen in quadrants, taking care to palpate areas of highest pain intensity last. The skin is palpated in areas of pain to assess for areas of allodynia and hyperalgesia. This can be performed with both the soft edge of a cotton-tipped applicator as well as the wooden edge. Particularly for women with low or lateral abdominal wall incisions, the authors evaluate the pathways of the ilioinguinal and iliohypogastric nerves for evidence of neuropathy [3].

Patients with ilioinguinal neuralgia complain from pain (mostly postsurgical) in the lateral aspect of the iliac fossa, lower abdomen, and upper thigh, as well as abnormal sensation in the cutaneous distribution of the nerve (hyperesthesia or hypoesthesia) [5]. On examination, there is tenderness on palpation 1 inch medial and inferior to the anterior superior iliac spine and impaired sensation along the sensory distribution of the nerve. Complete neurological examination may be helpful to exclude genitofemoral neuralgia, lumbosacral radiculopathy, and plexopathy [5]. This may be evaluated by a physiatrist. Both the iliohypogastric and ilioinguinal nerves originate from the T12–L2 spinal nerve roots. There is some overlap in the clinical presentation as the nerves emerge from the lateral border of the psoas major muscle, under the peritoneum, and travel around the abdominal wall, between the layers of the transversus abdominis muscles and the internal oblique muscles, emerging superficially at a point about 2–3 cm medial to the anterior superior iliac spine [6].

Genitofemoral neuralgia is a cause of neuropathic pain that is often debilitating in nature. It is characterized by chronic neuropathic groin pain that is localized along the distribution of the genitofemoral nerve. The symptoms include groin pain, paresthesias, and burning sensation spreading from the lower abdomen to the medial aspect of the thigh. It may present as pain radiating to the labia majora and mons pubis. Genitofemoral neuropathy has been attributed to iatrogenic nerve injury occurring during inguinal and femoral herniorrhaphy, with cases developing after both open and laparoscopic techniques. Diagnosis of genitofemoral neuralgia

can be challenging, due to the overlap in sensory distribution the nerve shares with the ilioinguinal and iliohypogastric nerve. Differential nerve blocks are recommended in an effort to differentiate the nerves when patients present with lower abdominal and groin pain [7]. Pudendal nerve pain, including physical examination, is discussed in great detail in Chapter 15.

Next, Carnett's test should be performed. Carnett's test was first described in 1926, by JB Carnett, an American surgeon [8], as a tool to evaluate abdominal wall pain and help differentiate it from visceral sources of abdominal pain. While supine, the patient is asked to perform either a straight-leg-raising maneuver while the examiner's hand touches the painful site or raise only the head (performing a sit-up). These maneuvers tighten the rectus abdominis muscles, increasing the pain when it originates from the abdominal wall structures: myofascial and/or nerve. True visceral sources of pain are associated with unchanged or less tenderness with this maneuver [9]. It has been suggested to consider blocking any trigger points of the abdominal wall before performing the pelvic examination [10].

The technique for detecting the obturator sign, called the obturator test, is carried out on each leg in succession. The patient lies on her or his back with the hip and knee both flexed at ninety degrees. The examiner holds the patient's ankle with one hand and knee with the other hand. The examiner internally rotates the hip by moving the patient's ankle away from the patient's body while allowing the knee to move only inward. This is flexion and internal rotation of the hip [11].

The technique for detecting the psoas sign is carried out on the patient's right leg. The patient lies on his or her left side with the knees extended. The examiner holds the patient's right thigh and passively extends the hip. Alternatively, the patient lies on their back, and the examiner asks the patient to actively flex the right hip against the examiner's hand [12].

The traditional components of the abdominal exam include auscultation, percussion, and palpation in all four quadrants to assess for masses, fluid, and vascular bruits. Although it is an important aspect of the abdominal exam, it may not be necessary. This portion of the exam should be undertaken as dictated by the history. Also, it may not be achievable on the same day as the remainder of the exam. It may be reasonable, particularly based on patient comfort or pain, to perform this, or other portions of the exam, on a subsequent visit.

External Genitalia

Once the abdominal exam is complete, both internal and external evaluation of the vagina should be performed in the lithotomy position. Visual inspection of the external genitalia should be performed, noting redness, discharge, abscess formation, excoriation, fistulas, fissures, ulcerations, pigment changes, condylomata, atrophic changes, or signs of trauma [3]. A cotton-tipped applicator may be used to assess for areas of allodynia and hyperalgesia. Evaluation of vulvar pain and its distinguishing characteristics is more thoroughly discussed in Chapter 12.

Manual and Bimanual Exam

A standard speculum is recommended to be performed at some point of the physical evaluation, to assess for intravaginal lesions, discharge, and cervical lesions/masses/tenderness, as well as obtain any indicated specimens for laboratory testing. The need for this aspect of exam is dictated, again, by the clinical history. It is important to note, however, that some patients may have high anxiety with this portion of the exam due to poor past experiences compounded by high levels of pain. In this case it may be reasonable to defer to a later visit. However, the manual exam can be quite illuminating and should be performed so long as the patient is comfortable.

While the patient is resting in lithotomy, these authors suggest discussing two items with the patient, prior to initiating the manual exam. The first is to establish the degree of pressure the examiner will apply during the vaginal exam. We suggest lightly palpating the patient's leg, with a single digit. This degree of pressure should be defined, and referred to by both patient and examiner during the exam, as "pressure." Should the patient experience any amount of pain or discomfort above this jointly established baseline, it will be referred to, again by both patient and examiner, as "pain." These binary choices allow both the patient and examiner to establish common language and understanding. During the exam, if "pain" is palpated, it can then be stratified to mild, moderate, severe, or exquisite.

Single-digit manual exam should be performed after establishing these guidelines. Single-digit exam is also referred to as "monomanual-monodigitial" in

that only one finger of one hand is used by the examiner, and no abdominal palpation is involved [3]. The exam begins with circumferential palpation of the introitus. "Pain" here can be due to muscle spasm as well as vulvar vestibulitis. Next palpation of the anterior vagina, urethra, and bladder is performed. Urethral tenderness, discharge, or thickening can suggest urethral inflammation or even a diverticulum, if a tender mass is noted. Thereafter, any bladder tenderness may be suggestive of either painful bladder syndrome or muscle spasm, particularly if the pain is noted on the lateral borders of the bladder. Next, the pelvic floor muscles should be palpated with a single digit. The levator ani complex is best evaluated on the lateral vaginal wall, approximately 1 cm proximal to the hymenal ring, from 7 to 11 o'clock on the right and 1 to 5 o'clock on the left. "Pain" experienced here is suggestive but not indicative of pelvic floor spasm (see Chapter 5). Although the examiner can ask the patient to perform a Kegel exercise, so as to better localize this muscle complex, doing so may cause aggravation of the spasm. These authors therefore recommend avoiding this approach in patients with history suggestive of pelvic floor spasm. The obturator internus should be gently palpated anterior and proximal to the levator complex, located just above the 3 and 9 o'clock positions. While in lithotomy position, the examiner may ask the patient to externally rotate her hip, against the examiner's free hand, which is placed on the outer aspect of the patient's knee, in order to bulge the obturator internus muscle into the vagina. This maneuver typically does not aggravate baseline pain, unlike the Kegel maneuver, and therefore may be performed for improved localization of the pain. Next, the examiner can apply gentle pressure along the ischial spines. Sensation of pain or paresthesia is suggestive of pudendal neuralgia and is discussed further in Chapter 5. These authors suggest performing this muscular and ischial spine exam, in entirety, on one side of the vagina, before proceeding to the contralateral side, so as to avoid aggravating baseline pain that may stem from examiner hand rotation. The single-digit exam may now be converted to a traditional bimanual exam at this point.

The bimanual exam should assess the posterior fornix, cervix, uterus, and adnexa, and should be performed after the monomanual exam. Should the patient need to postpone this portion of the exam, a discussion can take place at this point. During bimanual exam, "pain" and masses here can be suggestive of a plethora of causes such as endometriosis, leiomyomata, or adenomyosis, among many others.

Rectal Exam

These authors do not recommend routine examination of the rectovaginal septum and/or rectal sphincter. It should be performed in cases where the clinical history is suggestive of endometriosis, pelvic floor spasm, or contributory gastrointestinal pain.

After the Examination

Once the physical examination is complete, the patient should be allowed to dress and rest comfortably. At this point the authors suggest inquiring whether the patient's pain was reproduced or worsened as compared to typical circumstances. This question is a key discussion point, as the physical exam is an extension of the clinical history and therefore the history should guide the focus of the examination. A consultation between the clinical history and exam ultimately reveals diagnosis and treatment options.

Five Things You Need to Know

- Establish a trusting rapport, so that the patient feels safe telling you her story.
- Obtain the patient history in a chronological fashion.
- Physical exam findings are the extension of the history. Let the history dictate your examination.
- Systematic and gentle examination will reveal the diagnosis as pain triggers are identified.
- Always screen for intimate partner violence and sexual abuse.

References

1. Castellanos M, King L. Pelvic pain. In Norwitz E (ed), *Scientific American Obstetrics & Gynecology.* Hamilton: Decker; 2018.

2. Hassan S, Muere A, Einstein G. Ovarian hormones and chronic pain: a comprehensive review. *Pain.* 2014;**155**(12):2448–60.

3. ACOG Committee Opinion No. 777: Sexual Assault. *Obstet Gynecol.* 2019;**133**(4):e296–302.

4. Lamvu G, Carillo J, Witzeman K, Alappattu M. Musculoskeletal considerations in female patients with chronic pelvic pain. *Semin Reprod Med.* 2018;**36**:107–15.

5. Mieritz RM, Thorhauge K, Forman A, Mieritz HB, Hartvigsen J, Christensen HW. Musculoskeletal dysfunctions in patients with chronic pelvic pain: a preliminary descriptive survey. *J Manipulat Physiol Ther.* 2016;**39**(09):616–22.

6. Howard FM. Chronic pelvic pain. *Obstet Gynecol.* 2003;**101**(3):594–611.

7. Amerson JR. Inguinal canal and hernia examination. In Walker HK, Hall WD, Hurst JW (eds), *Clinical Methods: The History, Physical, and Laboratory Examinations*, 3rd ed, Chapter 96. Boston: Butterworths; 1990.

8. ter Meulen BC, Peters EW, Wijsmuller A, Kropman RF, Mosch A, Tavy DL. Acute scrotal pain from idiopathic ilioinguinal neuropathy: diagnosis and treatment with EMG-guided nerve block. *Clin Neurol Neurosurg.* 2007;**109**(6):535–7.

9. Amin N, Krashin D, Trescot A. Ilioinguinal and iliohypogastric nerve entrapment: abdominal. In Trescot AM (ed), *Peripheral Nerve Entrapments: Clinical Diagnosis and Management.* New York: Springer Science+Business Media; 2016, 413–24.

10. Cesmebasi A, Yadav A, Gielecki J, Tubbs RS, Loukas M. Genitofemoral neuralgia: a review. *Clin Anat.* 2015;**28**(1):128–35.

11. Carnett JB. Intercostal neuralgia as a cause of abdominal pain and tenderness. *Surg Gynecol Obstet.* 1926;**42**:625–32.

12. Tu F, As-sanie S. Evaluation of chronic pelvic pain in women. Uptodate.com. August 2019.

13. Matsunaga S, Eguchi Y. Importance of a physical examination for efficient differential diagnosis of abdominal pain: diagnostic usefulness of Carnett's test in psychogenic abdominal pain. Intern Med. 2011;**50**:177–8.

14. Huang IP, Smith DC. *Cope's Early Diagnosis of the Acute Abdomen*, 21st ed (book review). *Ann Surg.* 2006; **244**(2):322.

15. Bickley, LS. *Bates' Guide to Physical Exam and History Taking*, 9th ed. Philadelphia: Lippincott, Williams, and Wilkins; 2007, 390.

16. Slocumb JC. Neurologic factors in chronic pelvic pain: trigger points and the abdominal pelvic pain syndrome. *Am J Obstet Gynecol.* 1984;**149**:536–43.

Psychological Assessment of a Female Patient with Chronic Pelvic Pain

Dean A. Tripp, Katherine M. Fretz, and J. Curtis Nickel

Editor's Introduction

Patients with pelvic pain are often told that their pain is "all in their head." In many years of seeing patients for pelvic pain I have never seen one who did not have an organic reason for pain. Often patients with chronic pain, especially pelvic pain, may develop secondary depression and anxiety but neither of these conditions alone is responsible for their pain. Patients who are unable to have intercourse because of pain fear loss of the partner and become especially anxious. Additionally, because of the very personal nature of their pain they are often not able to discuss their condition with any friends or family members. It is very important to believe that the patient's pain is real and not voice any doubts, especially in the presence of a partner. Treatment of coexisting psychological disorders such as anxiety or depression it is very important in patients with pelvic pain.

Introduction

Chronic pain is a serious public health concern that is defined by its therapeutic challenge. Pain is devastating, estimated to be one of the leading global causes of diminished patient quality of life [1]. It is well known that multiple pain mechanisms and psychosocial patient characteristics are often involved in the different patient presentations found within any one disease. This individuality is important because it may affect treatment efficacy, thus leading to the suggestion of precision or tailored medicine. As such, there has been a push in the field of chronic pain for a multidimensional, evidence-based taxonomy system that acknowledges the myriad "biopsychosocial" mechanisms that commonly underlie these conditions. The Analgesic, Anesthetic, and Addiction Clinical Trial Translations Innovations Opportunities and Networks (ACTTION) partnered

with the US Food and Drug Administration (FDA) and the American Pain Society (APS) to develop a biopsychosocial taxonomy system for chronic pain conditions called ACTTION-APS Pain Taxonomy (AAPT; [2]). The AAPT system is designed to provide a multidimensional framework for healthcare providers to conceptualize chronic pain conditions using the following dimensions: "1) core diagnostic criteria; 2) common features; 3) common medical comorbidities; 4) neurobiological, psychosocial, and functional consequences; and 5) putative neurobiological and psychosocial mechanisms, risk factors, and protective factors" (p. 242).

Chronic pelvic pain is difficult to diagnose and treat because the discomfort can be indicated by more than one health concern. Examples of pelvic pain syndromes are interstitial cystitis/bladder pain syndrome (IC/BPS), inflammatory bowel disease (IBD, consisting of Crohn's disease and ulcerative colitis), pelvic inflammatory diseases (often associated with sexually transmitted infections), endometriosis, pelvic congestion syndrome, bacterial vaginosis, pelvic floor tension myalgia, vulvodynia (chronic vulvar pain), and ovarian cysts. Given the wide range of etiological and comorbid psychosocial factors, chronic pelvic pain is described as complex [3]. Indeed, research on pain and psychological characteristics of women waiting for gynecological surgery has shown that 18% reported high anxiety, 37% reported depressive symptoms, 47% had two or more symptoms of somatization, and 40% reported elevated pain catastrophizing [4]. Further, just over 30% reported moderate to severe pain intensity and interference due to pain. Of those in pain, depressive symptoms, somatization, and catastrophizing were associated with elevated pain intensity and interference. As such, a comprehensive multidisciplinary and biopsychosocial approach to assess and manage chronic pelvic pain is widely supported [e.g., 3, 5, 6].

Our collaborative pelvic pain clinical research group has taken a biopsychosocial, multidimensional approach, similar to the AAPT system, and applied it to urological pelvic pain conditions. The UPOINT system considers six domains when classifying a patient's symptoms: urinary, psychosocial, organ specific, infection, neurological/systemic, and tenderness (i.e., muscle) [7, 8]. While the UPOINT system is focused on urological pelvic pain, the AAPT system considers very similar principles in the assessment and management of pain conditions in that they consider factors beyond biology, such as psychosocial variables. While these variables are an often overlooked aspect of the biopsychosocial model, psychological factors are gaining more attention in the literature for their key role in effective pain management [9, 10]. As one recent example, our group has suggested that an optimal management of IC/BPS requires more personalized data than that obtained with symptom questionnaires and standard urological assessment [11]. We used a qualitative approach to develop a best evidence series of questions to explore the IC/BPS patient's total "clinical picture," suggesting that examining what is important to the patient has value.

Applying the biopsychosocial approach provided by the AAPT and UPOINT frameworks and our clinical experiences, this chapter briefly reviews psychosocial risk factors and functional consequences of chronic pelvic pain and suggests interview questions and tools (i.e., brief and valid questionnaires) for their assessment. These assessment recommendations for psychosocial factors are analogous to previous efforts [12, 13], but here the focus is on female chronic pelvic pain.

Overview of Pertinent Risk Factors and Functional Consequences

We know that women suffering from IC/BPS may perceive real improvement in their life situation with a multidisciplinary team applying an individually developed phenotype specific treatment plan, yet change in self-reported pain, urinary frequency, and urgency is often not significant [14]. These findings highlight the improvements that can be made when psychosocial factors are indirectly addressed through a caring environment. There are several important areas of research that support specific assessments. In the text that follows we outline specific disease-associated variables that we believe are important in capturing the patient experience.

Pain. Pain, and chronic pain in particular, is a complex phenomenon comprising physical, social, and psychological factors. Thus, a thorough patient assessment of pain must also include psychological evaluation. Women with chronic pelvic pain are at risk for extended periods of pain and psychological symptoms, with some samples of women with chronic pelvic pain experiencing their pain symptoms for more than 2 years [5]. Research has also shown that pain and urinary symptoms in women with IC/BPS are important factors in promoting maladaptive coping responses and diminished quality of life [15]. In another study, 73% of IC/BPS patients sampled reported numerous systemic pains outside the typical body areas associated with the bladder/pelvic region, with increased numbers of body pain sites being associated with greater pain severity and depression [16]. Thus, documenting and understanding comorbid pain is recommended.

Disability. Experiencing chronic pain results in disability in many of its sufferers [13]. Women with chronic pelvic pain experience limitations in a variety of daily living activities [17]. As well, physical disability can be worsened by a patient's negative perception of her illness, attempts to cope using illness-focused coping, and poorer emotional regulation in IC/BPS [15]. Given these findings, assessing disability holistically is important for patients with chronic pelvic pain in order to elucidate how their pain affects their functioning in a variety of contexts.

Quality of Life. Poor health-related quality of life is a common functional limitation for patients experiencing chronic pain [13]. Chronic pelvic pain sufferers report significant negative effects of the condition on their quality of life [5, 17]. This psychological variable is particularly important to assess, as it is likely a major factor underlying treatment-seeking given that it plays a major role in patients' well-being.

Catastrophizing. Pain catastrophizing (i.e., negative thoughts and emotions associated with actual or anticipated pain; [18]) plays a significant role in the development [12] and maintenance [13] of many pain conditions. Shoskes and colleagues [8] identified catastrophizing as an important maladaptive coping strategy to consider among patients with pelvic pain conditions. In a sample of women with pelvic pain, catastrophizing was significantly correlated with mental health and functioning, suggesting that it plays a role in many important disease-related outcomes [5]. In a recent unpublished study, catastrophizing and difficulties in emotion regulation were found to mediate the relationship between pain and depression/pain-related disability in women suffering from IC/BPS [19]. Further, catastrophizing and depression have both been found to be predictors of patient distress in IC/BPS, with more than one in five patients reported having had suicidal thoughts [20]. This study was important because it suggested that psychosocial risk factors were worrisome over and above IC/BPS-specific symptoms and patient pain experience in predicting suicidal thinking in IC/BPS.

Depression. While there is evidence that depressive symptomology is a consequence of experiencing chronic pain, it has also been shown to be a critical risk factor for the development of chronic pain conditions [12, 13]. Women with chronic pelvic pain experience significant levels of depression, with one study reporting more than 50% of their sample scoring above a clinical cutoff point [5]. Indeed, in a review of the research, depression was identified as an important risk factor among women experiencing recurrent pelvic pain [21]. Another study found that depression was the strongest multivariable predictor of suicidal ideation over and above IC/BPS pain and symptoms [20].

Anxiety. Similar to depression, anxiety can be conceptualized as both a risk factor for, and consequence of chronic pain [12,13], with a similar pattern found for chronic pelvic pain. Anxiety symptoms have been identified as a key risk factor for the development of noncyclical pelvic pain [21]. Further, the majority of a sample of women with chronic pelvic pain experienced anxiety symptoms that fell in the moderate to severe range [5].

Coping Style. One's pain coping style can either serve to be adaptive or maladaptive, playing an important predictive role for a patient's prognosis [12, 13]. A sample of women with chronic pelvic pain reported low levels of pain self-efficacy and low confidence in their coping skills in areas such as their ability to manage without medication [5]. IC/BPS research on coping has shown that disability is mediated by the effect of depressed mood and catastrophizing, which are precursors of illness-focused coping [22]. Women's negative thoughts about their illness in IC/

BPS have been found to be associated with behavioral illness-focused coping (e.g., pain guarding, pain induced resting, asking for assistance), while thoughts that one is in control of their illness and treatment (e.g., illness self-efficacy) has been found to be associated with using wellness-focused coping for pain (e.g., exercising/stretching, positive coping self-talk, and relaxation) [15]. Based on these findings, coping style is crucial to assess, as it could play a major role in treatment success; thus, having an understanding of how patients cope with their pain could help guide effective symptom management plans.

Social Support. In general, individuals with chronic pain who report greater levels of perceived social support tend to fare better [12]. However, individuals who receive solicitous support (i.e., someone takes over an activity and does it for them) actually tend to fare worse than those who do not receive this type of pain-behavior reinforcement [23]. In IC/BPS, women who receive "distraction" from their spouses when in pain report that distraction actually acts to "buffer" the deleterious effects of pain on their mental quality of life [24]. In an IBD sample, greater negative spousal responses and less perceived spousal support predicted poorer IBD-quality of life [25]. In this study, helplessness catastrophizing was a mediator, acting as a mechanism between both negative spousal responses and perceived spousal support with IBD-quality of life in two separate models. Thus, social interaction variables were associated with IBD-quality of life, but patients' experience of helplessness reduced their ability to benefit from social support [25]. Disentangling the type and amount of social support a patient is receiving can have important clinical implications for their pain management.

Sexual Functioning. Another functional consequence of chronic pelvic pain is sexual functioning difficulties [5]. Given the high prevalence and associated distress that comes along with sexual difficulties, it is a critical area of assessment for patients with chronic pelvic pain. In one sample, a majority of these women experienced pain during intercourse ranging from at least half of the time to almost always [5]. Of note, nearly half of their sample did not even attempt intercourse. Further, our group has found that sexual functioning, employment, and pain predicted mental and physical quality of life. In particular, sexual functioning was a primary predictor of mental quality of life in women with long-standing IC/BPS, suggesting that sexual functioning may be a salient therapeutic target in the multifaceted treatment of patients with IC/BPS [26]. These findings highlight the significant impact chronic pelvic pain has on women's sexuality.

Taken together, the reviewed research highlights many pertinent psychosocial risk and maintenance factors that are important to consider in the assessment of patients with chronic pelvic pain. The purpose was to highlight the significant impact that these factors have on how patients feel and function, as well as how central these factors can be in the case conceptualization of a patient's disease and prognosis. Proper assessment of these factors can contribute to better clinical outcomes for patients who suffer from chronic pelvic pain.

Methods to Assess Psychosocial Variables

The following sections outline two methods to assess the psychosocial risk factors and functional consequences for chronic pelvic pain. First, a series of interview questions that "tap into" the content areas reviewed earlier are provided. These questions can be used in a semistructured interview format to provide a base patient interview. Second, a listing and description of several brief, valid, and reliable questionnaires representing the factors described earlier are provided.

As shown in Table 4.1, there are several types of questions that could be asked in a patient interview to query each of the psychosocial domains. The questionnaires are meant to supplement a patient interview, in order to provide detailed, quantitative information on areas identified in the interview as being be of particular concern. Following a theme of discovery in the patient engagement, the assessment tools provide a quick and empirically validated way to gather further information about a patient's psychosocial functioning and easily gather information that can be used to track patient progress on several topics. If used in concert, these methods will provide clinicians insight into the psychosocial domains as suggested by the AAPT and UPOINT systems. Finally, this assessment method also allows for an effective way to communicate to other healthcare providers, such as psychologists or other mental health professionals, about what types of psychosocial issues for which a patient may require remediation. This information is invaluable in guiding multidisciplinary

treatment plans for patients and is a strategy considered the gold standard for those suffering from chronic pelvic pain.

Semistructured Interview

The first step is to remember to let the patient report about her "pain story" to you in her own words before asking more focused questions. When you are listening to the patient's experience you can expect her to cover areas of her social, personal, and emotional lives. This is important to keep in mind when establishing good patient rapport and when gathering information about a patient's psychosocial problems.

The basic framework of the interview, if you follow down the left side of Table 4.1, is to examine the impact and promoters of poor quality of life in our patients. Thus, the initial questions seek to determine whether their pain is acute, chronic, or follows a cycle. Asking the patient to characterize her pain is important. Cardinal symptoms queried can include the pain onset, duration and frequency, descriptions of the pain, and bodily locations (i.e., map out the areas on a body diagram with an X). Patients can also be asked about pain precipitating and alleviating factors (e.g., stress, physical exertion), and whether there have been any changes in the frequency or quality of their pain over time.

As shown in Table 4.1, there are several suggested questions that can be used to query the psychosocial factors described in this chapter. These questions can be used in full or partially based on the patient presentation and the previous knowledge of the patient's medical and psychosocial history. There are several single-item queries that have been supported by research in showing utility to quickly probe for patient characteristics (e.g., [27]). Though single-item queries do not provide incremental benefit above what is obtained in the full use of a questionnaire in many cases, a single question may seem more natural and efficient within the clinical interview. One good example is assessing social support. Although the question in Table 4.1 for social support assesses a component of functional social support, other forms of support such as structural social support or community engagement and attachment might be used as desired by the clinician.

Assessment Tools

Pain. As shown in Table 4.1, patients' pain can be assessed using the short form of the McGill Pain

Table 4.1 Overview of suggested measures for the assessment of psychosocial domains

Psychosocial Factor	General Interview Questions	Measure	Description	No. of Items
Pain	Please tell me something about your pain. Is this pain the same that you have had before, or has it changed in some way? When did your pain start? Do you ever get a break from your pain? If so, when? Have you ever had your pain and how it feels described or assessed? What would be some of the words you would use to describe your pain? Do you have pain during intercourse, bowel movements, sitting? On a scale of 1–10, with 10 being the worst pain you ever had, how severe is your pain?	McGill Pain Questionnaire-Short Form (SF-MPQ; [28])	Assesses emotional and sensory aspects of respondent's pain experience	15
Disability	Do you find that your pain makes it difficult to do things around the house, work, or other areas of your life?	Pain Disability Index (PDI; [29])	Measures pain-related disability in seven broad areas of functioning	7
Quality of life	Please rate your health as "excellent, good, fair, or poor"	Short-Form Health Survey (SF-12; [30]) WHOQOL-BREF [31]	Assesses health-related quality of life Assess quality of life	12 26
Catastrophizing	When you feel pain, do you have the thought that it is terrible and feel that it is never going to get any better?	Pain Catastrophizing Scale (PCS; [32])	Assesses thoughts and feelings that may be associated with pain	13
Depressive symptoms	Over the past couple of weeks, how much have you been bothered by feeling sad, down, or uninterested in life? [41]	Patient Health Questionnaire-9 (PHQ-9; [33]) The Center for Epidemiologic Studies Depression Scale (CES-D; [34])	Assesses symptoms based on the DSM-IV criteria for major depression Assesses depressive symptomology	9 20
Anxiety symptoms	Over the past couple of weeks, how much have you been bothered by feeling anxious or nervous? [41]	Generalized Anxiety Disorder 7-item scale (GAD-7; [35]) State-Trait Anxiety Inventory (STAI; [36])	Assesses symptoms of anxiety One scale assesses state anxiety, the other assesses trait anxiety	7 20 (for one subscale)
Coping style	Do you find that you cope with your pain by stopping and resting or do you try to get active?	Chronic Pain Coping Inventory (CPCI; [37])	Assesses illness- and wellness-focused coping strategies	Two versions – 8 or 16 items

Table 4.1 (cont.)

Psychosocial Factor	General Interview Questions	Measure	Description	No. of Items
Social support	Is there someone you can talk to about things that are important to you – someone you can count on for understanding or support? If yes, how many people?	Multidimensional Scale of Perceived Social Support (MSPSS; [38]) West Haven–Yale Multidimensional Pain Inventory (WHYMPI; [39])	Measures participant's perceived social support from family, friends, and significant others Part of a larger questionnaire, one subscale measures amount and type of support from significant others	12 14
Sexual functioning	Do you have any sexual problems or concerns associated with your pain or otherwise?	Female Sexual Function Index (FSFI; [40])	Assesses different facets of female sexual functioning	19

Questionnaire [28]. This brief scale includes sensory and affective descriptors of pain that respondents rate on a 4-point severity scale. This measure also includes a visual analog scale, a present pain index to determine overall pain intensity, and in some versions, a body map for pain locations.

Disability. Pain-related disability can be measured using the Pain Disability Index [29]. This questionnaire assesses disability in a holistic way, as it has respondents rate the extent to which various areas of daily living are interfered with. These areas are as follows: family/home responsibilities, recreation, social activity, occupation, sexual behavior, self-care, and life-support activity.

Quality of Life. The Short-Form Health Survey-12 is a brief tool that can be used to assess health-related quality of life [30]. This measure consists of two summary scales – physical and mental – that assess areas such as vitality, physical functioning, social functioning, general health, mental health, bodily pain, as well as physical and emotional role limitations because of one's health problems. However, this scale involves a complicated scoring procedure. While this procedure is outlined by the authors in their paper, a simpler tool that also assesses quality of life and can be scored in a simpler fashion is the shortened version of the World Health Organization Quality of Life scale, called the WHOQOL-BREF [31]. This scale assesses the following domains: physical health, psychological, social relationships, and environment. Respondents rate the extent to which they have experienced various statements in the past two weeks.

Catastrophizing. Pain catastrophizing can be measured using the Pain Catastrophizing Scale [32]. This measure has respondents rate the extent to which they experience certain thoughts and emotions when they are in pain. There are three subscales that capture different aspects of catastrophizing – rumination, magnification, and helplessness.

Depressive Symptoms. There are two popular options for depressive symptoms. Patient's depressive symptoms can be measured using the Patient Health Questionnaire-9 [33]. This questionnaire is based on the DSM-IV (*Diagnostic and Statistical Manual of Mental Disorders*, fourth edition) criteria for major depression, in which respondents rate the degree to which they have been bothered by various symptoms in the past two weeks. Another option is the Center

for Epidemiologic Studies Depression scale, which assesses the frequency of depressive symptoms endorsed for the previous week [34].

Anxiety Symptoms. The Generalized Anxiety Disorder 7-item scale [35] is an instrument that can be used to assess anxiety symptoms and is based on the symptoms for generalized anxiety disorder in the DSM-IV. To assess state anxiety, one of the subscales from the State-Trait Anxiety Inventory can be used [36]. When answering these questions, participants must take into consideration how they feel at that moment (i.e., their present state).

Coping Style. The degree to which patient's use illness- and wellness-focused coping strategies can be measured using the Chronic Pain Coping Inventory (shortened versions; [37]). This measure asks respondents to indicate how many days of the week they used a variety of strategies to cope with their pain.

Social Support. A patient's level of perceived social support from family, friends, and significant others can be assessed using the Multidimensional Scale of Perceived Social Support [38]. To get a measure of the type of social support a patient is getting (e.g., solicitous, punishing, distracting), which, as described earlier, could have important clinical outcomes, the social support section of the West Haven–Yale Multidimensional Pain Inventory [39] can be used. This section of the questionnaire asks respondents to indicate how often a significant other would respond to them in a particular way when they are in pain.

Sexual Functioning. To get a comprehensive look at a patient's sexual functioning, the Female Sexual Function Index [40] can be used. This relatively brief tool assesses a variety of areas, including desire, subjective arousal, lubrication, orgasm, satisfaction, and pain.

Conclusions

The bottom line in assessing patients may be that asking "questions" is an important feature of comprehensive clinical engagement. Indeed, based on patients' responses to specific questions of value to the patients themselves, a patient-driven clinical picture has emerged for chronic pelvic diseases such as IC/BPS [11]. Bladder pain and urinary symptoms are the primary concerns of IC/BPS patients, but other domains related to associated nonurological conditions such as poor sleep/persistent fatigue, IBS-like symptoms, low back and general muscle pain, inter-ference/impact (e.g., sleep, diet, travel, activities, sexual functioning), positive and negative beliefs/attitudes, and favorable and maladaptive coping mechanisms, compose the comprehensive clinical picture for patients. This wide range of patient responses observed in focus group work and interviews leads to the conclusion that although the major themes are of value in patient assessment, there is much more variability than similarities in the individual clinical picture [11].

Chronic pelvic pain is a problematic and often difficult to manage condition that has a significant negative impact on patient quality of life. The biopsychosocial model of care has been widely lauded as the go-to model in disease management, especially when pain is a central complaint, and is being pushed by current research [11]. There are several validated screening and diagnostic scales that are routinely used in the assessment of patient pain and psychosocial domains. Nevertheless, standard medical care rarely utilizes personalized questions or psychosocial assessments in practice. A timely assessment of patients' pain and the contributing factors can aid physicians in the development of appropriate treatment maps, helping them create specific actions to address the patient's troubles. As such, we suggest that the assessment of pain and psychosocial risk and maintenance factors in patients with chronic pelvic pain should involve a basic semistructured questioning approach that can be followed up with specific questionnaires.

In this chapter, we stress that the fundamental discussion of the patients' psychosocial well-being is an essential starting point in adhering to a biopsychosocial medical model. The use of disease-specific scales and some of the more generalized scales mentioned here will work well together, creating a battery for clinical use. Finally, there is little doubt that psychosocial assessment is a critical part of understanding your patient and thus guiding your approach, particularly when the research shows such a strong and reliable impact from psychosocial factors on patient well-being and disability.

Your patient needs to know that "finding" the underlying cause and/or the maintaining factors of chronic pelvic pain can be a difficult and lengthy process, and well-defined explanations for pain cause and cure may be impossible to provide. However, with patience and open communication

with your patients, you will be able to develop a relationship and treatment plan that helps them live as full a life, with as little discomfort as possible.

Five Things You Need to Know

- The assessment of pain, psychosocial risk, maintenance factors, and sexuality may be best accomplished by using a semistructured questioning approach, followed by specific questions based on their particular presentation.
- In providing a caring culture, you may make some emotional gains for your patients. For example, patients report that improvements in life situations are made when psychosocial factors are addressed through a caring clinical environment, even without specific intervention.
- Pain outside of the affected body area is important to ask about and document. Many patients report other pains (e.g., >75% of pelvic pain samples), creating the need for a "whole pain" picture for the patient.
- Catastrophizing (i.e., negative thoughts and emotions associated with actual or anticipated pain) and feelings of being helpless are key drivers of depression, and both factors been found to be predictors of increasing levels of patient distress.
- More than one in five patients with pelvic pain (i.e., IC/BPS) report having had suicidal thoughts. Do not be afraid to ask this important question, "Over the last 2 weeks, have you been bothered by any thoughts that you would be better off dead or of hurting yourself in some way."

References

1. Global Burden of Disease Study 2013 Collaborators. Global, regional, and national incidence, prevalence, and years lived with disability for 301 acute and chronic diseases and injuries in 188 countries, 1990–2013: a systematic analysis for the Global Burden of Disease Study 2013. *Lancet.* 2015;**386**: 743–800.
2. Fillingim RB, Bruehl S, Dworkin RH, et al. The ACTTION-American Pain Society Pain Taxonomy (AAPT): an evidence-based and multidimensional approach to classifying chronic pain conditions. *J Pain.* 2014;**15**:241–9.
3. Ghaly AF, Chien PF. Chronic pelvic pain: clinical dilemma or clinician's nightmare. *Sex Transm Infect.* 2000;**76**:419–25.
4. Walker S, Hopman WM, Harrison MB, Tripp D, VanDenKerkhof EG. Pain and psychological characteristics in women waiting for gynaecological surgery. *J Obstet Gynaecol Can.* 2012;**34**:543–51.

5. Bryant C, Cockburn R, Plante AF, Chia, A. The psychological profile of women presenting to a multidisciplinary clinic for chronic pelvic pain: high levels of psychological dysfunction and implications for practice. *J Pain Res.* 2016;**9**:1049–56.

6. Passavanti MB, Pota V, Sansone P, Aurilio C, De Nardis L, Pace MC. Chronic pelvic pain: assessment, evaluation, and objectivation. *Pain Res Treat.* 2017;**2017**:1–15.

7. Nickel JC, Shoskes D, Irvine-Bird K. Clinical phenotyping of women with interstitial cystitis/ painful bladder syndrome: a key to classification and potentially improved management. *J Urol.* 2009;**182**:155–60.

8. Shoskes DA, Nickel JC, Rackley RR, Pontari MA. Clinical phenotyping in chronic prostatitis/chronic pelvic pain syndrome and interstitial cystitis: a management strategy for urologic chronic pelvic pain syndromes. *Prostate Cancer Prostatic Dis.* 2009;**12**:177–83.

9. Gatchel RJ, McGeary DD, McGeary CA, Lippe B. Interdisciplinary chronic pain management: past, present, and future. *Am Psychol.* 2014;**69**:119–30.

10. Jensen MP, Turk DC. Contributions of psychology to the understanding and treatment of people with chronic pain: why it matters to ALL psychologists. *Am Psychol.* 2014;**69**:105–18.

11. Nickel JC, Tripp DA, Beiko D, et al. The interstitial cystitis/bladder pain syndrome clinical picture (IC/ BPS): a perspective from patients' life experience. *Urol Pract.* 2018;**5**(4):286–92.

12. Edwards RR, Dworkin RH, Sullivan MD, Turk DC, Wasan AD. The role of psychosocial processes in the development and maintenance of chronic pain. *J Pain.* 2016;**17**:T70–T92.

13. Turk DC, Fillingim RB, Ohrbach R, Patel KV. Assessment of psychosocial and functional impact of chronic pain. *J Pain.* 2016;**17**:T21–T49.

14. Nickel JC, Irvine-Bird K, Jianbo L, Shoskes DA. Phenotype-directed management of interstitial cystitis/bladder pain syndrome. *Urology.* 2014;**84**:175–9.

15. Katz L, Tripp DA, Carr LK, Mayer R, Moldwin RM, Nickel JC. Understanding pain and coping in women with interstitial cystitis/bladder pain syndrome. *BJU Int.* 2017;**120**:286–92.

16. Tripp DA, Nickel JC, Wong J, et al. Mapping of pain phenotypes in female patients with bladder pain syndrome/interstitial cystitis and controls. *Eur Urol.* 2012;**62**:1188–94.

17. Danielsss JP, Khan KS. Chronic pelvic pain in women. *BMJ.* 2010;**341**:772–5.

18. Sullivan MJ, Thorn B, Haythornthwaite JA, et al. Theoretical perspectives on the relation between catastrophizing and pain. *Clin J Pain.* 2001;**17**:52–64.

19. Crawford A. The role of emotion regulation in the relationship between pain, catastrophizing, depression, and disability in women with interstitial cystitis/bladder pain syndrome. Master's thesis. 2017. ProQuest Dissertations and Theses database (UMI No. 10671787).

20. Tripp DA, Nickel JC, Krsmanovic A, et al. Depression and catastrophizing predict suicidal ideation in tertiary care patients with interstitial cystitis/bladder pain syndrome. *Can Urol Assoc J.* 2016;**10**:383–8.

21. Latthe P, Mignini L, Gray R, Hills R, Khan K. Factors predisposing women to chronic pelvic pain: systematic review. *BMJ.* 2006;**332**:749–55.

22. Katz L, Tripp DA, Nickel JC, Mayer R, Reimann M, van Ophoven A. Disability in women suffering from interstitial cystitis/bladder pain syndrome. *BJU Int.* 2013;**111**:114–21.

23. Turk DC, Kerns RD, Rosenberg R. Effects of marital interaction on chronic pain and disability: examining the down side of social support. *Rehabil Psychol.* 1992;**37**:259–74.

24. Ginting JV, Tripp DA, Nickel JC, Fitzgerald MP, Mayer R. Spousal support decreases the negative impact of pain on mental quality of life in women with interstitial cystitis/painful bladder syndrome. *BJU Int.* 2011;**108**:713–7.

25. Katz L, Tripp DA, Ropeleski M, et al. Mechanisms of quality of life and social support in inflammatory bowel disease. *J Clin Psychol Med Settings.* 2016;**23**:88–98.

26. Nickel JC, Tripp D, Teal V, et al. Sexual function is a determinant of poor quality of life in women with treatment refractory interstitial cystitis. *J Urol.* 2007;**177**:1832–6.

27. Flynn KE, Lindau ST, Lin L, et al. Development and validation of a single-item screener for self-reporting sexual problems in U.S. adults. *J Gen Intern Med.* 2015;**30**:1468–75.

28. Melzack R. The short-form McGill pain questionnaire. *Pain.* 1987;**30**:191–7.

29. Pollard CA. Preliminary validity study of the pain disability index. *Percept Mot Skills.* 1984;**59**:974.

30. Ware JE, Kosinski M, Keller SD. A 12-item short-form health survey: construction of scales and preliminary tests of reliability and validity. *Med Care.* 1996;**34**:220–33.

31. WHOQOL Group. Development of the World Health Organization WHOQOL-BREF quality of life assessment. *Psychol Med.* 1998;**28**:551–8.

32. Sullivan MJ, Bishop SR, Pivik J. The pain catastrophizing scale: development and validation. *Psychol Assess*. 1995;7:524–32.

33. Kroenke K, Spitzer RL, Williams JB. The PHQ-9. *J Gen Intern Med*. 2001;16:606–13.

34. Radloff LS. The CES-D scale: a self-report depression scale for research in the general population. *Appl Psychol Meas*. 1977;1:385–401.

35. Spitzer RL, Kroenke K, Williams JB, Löwe B. A brief measure for assessing generalized anxiety disorder: the GAD-7. *Arch Intern Med*. 2006;166:1092–7.

36. Spielberger CD, Gorsuch RL, Lushene R, Vagg PR, Jacobs GA. *Manual for the State-Trait Anxiety Inventory*. Palo Alto, CA: Consulting Psychologists Press; 1983.

37. Jensen MP, Keefe FJ, Lefebvre JC, Romano JM, Turner JA. One- and two-item measures of pain beliefs and coping strategies. *Pain*. 2003;104:453–69.

38. Zimet GD, Dahlem NW, Zimet SG, Farley GK. The multidimensional scale of perceived social support. *J Pers Assess*. 1988;52:30–41.

39. Kerns RD, Turk DC, Rudy TE. The West Haven-Yale multidimensional pain inventory (WHYMPI). *Pain*. 1985;23:345–56.

40. Rosen R, Brown C, Heiman J, Leiblum S, Meston C, Shabsigh R, et al. The female sexual function index (FSFI): a multidimensional self-report instrument for the assessment of female sexual function. *J Sex Marital Ther*. 2000;26:191–208.

41. Young QR, Nguyen M, Roth S, Broadberry A, Mackay MH. Single-item measures for depression and anxiety: validation of the screening tool for psychological distress in an inpatient cardiology setting. *Eur J Cardiovasc Nurs*. 2015;14:544–51.

Chapter 5

Musculoskeletal Assessment for Patients with Pelvic Pain

Lauren Hill and Karen Brandon

Editor's Introduction

Pelvic floor assessment is probably the most important part of the physical examination in patients with chronic pelvic pain and this exam is best performed by a skilled pelvic floor physical therapist. Physicians who see a large number of patients with pelvic pain should probably partner with a physical therapist and refer those patients for assessment. Some of the red flags on the history part of the assessment for pelvic floor dysfunction are urinary hesitancy (delayed onset of urine flow when trying to urinate) and pain after intercourse, or pain with physical activity (post exertion muscle soreness). Patients with pelvic floor muscle spasms also often have discomfort and pain with use of tampons, vaginal probe ultrasound, and pelvic exam. On pelvic exam when palpating with one finger muscles may feel tight and tender, often to the point where the examiner is not able to insert one finger. The obturator internus muscle is best palpated during the pelvic exam in the lithotomy position with the patient pushing with her knee against the examiner's external hand.

Introduction

Chronic pelvic pain (CPP) is a widespread disabling condition that is partly misunderstood because it is mostly a diagnosis of exclusion. In addition, viewing the problem as having a single etiology has created a dilemma regarding the assessment, classification, and management of CPP [1]. Most often a primary allopathic approach has excluded the possibility of the musculoskeletal/somatic and myofascial systems' contribution to initiating or maintaining impairments that are found in patients with pelvic pain. In fact, the pathophysiology of chronic pelvic pain can arise from the pelvic viscera, peripheral or central nervous system, pelvic joints, muscles, and connective tissue. It is also evident that as the body attempts to manage a local disturbance there are interactions between the other systems that can further complicate the clinical picture.

To best understand the musculoskeletal system, we must start with some physical medicine tenets. The purpose of the musculoskeletal structures of the pelvis is for "form and function": to house and protect the vital organs of the reproductive, gastrointestinal, and urological systems and thus allow for normal supportive and dynamically controlled (both reflexive and volitional) activities of evacuation, penetration, and pleasure to be achieved for the individual. Another tenet is that generally the musculoskeletal system responds to injury, trauma, or perceived threat in a predictable way [2, 3]. The final tenet is that the response of the musculoskeletal system is decided by the brain, which can not only modulate somatic activation and inhibition continuously but also interpret the function of the system based on the current context of the individual [4]. Because of these understandings, we recognize that while we must adequately assess local impairments and global relationships, we also have to understand the psychosocial implications of a history of pain or what pelvic pain means to the person's role, vocation, and abilities.

According to Wall and DeLancey, pelvic floor dysfunction as it relates to pelvic pain is poorly addressed partly due to "professional compartmentalization of the pelvic floor" [5]. This again speaks to the importance of integrated and coordinated care among multiple providers as well as treatment planning that recognizes the pelvic floor as a dynamic system that interacts with the rest of the body. Pelvic health physical therapy has a role in the integrated care and effective treatment of musculoskeletal causes of pelvic pain [6–8].

In this chapter we will outline screening for myofascial and mechanical impairments and describe a complete pelvic physical therapy clinical evaluation associated with musculoskeletal involvement in women with CPP.

Function-Based Approach

When addressing CPP from a musculoskeletal standpoint, establishing the goal of the intervention is important. Many factors contribute to determine the ultimate prognosis for the individual but usually fall within curative (recovery), improvable (rehabilitative), and manageable (adaptive) outcomes. This is most easily understood when looking at typical neurological or orthopedic conditions [9]. When someone sustains a femur fracture he or she can recover completely with no limitations; require rehabilitation and have some form of persisting impairment like a limp or impaired endurance; or always require some adaptation, such as a cane, and have limitations to participation in some physical activities. Similarly, in patients with CPP, for functional limitations such as sitting intolerances, impaired participation in sexual activities, and interruptions in daily tasks, we have similar expectations. Setting a baseline to understand the current status requires information to be collected on the patient's reported previous function. This must include assessment from the different roles the patient participates in. Patients with CPP can experience limitations in self-care, vocational, relational, and recreational domains [10]. While they are all important, patients' value of each area determines how it affects their quality of life and what their priorities are for treatment. Often it is helpful for the clinician to guide the patient through the process of identifying the limitations and the physical therapist can further describe the physiological elements required to complete the activity, and those that may be rehabilitated or adapted. This approach is focused not on pain level, but on capability of doing the activity to satisfaction [11]. The principle is to encourage patients to use their ability as a guide to improvement and not be limited by what they think their pain will stop them from doing. In addition, physical therapists can guide patients in managing their pain symptoms by using graded exposure techniques and imagery where useful, and to identify where they can stretch their tolerances by doing edgework but minimizing "flare ups" of their pain with pacing activities [12]. By creating an initial biopsychosocial perspective with CPP, clinicians can help patients achieve their activity goals by introducing variety to previously challenging tasks, and not being limited to linear progression based on their pain score.

Subjective Intake

Chronic pain studies in the last few decades have been critical about measurement of more than just a single measure of the impact of pain on the individual [13]. Not only does it poorly correlate with their disability or their functional loss, but in chronic pain it does not serve as an adequate marker for systemwide improvements.

In addition, the style of a typical single-symptom /single-system–based assessment is often too narrow of a net to capture the complexities of the patient with chronic pelvic pain [14].

Patient intake can have several components. It is important that the patient be informed that to adequately assess her problem, you will need to look at it from many angles, and this requires a few forms asking different questions and time with you to go over her answers.

First, a collection of medical history can detail injuries, surgeries, and early diseases; ongoing chronic conditions; and former and current interventions. For women, include gestation and parity history as well as any specifics about delivery methods or complications. It is also important to note which conditions are now stable and to identify overlapping conditions. It is recommended that there be clear inclusion of lumbar spine and hip pain in the questionnaire [15, 16]. Next, it is important to clarify the patient's primary complaint, which can be a single symptom, or many that limit participation in a particular function. A McGill Pain Questionnaire with body chart can be helpful in identifying where the patient localizes different pain complaints and descriptions and reminds the clinician to look for drivers or relationships outside the pelvis.

In addition to the completion of a pain questionnaire the patient should also complete the short screening for pain catastrophizing (PCS)[17], central sensitization (CSI)[18], and kinesiophobia (TSK)[19] (Table 5.1). This information is significant and is not easily ascertained by interview or even on follow-up visits, as it reflects the patient's perceptions about her condition that can impact the magnitude of her pain experience and her rehabilitation and recovery, and highlights nonvisceral and nonsomatic sources of persistent pain that need to be addressed with a specific inclusive neuropathic approach.

Table 5.1 Sample of standardized tools for chronic pain assessment

Measure	Domain Assessed
Verbal Rating Scale (VRS)	Pain intensity using verbal descriptors (e.g., mild, moderate, severe)
Visual Analog Scale (VAS)	Pain intensity using a 10- or 100-mm line, anchored by no pain and worst possible pain
McGill Pain Scale	Pain quality, location, exacerbating and ameliorating factors
Pain Disability Index (PDI)	Pain disability and interference of pain in functional, family, and social domains
Pain Catastrophizing Scale (PCS)	Catastrophic thoughts related to pain
Tampa Kinesiophobia Scale (TKS)	Fear of movement or limited activity
Central Sensitization Inventory (CSI)	Measure of somatic and emotional symptoms of CS
Vulvar Questionnaire (VQ)	Questions regarding vulvar pain symptoms
Pain Urination and Frequency (PUF)	Questions regarding bladder symptoms
GI Symptom Rating Scale (GSRS-IBS)	Questions regarding abdominal/bowel symptoms
Marinoff Scale	Tolerance to sexual intercourse activity

Finally, the patient's demographic information is valuable to put together the lifestyle and functional demands of the individual. Clarification of support systems available with regard to their relationship to the patient, and who the patient lives with is important. Determine the patient's job status, including the demands as well as the tasks and tolerances required. If the patient has been on leave from work, establish when she was placed on leave and for which condition and if she is scheduled to return. Information about the patient's general health can be initially determined by self-report about diet, exercise, sleep, and stress control.

Once those forms are collected and scored, a patient-centered interview can begin [20]. First, the provider invites the patient to tell the purpose of her visit in her own words. The provider can practice reflective listening at moments in the patient's story to clarify and direct the interview. Once the reason for the visit is established, the provider may want to clarify what the patient's understanding is of the problem, what she believes is the etiology, and what she thinks will improve her condition. If it is clear what the patient's belief system is concerning her problem, it will be easier to educate or motivate her for health behavior changes.

Next is a brief review of the medical history to clarify the timeline or any unclear information. In addition, a function-based review of systems includes questions about bowel regularity, continence, and consistency; bladder continence, frequency, voiding; and sexual function for pain report, impact on desire, arousal, and orgasm. Questions have been included in Table 5.2.

When reviewing the reported pain, on either the VAS or McGill Pain Questionnaire, the provider should include follow-up questions about easing factors and aggravating factors. He or she should ask the patient to quantify pain at rest, average, and maximum on the VAS. It is important to determine if the pain has a pattern that is hormonally cyclic, episodic by physical activity, related to sleep/rest cycles, or to bowel and bladder activity. If the patient reports episodes of pain that are intermittent the provider can have her quantify how many she has had within a time period. If she reports constant pain, the provider can have her describe the daily range on the VAS. The Pain Disability index (PDI)[21] can be helpful for categorizing areas of impairment that affect the patient's lifestyle and to what degree. For specific vulvovaginal pain the Vulvar Questionnaire (V-Q)[22] can be used, and for bladder-related symptoms as a primary tool the PUF[23] questionnaire, and Gastrointestinal Symptom Rating scale (GSRS-IBS)[24] for bowel-related pain. The Marinoff Scale is used to assess tolerance to sexual penetrative activities (Table 5.1).

Initiating a musculoskeletal assessment includes gathering information about many systems that interact with muscles, ligaments and bones. It is also important for the provider to clarify the patient's primary concern, how she is currently functioning or her limits of function, to direct the next part of the evaluation, the physical assessment.

Objective Assessment

Clinical Anatomy Overview

The pelvic floor is made up of superficial and deep muscles that contribute to numerous systems

Table 5.2 Screening questions for pelvic pain in pelvic physical therapy

Age: Gravida: Para:

Did you have any trouble with the deliveries?

Occupation and demands?

Live with? Stairs at home or work?

Any hip pain? Low back pain?

Difficulty standing? If so, how long? Difficulty sitting? If so, how long? Difficulty walking? If so, how long/far?

Do you have regular periods? Perimenopausal? Menopausal?

On birth control? If yes, method?

Any urine leaking? Any frequency of urine, needing to urinate more than every 2 hours?

Night waking to urinate? Any trouble emptying bladder?

Any bowel difficulty or pain on emptying? Bowel movement every 1–3 days? What is the consistency?

Pain symptoms found where: Location?

24-Hour pattern?

If episodic how many a day/week? If constant what is range of pain experienced?

Easing factors? Aggravating factors?

Sleep disturbance? Falling asleep or waking with pain?

Takes medication for pain: if yes, how much and how often? What is its effect?

What home activity does this pain keep you from doing?

Does this activity keep you from work-related responsibilities?

Does this activity keep you from leisure or fitness activities?

If the pain score goes up by 2–3 points, what do you find you have difficulty doing?

If the pain score goes down by 2–3 points, what do you find you are able to do?

Do you have pain or discomfort or problems with sex?

If yes: When did sex pain start?

Was this the first sexual encounter?

Have you tried a lubricant? What kind?

Does it limit penetration completely?

Does it hurt at entry or deep? Does it change with certain positions?

Describe if it hurts at the beginning, all the way through, or is there pain afterwards?

Do you have trouble with the last vaginal exam by a physician or nurse?

Do you use tampons? If yes, are you still able to use them?

Since the pain problem, has desire for sexual activity changed to higher, lower, or stayed the same?

Since the pain problem, are you able to do other physically intimate things besides intercourse?

Is your partner aware of your pain and accommodating?

throughout the body including musculoskeletal, respiratory, reproductive, lymphatic, gastrointestinal, and urological. They function to provide sphincter control and support to maintain continence and prevent prolapse of pelvic organs [25]. By way of their connections to the pelvis, hips, and other abdominal and back musculature, they help stabilize the sacro-iliac (SI) joints, lumbar spine, sacrococcygeal joint, pubic symphysis, and hips to allow for load transfer from the lower extremities to the pelvis and postural stability during functional tasks and movements. They are synchronized with the deep core musculature to allow for appropriate intraabdominal pressure fluctuations and optimal respiratory function [26]. Through appropriate contraction and relaxation of the pelvic floor muscles, they allow for optimal sexual function [27]. Additionally, similar to the calf muscles in the lower extremities, they contribute to the flow and return of blood and lymphatic fluid to prevent congestion.

More specifically, the pelvic floor is composed of three layers: superficial, intermediate, and deep. The superficial muscles of the pelvic floor consist of the bulbocavernosus, ischiocavernosus, superficial transverse perineal, and external anal sphincter. The intermediate or second layer includes the deep transverse perineal, sphincter urethrovaginalis, compressor urethra, and external urethral sphincter. The third and deepest layer includes the levator ani group (puborectalis, pubococcygeus, and iliococcygeus) and coccygeus. The third layer is connected to the obturator internus muscle through the arcus tendinous levator ani (ATLA), a fascial band formed by the obturator internus and extending from the ischial spine to the posterior pubic symphysis. The piriformis muscle, along with the obturator internus, are hip muscles that attach within the pelvis and contribute to the musculature of the posterior and lateral pelvic walls respectively. All these muscles are housed within the boundaries of the pubic bone anteriorly, ischiopubic ramus and ilium laterally, and the sacrum and coccyx posteriorly.

Because of the anatomical relationships between intrapelvic and extrapelvic muscles, biomechanical dysfunctions and imbalances can result in pain and impairments throughout the entire pelvic girdle. Overactive pelvic floor muscles can be the causative agent in musculoskeletal conditions due to anatomical and functional relationships related to the respiratory diaphragm, abdomen, spine, sacrum, coccyx, and hips. Alternatively, malalignment; impaired biomechanics; or injury and pain in the trunk, pelvis, or lower quarter can impact the pelvic floor due to faulty load transfer, gait dysfunctions, and other suboptimal movement patterns causing overuse and overactivity in the pelvic floor muscles [28]. Musculoskeletal structures of the low back, abdomen, pelvis, and hips are also neurologically connected to the pelvic floor through shared innervation. Studies show that in patients with pelvic floor muscle pain or abnormality it is common to find tender points or abnormality in the obturator internus, iliopsoas, gluteus, quadratus lumborum, and piriformis muscles [29]. Abnormal musculoskeletal findings were found in patients with chronic pelvic pain 37% of the time compared to controls without pelvic pain only 5% of the time [30].

The bony structure of the pelvic girdle is formed by the ilium, ischium, and pubis, which fuse to form the innominate bones. The pelvic girdle is a supportive yet dynamic link between the thorax, spine, and lower extremities [28]. The two sides of the bony pelvis are joined through the connection between the ilia and sacrum posteriorly and the superior pubic rami forming the fibrocartilaginous pubic symphysis joint anteriorly. In optimal pelvic movement, the motion of the sacrum is correlated and synchronized with motion at the sacrococcygeal and lumbosacral joints. As the sacrum extends, the apex of the coccyx flexes and as the sacrum flexes, the apex of the coccyx extends. Lastly, the femoral head articulates with the acetabulum of the innominate bones and couples with ilium movement. As the hip flexes, the ilium rotates posteriorly, and as the hip extends the ilium rotates anteriorly. Through these various joints, connections, and the synchronization of movement, one can appreciate how optimal or suboptimal movement at the spine, sacrum, coccyx, and hips can influence the pelvis and its musculature [28].

Sacroiliac Joint

The main function of the pelvic girdle joints is to provide stability and transfer forces to the lower extremities. Ligamentous support to the SI joint is provided by some of the strongest ligaments in the body. The anterior or ventral sacroiliac ligament is a thickening of the fibrous capsule of the SI joint and is the weakest of the supports. The interosseus sacroiliac ligament forms the major connection between the sacrum and innominate and is the strongest of the ligamentous group spanning from the lateral sacral crest to the iliac tuberosity. It resists anterior and inferior movement of the sacrum. The long dorsal sacroiliac ligament connects the posterior superior iliac spine (PSIS) with the lateral aspect of the third and fourth segments of the sacrum. Nutation, or anterior motion of the sacrum, places slack on the ligament. This ligament can be palpated directly below the PSIS, felt as a thick band, and can often be a source of pain or reproduce SI joint pain. The long dorsal ligament is connected to the gluteus maximus muscle through shared fascia, and connections have been found to the multifidi muscles as well. The sacrotuberous ligament is formed by lateral, medial, and superior bands. The superior fibers combine with the long dorsal ligament. The lateral band connects the ischial tuberosity and posterior inferior iliac spine and receives some fibers from the piriformis. The medial fibers span from the lateral lower sacrum and coccyx and run toward the ischial tuberosity. Muscular attachments from the gluteus maximus muscle also insert onto the sacrotuberous ligament, therefore increasing tension during muscular contraction. The sacrotuberous ligament stabilizes against nutation of the sacrum. The perforating cutaneous nerve travels through the sacrotuberous ligament to supply the skin covering the inferior and medial aspects of the buttocks. Lastly, the sacrospinous ligament spans from the lateral part of the sacrum and coccyx and onward to the ischial spine and is connected to the coccygeus muscle. SI joint disorders can be a common finding in patients with pelvic floor muscle dysfunction, with concomitant observation or history reporting including faulty biomechanics, degenerative changes, habitual postures, and pregnancy-related SI joint pain. SI joint pain is typically noted with palpation over the SI joint as well as possible referral of pain into the iliac crest, low back, groin, buttocks, and down the back of the thigh. Compression of the SI joints due to increased tension into the pelvic floor can lead to poor motor control; impaired lumbopelvic stabilization; posturing into a posterior pelvic tilt; hip restrictions into flexion, adduction, and internal rotation; and tender point in the obturator internus, piriformis, and coccygeus [31]. Patients may report pain with palpation of the posterior superior iliac spine (PSIS) that is worsened with prolonged sitting, standing, walking, or lying down and walking up hills or stairs, radiating pain into the buttocks with some alleviation of pain in side-lying.

Assessment of the SI joint can include posterior palpation of the long dorsal SI ligament (or Fortin's finger sign). There are passive and active tests that demonstrate SI dysfunction. If the patient is standing a single limb stance can elicit pain on the ipsilateral SI joint, as well as demonstrate weakness or impaired ligamentous integrity. Supine the examiner is standing at the side of the patient. The examiner crosses his or her arms and places them at the medial aspects of the patient's anterior superior iliac spines. A gapping pressure is applied in an outward direction bilaterally and simultaneously. The examiner then uncrosses his or her arms and places his or her hands on the iliac crests to apply an inward/downward force. Pain indicates a positive test. While the patient is in the supine position one can add the posterior provocation test, bringing the ipsilateral knee up to the patient's chest and crossing midline and applying a long axis compression into the femur. Hip pain may be present but is positive for SI dysfunction if the posterior pelvic girdle pain is elicited.

Pubic Symphysis

Pain and dysfunction into the anterior bony pelvis can also contribute to overall pelvic pain. Dysfunction into the pubic symphysis can refer pain into the low abdomen and groin that can be mistaken for bladder or other visceral pain. Osteitis pubis is characterized by a sharp or aching anterior pelvic pain over the pubic symphysis, lower abdominal muscles, or perineum due to infection, inflammation, trauma during contact sports, or repetitive trauma due to increased shearing such as during pregnancy as a result of ligamentous laxity. The pain may also radiate into the adductors, leading to spasm in these muscles [32]. Muscle dysfunctions and imbalances between the hip adductors, abdominals, and pelvic floor can also cause excessive or inappropriate shearing of the pubic symphysis, leading to pain symptoms [33]. Osteitis pubis has also been reported to complicate a variety of pelvic surgeries including abdominoperineal resection, inguinal herniorrhaphy, anterior colporrhaphy, retropubic urethropexy, and periurethral collagen injection. Patients may report pain that worsens with running, climbing stairs, transitional movements such as sit to stand, rolling in bed, or getting out of the car. Although pubic symphysis pain disorders can refer to the pelvic girdle, labia, and perineum, often the pelvic floor muscles are overlooked as possible contributors to the pain, particularly the superficial

layer of the pelvic floor. The bulbocavernosus and ischiocavernosus muscles directly attach to the pubic symphysis, as does the deeper anterior aspect of the pubococcygeus, and these should be assessed for pain reproduction during palpation, particularly for unilateral tension. Diagnosis can be based on radiological examination including x-rays; palpation that would include pain at the pubic symphysis; and likely observation of difficulty during gait including a waddling gait, hip stiffness, and pain with transitional movements.

A lateral compression test can be performed with the patient side-lying while applying a downward force at the lateral iliac crest and considered positive with reproduction of pain in the pubic symphysis area. The symphysis gap test is also performed and includes having the patient supine with bilateral hips and knees flexed to 90 degrees, legs supported by the examiner. The patient then performs an isometric adductor contraction against the fist of the examiner placed between the knees. A painful isometric muscle contraction with pain into the pubic symphysis is considered positive.

Coccyx

The coccyx can also be a location of pain and dysfunction in combination with pelvic floor muscle hyperactivity. The coccyx is stabilized through the sacrotuberous, sacrospinous, and long dorsal ligaments which can all be concomitant pain referral areas in conjunction with coccyx pain. The coccyx also acts as an insertion site for the deep pelvic floor muscles (pubococcygeus, iliococcygeus, and coccygeus), and gluteus maximus and contraction or relaxation of these muscles can influence coccygeal movement [28]. Coccyx pain can be the result of direct injury to the coccyx including a fall or during childbirth, repetitive compression or poor posturing of the coccyx such as in cycling and horseback riding, or pelvic malalignments due to leg length discrepancy or indirectly through pelvic floor muscle tension or surgery involving the sacrospinous ligaments. The subjective interview might include symptoms such as pain during/after sitting with the length of sitting being a factor; acute spike of pain during transitional movements such as sit to stand; greater difficulty sitting on soft surfaces than on firm; pain with bowel movements; and possible referral of pain into the sacrum, low back, rectum, and lower extremities.

Assessment would include palpation of the coccyx in standing as well as while prone to determine available movement, pain reproduction, or deviation laterally as well as palpation of the ligamentous and muscular attachments that influence the coccyx as described earlier. The movement of the coccyx may be better appreciated through rectal examination if this seems to be a large source of the patient's pain.

Assessment of the involvement of the lumbar spine includes standing passive flexion and extension of the trunk as well as side bending and rotation. Pain elicited that reproduces radicular pain into the pelvis or lower extremity and pain that occurs at spine with specific motions should be further assessed with a spinal accessory motion exam and evaluation of neural system.

Lumbar Spine

The lumbar spine can also influence, and be influenced by, the pelvic floor muscles. As discussed earlier, the lumbar spine is connected via muscular and ligamentous attachments to the pelvic girdle, and the transfer of loads from the lower extremities to the spine is routed through the pelvic girdle. Lumbopelvic posturing into either excessive lumbar lordosis or lumbar flexion can impact recruitment and coordination of abdominal as well as pelvic floor muscles, impacting resting tone of the pelvic floor and maintenance of continence [34]. Pelvic floor muscle hyperactivity can refer pain into the low back area and can be a source of impairment related to spinal stability and mobility through connections between the gluteal muscles, transversus abdominis, and psoas. Low back pain has also been found to alter the anticipatory recruitment of the transversus abdominis muscle, therefore altering the synchronization of the deep core muscles including the pelvic floor muscles. The deep core feedforward impairments related to low back pain are shown to persist even once pain is resolved [35]. Muscle imbalances or dysfunctions can lead to compression and irritation of nerves exiting the lumbar spine, therefore contributing to radiating symptoms into the pelvis and lower extremities. This can include compression on the iliohypogastric (T12–L1), ilioinguinal (L1), lateral femoral cutaneous (L2–L3), femoral (L2–L4), genitofemoral (L1–L2), and obturator (L2–L4) nerves. These nerves innervate areas including the mons pubis, inguinal regions, groin, medial and anterior thighs, and genitals [36]. Studies have shown significant correlations between low back pain and pelvic floor issues, with up to 95.3% of participants in one study with low back pain found to have some form of pelvic floor dysfunction and 71% of those demonstrating hypertonicity or tenderness of the pelvic floor muscles [15].

If a patient reports pain or genital/sexual dysfunction a screening of S2–S4 be included to rule out impairment from the lumbosacral nerves that control pelvic floor sensory and motor functions.

Transverse Abdominus

The pelvic floor is also intimately linked to what is referred to as the deep core. The deep core is thought of as a canister that includes the pelvic floor muscles at the base, respiratory diaphragm at the top, transversus abdominals in the front, and multifidi spinal stabilizers in the back. This deep core canister provides proximal stability upon which more distal mobility can occur and helps to prepare the body for load transfer [28]. Research shows this group of locally functioning deep core muscles activate as a unit and have anticipatory function in that they fire prior to initiation of movement [37]. The more globally functioning superficial abdominal muscles include the rectus abdominis, obliques, and erector spinae muscles. Patients with pelvic pain may tend to overuse these global stabilizers due to dysfunction with the synchronization pattern with the deep core stabilizers because of weakness and/or overactivity in the pelvic floor muscles. When this occurs, faulty movement patterns and suboptimal muscle activation ensues that, over time, likely contribute to a patient's continued pain. Research has found that increased activation of the deep muscles and/or decreased activity in the global muscles during movement tasks can help to improve movement patterns and decrease patient symptoms [38].

Assessment of the transverse abdominus is typically with ability to draw in the navel but also for endurance in tonic postures such as ability to maintain neutral thoracolumbar and lumbopelvic spine with demands such as a plank start position for a push up. Activation can also be assessed with dynamic rehabilitative ultrasound.

Piriformis Muscle

The piriformis muscle connects to the pelvic girdle through its attachment to the anterior surface of the sacrum and inserts onto the greater trochanter of the hip with additional attachments to the sacrotuberous ligament. The tendon of the piriformis then joins with other hip rotator tendons including the superior and inferior gemelli and obturator internus and externus tendons. The function of the piriformis muscle is to extend, abduct, and externally rotate the hip; stabilize the SI joint; and control innominate anterior rotation. Tenderness and pain into the piriformis can be a common symptom for patients with pelvic floor muscle hyperactivity because of these connections and the resultant muscle imbalances that can occur due to dysfunction and/or upregulation of muscles surrounding the pelvic floor muscles by way of fascial, neural, and anatomical connections [28]. Piriformis syndrome refers to pain and/or numbness in the buttock caused by spasm and therefore compression of the sciatic nerve, which runs beneath the piriformis muscle referring symptoms into the ipsilateral posterior thigh and possibly foot. The pudendal nerve can also become compressed as it exits the medial inferior surface of the piriformis. Spasm of the piriformis and sacral dysfunction can place tension on the sacrotuberous ligament with resultant compression on the pudendal nerve as well leading to neuralgia symptoms into the vulvar area. The patient with piriformis spasm may demonstrate increased external rotation of the ipsilateral hip noted as increased turning out at the foot during gait [39].

> During assessment, the patient rests supine with the testing hip in external rotation. The clinician asks the patient to bring the hip into internal rotation and a positive test elicits pain in the buttock/piriformis area. Pain can also be felt during passive internal rotation into the buttock area knows as the Freiberg sign.

Hip Joint

Due to the connection between the femoral head and acetabulum of the pelvis, hip impingement syndromes can occur as a result of pelvic girdle dysfunction. Abnormal contact between the femoral head and acetabulum can be due to increased tension or weakness within hip flexors, extensors, and deep rotators including the psoas, obturator internus/externus, piriformis, and gluteus maximus/medius misaligning the femoroacetabular junction. Patients may describe symptoms including groin, anterior or medial thigh pain, deep hip pain, and sensations of locking within the joint. Pain may be reproduced during turning or pivoting motions and/or passive, active, or resisted movement into hip flexion, adduction, or internal rotation. Restrictions are typically seen within the iliopsoas, quadriceps, tensor fascia lata, and external hip rotators in the form of decreased passive range of motion into hip extension, knee flexion, hip adduction, and hip internal rotation respectively [40].

If the femur continues to be malpositioned within the acetabulum, labral injuries can occur, although most labral tears are due to repetitive sports injuries that involve frequent pivoting or cutting type maneuvers. The most common patient complaint with labral tears is pain in the anterior hip or groin, less common into lateral and deep posterior buttock, lower abdominal quadrant, and knee. The pain may be described as a sharp or dull pain. Pain reports are often accompanied by mechanical complaints of clicking/catching or giving way. Development of labral tears is possible during twisting/pivoting injuries, posterior hip dislocations, hyperflexion or hyperextension movements, or idiopathically. Along with pain complaints, patients with hip labral tears may report decreased hip mobility and pain with prolonged sitting. Studies have shown a relationship between hip function and pelvic floor muscle function including a case series of patients with labral tears as a comorbidity of low back and pelvic girdle pain [41]. Labral tears in the hip have also been linked to vulvar pain syndromes such as vulvodynia and resultant hyperactive pelvic floor muscles [16].

> Assessment should include performance of the anterior hip impingement test, which is performed with the patient supine and the hip and knee at 90 degrees flexion. The hip is internally rotated while an adduction force is applied through the femur. A positive test would produce pain in the anterolateral hip or groin. McCarthy's sign is another test involving bilateral hip flexion, bringing the patient's knees to chest passively followed by extension with internal rotation of the affected hip and again extension with external rotation. Impingement testing includes passively taking the hip into flexion, adduction, and internal rotation. A positive test would be reproduction of pain or a clicking sensation. A labral tear can also be confirmed through MRI, MRA, or arthroscopy.

Endopelvic Fascia

This connection between the hip and pelvic floor muscles is mitigated through the fascia covering the pelvic floor muscles, as this is continuous with endo-pelvic fascia above, perineal fascia below, and obturator fascia laterally. Further, thickening of the obturator fascia becomes the arcus tendinous fascia pelvis which extends from the pubis anteriorly to the ischial spine posteriorly. From that point, the para-vaginal connective tissue attaches the anterior wall of the vagina to the arcus tendinous fascia pelvic and posterior vaginal wall to the levator ani and are considered an extension of the endopelvic fascia. The pubococcygeus originates on the fascia that surrounds the obturator internus. Extending superior to the arcus tendinous fascia pelvic is a thickening of the levator ani called the arcus tendinous levator ani, which is where the levator ani muscle originates [42]. While the endopelvic fascia is noncontractile it is subject to the contraction (or relaxation) of the attached muscles.

Psoas Muscle

The psoas muscle is another key player in the connection between the lumbar spine, pelvic girdle, and hip as it arises from the anterolateral aspect of T12–L5 vertebral bodies and transverse processes traversing through the pelvic cavity, crossing the hip, joining fibers with the iliacus, and inserting onto the lesser trochanter as the iliopsoas. The psoas has direct connections to the respiratory diaphragm superiorly and to the coccygeus inferiorly by way of fascial connections, demonstrating the intimate link this muscle has to contributing to the deep core and pelvic girdle [43].

The psoas functions to flex the hip and spine as well as mobilize the trunk into flexion, rotation, and side bending. Decreased flexibility, myofascial trigger points, or injury to the psoas can refer pain into the lumbar spine, superior iliac crest posteriorly, SI joint, abdomen adjacent to the umbilicus, or inside the ilium or lateral rectum region near the inguinal ligament and upper thigh [44].

Patients with psoas spasm may report pain into the low back area when sitting or standing, difficulty in attaining full upright posture, and pain in the contralateral gluteal region. Spasm in the psoas is typically associated with shortening of the ipsilateral quadratus lumborum abnormal pull on the ilium and increased tension into the pelvic floor muscles [45]. The iliohypogastric, ilioinguinal, and genitofemoral nerves pass over or through the psoas and can be compressed or irritated due to psoas spasm or dysfunction, thus radiating pain along the length of these nerves into the abdomen, pelvis, genitals, and lower extremities. The obturator nerve emerges at the medial border of the psoas and if compressed can radiate pain into the inner thigh.

> Assessment should include transabdominal palpation for tenderness, trigger points, or reproduction of pain and length tests including the Thomas Test. The Thomas Test is performed with the patient lying supine with the testing limb hanging over the side of the table, the opposite knee flexed toward the chest. The clinician passively flexes the knee of the hanging limb while simultaneously extending the same hip to assess flexibility of the psoas or reproduction of symptoms.

Rectus Abdominus

Superficial to the deep psoas muscle, the abdominal wall and related myofascia can develop tender points and be a common comorbidity of chronic pelvic pain. Myofascial trigger points above the pubis and within lower rectus abdominis and internal oblique can cause urinary urgency/frequency and bladder, buttock, perineal, and back pain. Palpation of these areas can also produce somatovisceral symptoms such as nausea, vomiting, and muscle spasm [44]. These myofascial trigger points are usually localized within a skeletal muscle fascia or in the muscle covering fascia and can again be classified as active or latent [46]. Along with tender points within the abdominal wall, connective tissue abnormalities have been found to be associated with the presence of tender points and refer to a thickening of the subcutaneous tissues with resistance to movement. Fitzgerald and Kotarinos described connective tissue abnormalities as frequent in women with overactive pelvic floors and identified commonly affected regions on the abdominal wall, thighs, low back, buttocks, and perineum. The reliability of connective tissue assessment warrants further research [47]. Restriction in the connective tissue as well as tender point formation can also be a result of poor posturing and lumbopelvic dysfunctions that could be further assessed via physical therapy referral and not covered within the scope of this chapter. In addition, superficial nerves can be affected by muscular or scar tissue that create localized burning and sharpness after trocar sites heal, or after local incisions such as Pfannenstiel incision or hernia repair. Palpation of the abdominal wall is crucial and the most common method used to determine if the abdominal wall is a possible source or contributor to pelvic pain [48].

> The assessment should include Carnett's sign, which helps to discriminate between parietal and visceral pain origins. The clinician applies pressure on the site of the abdominal pain while the patient performs a small curl up to contract the rectus abdominus muscle. If the pain worsens, it is considered positive for pain originating from abdominal muscle versus visceral origin.

Physical Examination of the Pelvic Floor

When the provider is prepared to start the palpation portion of the physical exam, approaching the patient with a clear explanation of what to expect, the purpose of the exam and consent for examination is imperative in this type of clinical care [49]. Owing to the nature of the condition being a pain syndrome, all efforts should be made to use only provocatory methods when necessary and not to create more emotional or tissue distress with excessive procedures. In addition, many patients have seen multiple providers, so clinicians should be mindful of the patient's tolerance level. Identifying potential yellow flags during the intake that include history of trauma is valuable for how to proceed with the examination. Using reflective listening and appropriate inquiry while both empathizing and normalizing the patient's experience allows the clinician to take time to note hesitations and nonverbal discomfort in areas of discussion during the consult.

Giving clear permission for the patient to stop any part of the physical exam is a way to allow control and also confer respect to the patient regarding her participation [49]. Several institutions require the presence of a chaperone for all pelvic exams to ensure the comfort level and safety of both the patient and provider.

Observation of Pelvic Muscle Activity

Visual observation is the first step in examining the superficial layer of the pelvic floor as well as the overall function of the muscles. Assessment is typically performed in the dorsal lithotomy position with consideration for the position of the patient's pelvis. It is optimal to have the patient in a neutral pelvic position, which places the pelvic floor muscles in an optimal position to assess for baseline functioning

due to changes in pelvic floor recruitment based on lumbopelvic position.

After brief inspection of the vulva, perineum, and anus for skin pathologies and/or anatomical abnormalities the examiner notes the resting position of the perineal body in relation to the bilateral ischial tuberosities. Typically, with normal pelvic floor muscle activity, the perineal body should appear in-line with the ischial tuberosities. Patients with overactive pelvic floor muscles may appear to have a perineal body that is elevated in the cranial direction or ascended compared to the ischial tuberosities [50]. By contrast, patients with underactive pelvic floor muscles may have a perineal body that appears lowered in the caudal direction or descended compared to the ischial tuberosities. The International Continence Society (ICS) classifies function or dysfunction of the pelvic floor into normal, overactive, underactive, or nonfunctioning conditions [51] (Table 5.3).

After the anatomy is explained using a model or an illustration, the clinician can also observe pelvic floor function that can later be compared to the function felt during internal palpation. The patient should be provided clear instructions to perform a pelvic floor contraction such as to "stop a flow of urine," "prevent gas from coming out," "nod the clitoris," or "pull up and in." The clinician should notice symmetrical movement inward or in a ventral and cephalad direction, likely seeing the greatest excursion of movement at the perineal body without compensatory use of accessory pelvic muscles such as the hip adductors, gluteals, or abdominals. The patient with hyperactive or hypoactive pelvic floor muscles may demonstrate limited excursion of movement either due to limited muscle range of motion from a shortened length–tension relationship of muscle fibers or due to limited muscle strength and coordination, respectively [36]. Patients with overactive pelvic floor muscles may report pain, or reproduction

Table 5.3 International Continence Society (ICS) definition of pelvic floor function

Normal pelvic floor muscles: pelvic floor muscles that can voluntarily contract
Overactive pelvic floor muscles: pelvic floor muscles that do not relax, or may even contract when relaxation is functionally needed, for example, during micturition or defecation
Underactive pelvic floor muscles: pelvic floor muscles that cannot voluntarily contract when this is appropriate
Nonfunctioning pelvic floor muscles: pelvic floor muscles where there is no action palpable

of symptoms, with contraction of the pelvic floor muscles. The clinician then observes if the patient is able to relax the pelvic floor muscles, seen as a descent or caudal movement of the perineal body back to or past the starting baseline. The patient should then be asked to perform a pelvic floor "bulge" or drop as if she is "passing a little gas" or "starting a flow of urine." This should be distinguished from a straining or Valsalva maneuver, which involves breath holding and maximal effort. A gentle pushing out or caudal movement of the perineal body should be noted without breath holding during a bulge. Patients with overactive pelvic floor muscles may likely demonstrate difficulty performing this maneuver, as an elevated resting tone and incomplete relaxation capacity are a common finding in women with chronic pelvic pain and pelvic floor muscle overactivity [52]. Impaired muscle coordination and/or lack of pelvic floor muscle awareness may also be noted and observed as a perineal descent when the patient is asked to perform a contraction indicating the patient is straining instead of contracting and likely contributing to symptoms of incontinence. Patients may also demonstrate a pelvic floor contraction when asked to bulge or gently push out their pelvic floor, which could be contributing to impaired voiding mechanics and incomplete and/or painful emptying of bowel and bladder [53].

Vaginal Assessment of Muscle Function

Once observation of the vulva and pelvic floor function has been performed, assessment should include palpation. After gaining consent for further assessment, the clinician can insert a single digit centrally in the vaginal introitus approximately 2 inches, and after asking if there is any pain, the clinician can assess the volitional contraction patient is able to generate with the same cues used to compress and draw the finger inward and upward. The contraction should be felt as a tightening, lift, and pull inward around the examination finger. While various grading scales have been proposed and are widely used clinically the intrarater reliability is limited for most of the subjective test. The two most recognized are the PERFECT scheme (Power, Endurance, Repetitions, Fast contractions, Every-Contraction-Timed) and the Modified Oxford scale (0–5). Laycock et al. found the ratings to be reliable and reproducible when testing pelvic floor muscle strength, coordination, and endurance; however, in other studies, the interobserver variability has been found to be high and intertester agreement to be fair [54]. The

Modified Oxford Scale is another quantitative assessment developed to determine pelvic floor muscle movement and strength during contraction. Ratings include 0 (zero) being no palpable contraction; 1 (trace) is a flicker of movement or pulsation; 2 (poor) is felt as a contraction without a lift; 3 (fair) is moderate contraction and lift felt more into posterior versus anterior aspects of the pelvic floor; 4 (good) is contraction and lift from anterior, posterior, and side walls of the pelvic floor; 5 (strong) is a full circumference squeeze pressure and displacement of the clinician's finger with an inward pull even with applied resistance. Owing to the variability in the reliability the ICS recommends the contraction can be identified as absent, weak, normal, or strong. Normal pelvic floor muscles should then relax back to their resting positioning voluntarily, which should be felt as a complete release of the squeezing/lifting pressure felt during the contraction and return of the pelvic floor back to or below baseline. A voluntary relaxation can be noted as absent (no relaxation is noted after contraction), partial (return of the pelvic floor to baseline), or complete (return of the pelvic floor beyond baseline). In some cases, a reflexive contraction or a descent of the pelvic floor can be observed by requesting a volitional clearing of the throat, which simulates what happens with the increased interabdominal pressure of a cough or squeeze.

Vaginal Assessment of Pelvic Floor Structures

Although subjective, digital palpation is widely used among clinicians as a method to determine the quality of muscular tissue. The clinician should be palpating with the intent to determine the tissue elasticity, texture, tone, sensation, scars, muscle symmetry, tenderness, pain reproduction, and/or intensification, keeping in mind symptoms may be unilateral. Pelvic floor muscle that is considered normal should not reproduce a painful sensation, should have appropriate tissue quality, and would likely be felt as a "pressure" sensation by the patient [55]. Kavvadias et al. found when performing internal palpation on asymptomatic, nulliparous women, overall low pain scores were found. This study also found there to be good to excellent interrater and test–retest reliability for palpation of the levator ani, obturator internus, and piriformis muscles as well as for pelvic floor muscle contraction [56]. Assessment of patients with overactive pelvic floor muscles may demonstrate a tissue quality that feels like a taut band or area with decreased extensibility and would likely be painful during palpation. The pain elicited during palpation may be localized to that specific area within the pelvic floor muscles or may reproduce/refer pain to adjacent areas. Patients with underactive pelvic floor muscles will likely demonstrate pain with palpation; however, the tissue quality will appear to be highly extensible. Palpation in all circumstances is best performed in a gentle fashion, as increased pressure is not necessary to produce a pain response in patients with overactivity. Further, in patients with chronic pelvic pain, it is possible that the palpation itself involving distension of the vaginal tissues could elicit elevated pelvic floor muscle tension due to protective guarding responses and elevated resting tone over time [57, 58]. Somatic activation is also present with anticipatory or perceived threat to the local area or the system. Van der Velde et al. demonstrated that in the absence of a local stimulus, pelvic floor muscle tension bias could be maintained in the muscle with a fear stimulus [59]. Overactive pelvic floor muscles, when shortened for prolonged periods of time due to subconscious tightening or muscle guarding due to pain, can also demonstrate a shortened length–tension relationship within the muscle fibers impacting the strength, flexibility, and recruitment patterns of these intrapelvic muscles [60]. The length–tension relationship refers to the force a muscle is capable of generating at various discrete lengths of overlap of the muscle fibers; thus increased overlap within overactive muscles would produce less tensile or strength capability. This can lead to impaired coordination with the surrounding muscles of the pelvic girdle and hip.

The combination of the clinicians' observation of the pelvic floor in terms of resting position, anatomical landmarks, and coordination of pelvic floor muscles during movement combined with what is appreciated through palpation will help to create the overall picture of the patients' pain symptoms.

Palpation should begin at the first layer of pelvic floor muscles including the bulbocavernosus, ischiocavernosus, and superficial transverse perineal muscles. These muscles may reproduce pain in the perineal area or around the urogenital structures. Superficial transverse perineal muscle hypertonicity may also be implicated as a source of, or contributing factor to, pain symptoms after episiotomy. The ischiocavernosus shares myofascial connections with hip adductor muscles at their proximal attachment to the pubic rami, and this muscle could be implicated in patient complaints of inner thigh pain. Patients with overactivity into the superficial layer of pelvic floor muscles may relate symptoms of dyspareunia, clitoral pain, and pain with orgasm [50, 61]. Pain may also be noted with palpation along pelvic floor muscle insertion sites including the pubic rami, ischial tuberosities, and coccyx. This external palpation may be what the clinician relies on for diagnosis and treatment planning if internal palpation is not possible.

Continued palpation into the second layer of pelvic floor muscles would include the deep transverse perineal, sphincter urethrovaginalis, compressor urethra, and external urethral sphincter. These muscles, particularly those toward the anterior aspect of the pelvic floor, in conjunction with anterior aspects of first- and third-layer muscles, can contribute to pain associated with bladder voiding, difficulty with bladder emptying, or interstitial cystitis/bladder pain syndrome [62].

The third and deepest layer of pelvic floor muscles including the levator ani group, obturator internus, and coccygeus can also cause, or contribute to, pelvic pain. The puborectalis muscle is palpated at the vaginal opening. The pubococcygeus is felt just lateral to midline with pressure posteriorly further into the vaginal canal. These two muscles can refer pain into the suprapubic area, urethra, bladder, and perineum and hypertonicity can contribute to dyspareunia and dysfunction such as increased urinary urgency and frequency [50]. The obturator internus is located laterally and can be confirmed by having the patient externally rotate the ipsilateral hip against resistance provided at the knee. The obturator internus can reproduce pain into the anal region, coccyx, vagina, rectum producing a sense of fullness, and thigh [62]. The obturator can also be a source of pain that is described as being within the hip joint laterally or into the medial thigh due to obturator nerve compression. The obturator internus can be followed posteriorly until the ischial spine is reached. The ATLA can also be palpated as a string-like presence just inferior to the obturator and tracking back toward the ischial spine where a Tinel's sign of the pudendal nerve can be performed [63]. Palpating along the posterior vaginal wall, the small coccygeus and larger piriformis can be palpated. The coccygeus can refer pain into the sacrococcygeal region and into the buttocks with the patient describing pain with sitting, anal pain/pressure, and pain during bowel movements. The piriformis can radiate pain into the sacroiliac region, buttock, posterior hip, and posterior thigh. Caudal to those muscles, the iliococcygeus can be palpated and when hypertonic can reproduce pain into the perineal, deep vaginal, rectal, and sacrococcygeal areas with reports of pain before, during, and after bowel movements and pain on deep penetration [44]. The examiner should also palpate the anterior aspect of the pelvic floor by rotating the palpating digit upward toward the back side of the pubic bone to appreciate the anterior attachment of the pubococcygeus. Anterior pelvic floor hyperactivity including second-layer pelvic floor muscles, as well as the anterior attachment of the pubococcygeus to the posterior aspect of the pubic rami, can reproduce pain into genital structures such as the bladder, urethra, and lower abdomen. The pain reported during internal assessment may also be poorly localized for the patient.

Internal pelvic floor palpation can be performed in a clockwise fashion or one side at a time depending on the patient's tolerance for palpation and limiting overall excessive movement within the vaginal canal that could trigger a guarding response and inaccurate assessment. Some patients are unable to tolerate internal assessment. Palpation of most pelvic floor muscles is possible to an extent through external tissue; however, this may diminish the ability to determine tissue quality. Assessment of the pelvic floor transrectally can also be an option if vaginal assessment is not possible; however, there are limitations in the ability to assess anterior aspects of the intermediate and deep muscle layers in this fashion.

As with strength testing, there is limited evidence regarding the validity and reliability of internal palpation assessment methods for pelvic floor muscle tone. Reissing et al. used an assessment in their study that measures tone based on a 7-point scale for assessing women with vulvar vestibulitis. The scale ranges from +3 (very hypertonic) to −3 (very hypotonic), with 0 for normal pelvic floor muscle tone. They found near perfect agreement (kappa statistic of 0.824 with $p < 0.0001$) between the two physical therapists performing assessments of the pelvic floor muscle tone using this scale within the study; however, further study of psychometric properties has not been performed.

Other tools to assess pelvic floor muscle tone and contractile properties are available including EMG, ultrasound, imaging manometry, and dynamometry; however, owing to its ease and low cost, digital palpation and observation are still the most widely used in the clinical setting. Digital palpation can provide invaluable information regarding the patient's awareness of her pelvic floor, contraction and relaxation ability, tender points, or impaired tissue extensibility present and how this could relate to overall dysfunction of the pelvic floor. This information is then used to help diagnose and guide optimal treatment.

Summary

Numerous muscle groups attach onto the pelvis and contribute to the coordination of movement through the pelvic girdle including the pelvic floor muscles, hip musculature, abdominals, and spine stabilizers. Dysfunction or imbalance due to overuse, weakness, or hypermobility in any one of these muscle groups can impact movement and function at the pelvis, and it is therefore easy to see how patients with pelvic pain may also describe symptoms above and below the pelvis that seem related to or contributing to their symptoms and overall pain presentation. A thorough assessment of palpation and measurement of muscle length, strength, and firing patterns with bilateral comparison can indicate impairments that may relate to the patient's pain complaint. For non–physical therapy clinicians a screening of the palpation of the abdominal wall, for SI joint or pubic symphysis/coccyx pain; active or passive range of motion tests of the lumbar spine; standing single-limb flexion testing; and hip mobility in the supine position would indicate if further assessment would be valuable. If the patient complains of any pain with those activities, it would be recommended that she be referred for physical therapy evaluation.

Classification of Pelvic Floor Muscle Dysfunction

There are many ways to describe and group conditions that include the pelvic floor. As described in previous chapters, musculoskeletal etiologies are one of many contributors. The European Urological Association (EUA) guidelines describe musculoskeletal pelvic pain as a phenotype of "Pelvic floor muscle pain syndrome." It is the "occurrence of persistent or recurrent episodic pelvic floor pain" [64].

Generally, the term pelvic floor dysfunction refers to symptoms that demonstrate impaired function of the pelvic floor as it relates to its multiple demands.

Overactive pelvic floor dysfunction is the current term utilized to indicate that there is an increase in activation and above necessary contraction for the resting state or particular demands of the pelvic floor. Overactive pelvic floor (OAPF) muscles are noted when the muscles do not relax or inappropriately contract when relaxation is attempted or required such as during voiding. Patients with overactive pelvic floor muscles relate symptoms such as difficulty completely emptying the bowel or bladder, urinary hesitancy, and dyspareunia. Overactivity in the pelvic floor can contribute to incontinence and may be due to multiple factors including muscle rigidity and shortened length–tension relationship of the muscle fibers and thus decreased maximal strength capacity to prevent leak with increased pressure or incomplete pelvic floor relaxation during micturition. Patients with an overactive pelvic floor would demonstrate resting activation above normal, may have limited contraction and difficulty returning to baseline, and palpable high tone.

Underactive pelvic floor muscles are noted when the muscles cannot perform a voluntary or involuntary contraction when this is necessary or appropriate due to reduced muscle fiber coordination, or strain from trauma. Patients with underactive pelvic floor muscles tend to relate dysfunction such as bowel or bladder incontinence or pelvic organ prolapse complaints. In this condition, pelvic floor muscles would demonstrate little to no palpable or observable muscle activity in terms of voluntary or involuntary contraction and low palpable tone.

Pelvic pain is often the result of increased tone, but pelvic pain can also be found in the presence of underactive pelvic floor muscles. Pelvic floor over-recruitment can slacken the posterior ligaments, making the SI joint less robust, and excessive recruitment in hip muscles including deep external rotators, long adductors, and iliopsoas can be concurrent in OAPF [65]. Pelvic floor muscle incoordination can cause lack of control against forces requiring pelvic girdle compression (force closure) during increased intraabdominal pressure or maintenance upright stability.

Assessment of these intricate muscular connections and movement patterns is likely not possible during a medical evaluation of a patient's pelvic pain; however, a general understanding of these interconnections can help the clinician piece together subjective patient reports, helping the patient understand her seemingly unrelated symptoms and ultimately direct treatment. An understanding of the physiological principles behind the mechanical deficits found is important when evaluating the broad picture of how to address the musculoskeletal system to restore function locally and globally. Normalizing the musculoskeletal system starting from the joints adjacent to the pelvic floor and restoring support of the pelvic girdle helps in bringing the pelvic floor muscles into homeostasis. Further thorough assessment can then be provided through referral to pelvic health physical therapy.

Conclusion

Chronic pelvic pain is a multifactorial condition, and thorough evaluation requires a systematic and comprehensive approach that very often cannot be left in the hands of a sole provider. In conjunction with primary care providers and gynecological specialists, pelvic floor physical therapists, physical medicine and rehabilitation doctors, and pain management specialists can help to create an overall picture of the patient presenting with pelvic pain. This whole person perspective with a shared understanding of the various body systems, including the musculoskeletal system, that may be contributing to and perpetuating the pain presentation can then help to better direct diagnosis and proposed treatment interventions.

Five Things You Need to Know

- When initiating intake on a patient with pelvic pain, the clinician should start with an understanding of how the patient's pain impacts her daily function, their role, and their desired recreation. This can be assessed with standardized questionnaires or simply open-ended interview style but must encompass more than just a pain number scale.

- Understanding the relationship between the optimal function of the lumbopelvic joints and the muscles that support them offers pelvic pain clinicians a comprehensive model with which to screen for drivers of pain that are not in the gynecological, gastrointestinal, or urological system but commonly generate pain in the same areas. Patients with musculoskeletal drivers often have positional or activity-based pain and also activity intolerances.

- A proper screening of symptoms in bowel, bladder, and sexual function can identify relationships of pelvic floor dysfunction. Knowing what the normal function of the pelvic floor muscles is within each system helps to clarify when there is a problem. Often pain creates a cascade of symptoms in an adjacent system.

- After careful palpation of pelvic floor muscles elicits tenderness, it is important to determine if the pain is localized or referred and if it provokes similar complaints of pain in the abdomen, vagino/rectal areas, or with intercourse. Evaluation of the patient's volitional ability to contract, relax, and elongate the pelvic floor muscles should also be included in the physical exam.

- The two most common classifications of pelvic floor dysfunction are the underactive and overactive pelvic floor. Both have mechanisms that can contribute to pain, but the most common classification contributing to chronic pelvic pain is the overactive pelvic floor.

References

1. Tu FF, Holt J, Gonzales J, Fitzgerald CM. Physical therapy evaluation of patients with chronic pelvic pain: a controlled study. *Am J Obstet Gynecol.* 2008;**198**(3):272e271-7.

2. Huard J, Li Y, Fu FH. Muscle injuries and repair: current trends in research. *JBJS.* 2002;**84**(5):822–32.

3. Järvinen TA, Järvinen M, Kalimo H. Regeneration of injured skeletal muscle after the injury. *Muscles Ligaments Tendons j.* 2013;**3**(4):337.

4. Miller J, MacDermid JC, Richardson J, Walton DM, Gross A. Depicting individual responses to physical therapist led chronic pain self-management support with pain science education and exercise in primary health care: multiple case studies. *Arch Physiother.* 2017;**7**:4.

5. Wall LL, DeLancey JO. The politics of prolapse: a revisionist approach to disorders of the pelvic floor in women. *Perspect Biol Med.* 1991;**34**(4):486–96.

6. FitzGerald MP, Anderson RU, Potts J, et al. Randomized multicenter feasibility trial of myofascial physical therapy for the treatment of urological chronic pelvic pain syndromes. *J Urol.* 2009;**182**(2):570–80.

7. FitzGerald MP, Payne CK, Lukacz ES, et al. Randomized multicenter clinical trial of myofascial physical therapy in women with interstitial cystitis/painful bladder syndrome and pelvic floor tenderness. *J Urol.* 2012;**187**(6):2113–18.

8. Goldfinger C, Pukall CF, Gentilcore-Saulnier E, McLean L, Chamberlain S. PAIN: a prospective study of pelvic floor physical therapy: pain and psychosexual outcomes in provoked vestibulodynia. *J Sex Med.* 2009;**6**(7):1955–68.

9. Mosqueda LA. Assessment of rehabilitation potential. *Clin Geriatr Med.* 1993;**9**(4):689–703.

10. Alappattu MJ, Bishop MD. Psychological factors in chronic pelvic pain in women: relevance and application of the fear-avoidance model of pain. *Phys Ther.* 2011;**91**(10):1542–50.

11. Ballantyne JC, Sullivan MD. Intensity of chronic pain: the wrong metric? *N Engl J Med.* 2015;**373**(22):2098–9.

12. Blickenstaff C, Pearson N. Reconciling movement and exercise with pain neuroscience education: a case for consistent education. *Physiother Theor Pract.* 2016;**32**(5):396–407.

13. Dansie EJ, Turk DC. Assessment of patients with chronic pain. *BJA: Br J Anaesth.* 2013;**111**(1):19–25.

14. Turk DC, Dworkin RH, Revicki D, et al. Identifying important outcome domains for chronic pain clinical trials: an IMMPACT survey of people with pain. *PAIN.* 2008;**137**(2):276–85.

15. Dufour S, Vandyken B, Forget MJ, Vandyken C. Association between lumbopelvic pain and pelvic floor dysfunction in women: a cross sectional study. *Musculoskelet Sci Pract.* 2018;**34**:47–53.

16. Coady D, Futterman S, Harris D, Coleman SH. Vulvodynia and concomitant femoro-acetabular impingement: long-term follow-up after hip arthroscopy. *J Lower Genit Tract Dis.* 2015;**19**(3):253–6.

17. Sullivan MJ, Bishop SR, Pivik J. The pain catastrophizing scale: development and validation. *Psychol Assess.* 1995;**7**(4):524.

18. Neblett R, Hartzell MM, Mayer TG, Cohen H, Gatchel RJ. Establishing clinically relevant severity levels for the central sensitization inventory. *Pain Pract.* 2017;**17**(2):166–75.

19. Lundberg MKE, Styf J, Carlsson SG. A psychometric evaluation of the Tampa Scale for Kinesiophobia: from a physiotherapeutic perspective. *Physiother Theor Pract.* 2004;**20**(2):121–33.

20. Smith RC, Marshall-Dorsey AA, Osborn GG, et al. Evidence-based guidelines for teaching patient-centered interviewing. *Patient Educ Counsel.* 2000;**39**(1):27–36.

21. Pollard CA. Preliminary validity study of the pain disability index. *Percept Motor Skills.* 1984;**59**(3):974.

22. Hummel-Berry KWK, Herman H. Reliability and validity of the Vulvar Functional Status Questionnaire (VQ). *J Womens Health Phys Ther.* 2007;**31**(3):28–33.

23. Brewer ME, White WM, Klein FA, Klein LM, Waters WB. Validity of Pelvic Pain, Urgency, and Frequency questionnaire in patients with interstitial

cystitis/painful bladder syndrome. *Urology*. 2007;**70**(4):646–9.

24. Wiklund I, Fullerton S, Hawkey C, et al. An irritable bowel syndrome-specific symptom questionnaire: development and validation. *Scand J Gastroenterol*. 2003;**38**(9):947–54.

25. Wei JT, De Lancey JO. Functional anatomy of the pelvic floor and lower urinary tract. *Clin Obstet Gynecol*. 2004;**47**(1):3–17.

26. Hodges PW, Sapsford R, Pengel LH. Postural and respiratory functions of the pelvic floor muscles. *Neurourol Urodyn*. 2007;**26**(3):362–71.

27. Rosenbaum TY. Musculoskeletal pain and sexual function in women. *J Sex Med*. 2010;**7**(2 Pt 1):645–53.

28. Lee D, Lee, L-J. *The Pelvic Girdle*. Edinburgh: Elsevier; 2011.

29. Itza Santos F, Zarza D, Serra Llosa L, Gómez Sancha F, Salinas J, Allona-Almagro A. [Myofascial pain syndrome in the pelvic floor: a common urological condition] (in Spanish). *Actas Urol Esp*. 2010;**34**(4):318–26.

30. Tu FF, As-Sanie S, Steege JF. Prevalence of pelvic musculoskeletal disorders in a female chronic pelvic pain clinic. *J Reprod Med*. 2006;**51**(3):185–9.

31. FitzGerald MP KR. Rehabilitation of the short pelvic floor I: background and patient evaluation. *Int Urogynecol J Pelvic Floor Dysfunct*. 2003;**14**:261–8.

32. Mehin R, Meek R, O'Brien P, Blachut P. Surgery for osteitis pubis. *Can J Surg*. 2006;**49**(3):170–6.

33. Ekci B, Tamam, C., Altinli, E. A rare clinical condition after pelvic surgery: osteitis pubis. *Anatol J Clin Invest*. 2009;**3**(4):259–61.

34. Sapsford RR, Richardson CA, Maher CF, Hodges PW. Pelvic floor muscle activity in different sitting postures in continent and incontinent women. *Arch Phys Med Rehabil*. 2008;**89**(9):1741–7.

35. Hodges PW, Moseley GL, Gabrielsson A, Gandevia SC. Experimental muscle pain changes feedforward postural responses of the trunk muscles. *Exp Brain Res*. 2003;**151**(2):262–271.

36. Padoa A, Rosenbaum TY. *The Overactive Pelvic Floor*. Cham, Switzerland: Springer; 2016.

37. Hodges PW, Richardson CA. Contraction of the abdominal muscles associated with movement of the lower limb. *Phys Ther*. 1997;**77**(2):132–42.

38. Hodges PW, Moseley GL. Pain and motor control of the lumbopelvic region: effect and possible mechanisms. *J Electromyogr Kinesiol*. 2003;**13**(4):361–70.

39. Boyajian-O'Neill LA, McClain RL, Coleman MK, Thomas PP. Diagnosis and management of piriformis

40. Bedi A, Dolan M, Leunig M, Kelly BT. Static and dynamic mechanical causes of hip pain. *Arthroscopy*. 2011;**27**(2):235–51.

41. Fonstad P, Hooper, R.A. Hip labral tears as a co-morbidity of low back and pelvic girdle pain following motor vehicle collisions: a case series. *J Back Musculoskel Rehabil*. 2008;**21**:245–51.

42. Yavagal S, de Farias TF, Medina CA, Takacs P. Normal vulvovaginal, perineal, and pelvic anatomy with reconstructive considerations. *Semin Plast Surg*. 2011;**25**(2):121–9.

43. Horton R. The anatomy, biological plausibility and efficacy of visceral mobilization in the treatment of pelvic floor dysfunction. *J Pelvic Obstet Gynaecol Physiother*. 2015;**117**:5–18.

44. Pastore EA, Katzman WB. Recognizing myofascial pelvic pain in the female patient with chronic pelvic pain. *J Obstet Gynecol Neonatal Nurs*. 2012;**41**(5):680–91.

45. Bogduk N, Pearcy M, Hadfield G. Anatomy and biomechanics of psoas major. *Clin Biomech*. 1992;**7**(2):109–19.

46. Montenegro ML, Gomide LB, Mateus-Vasconcelos EL, et al. Abdominal myofascial pain syndrome must be considered in the differential diagnosis of chronic pelvic pain. *Eur J Obstet Gynecol Reprod Biol*. 2009;**147**(1):21–4.

47. FitzGerald MP, Anderson RU, Potts J, et al. Randomized multicenter feasibility trial of myofascial physical therapy for the treatment of urological chronic pelvic pain syndromes. *J Urol*. 2009;**182**:570–80.

48. Suleiman S, Johnston D. The abdominal wall: an overlooked source of pain. *Am Fam Physician*. 2001;**64**(3):431–8.

49. Rosenbaum TY, Owens A. The role of pelvic floor physical therapy in the treatment of pelvic and genital pain-related sexual dysfunction (CME). *J Sex Med*. 2008;**5**(3):513–23.

50. Hartmann D, Sarton J. Chronic pelvic floor dysfunction. *Best Pract Res Clin Obstet Gynaecol*. 2014;**28**(7):977–90.

51. Haylen BT, Freeman RM, Swift SE, et al. An International Urogynecological Association (IUGA)/ International Continence Society (ICS) joint terminology and classification of the complications related directly to the insertion of prostheses (meshes, implants, tapes) & grafts in female pelvic floor surgery. *Int Urogynecol J*. 2011;**22**(1):3–15.

52. Laan EvL RHW. Overactive pelvic floor: sexual functioning. In Padoa A, Rosenbaum TY (eds), *The*

syndrome: an osteopathic approach. *J Am Osteopath Assoc*. 2008;**108**(11):657–64.

666666 no

Overactive Pelvic Floor. New York: Springer Science +Business Media; 2016.

53. Faubion SS, Shuster LT, Bharucha AE. Recognition and management of nonrelaxing pelvic floor dysfunction. Paper presented at Mayo Clinic Proceedings; 2012.

54. Laycock J, Jerwood D. Pelvic floor muscle assessment: the PERFECT scheme. *Physiotherapy*. 2001;**87**(12):631–42.

55. Loving S, Thomsen T, Jaszczak P, Nordling J. Pelvic floor muscle dysfunctions are prevalent in female chronic pelvic pain: a cross-sectional population-based study. *Eur J Pain*. 2014;**18**(9):1259–70.

56. Kavvadias T, Pelikan S, Roth P, Baessler K, Schuessler B. Pelvic floor muscle tenderness in asymptomatic, nulliparous women: topographical distribution and reliability of a visual analogue scale. *Int Urogynecol J*. 2013;**24**(2):281–6.

57. Reissing ED, Brown C, Lord MJ, Binik YM, Khalife S. Pelvic floor muscle functioning in women with vulvar vestibulitis syndrome. *J Psychosom Obstet Gynaecol*. 2005;**26**(2):107–13.

58. Glazer HI, Marinoff SC, Sleight IJ. Web-enabled Glazer surface electromyographic protocol for the remote, real-time assessment and rehabilitation of pelvic floor dysfunction in vulvar vestibulitis syndrome: a case report. *J Reprod Med*. 2002;**47**(9):728–30.

59. van der Velde J, Everaerd W. The relationship between involuntary pelvic floor muscle activity, muscle awareness and experienced threat in women with and without vaginismus. *Behav Res Ther*. 2001;**39**(4):395–408.

60. Montenegro ML, Vasconcelos EC, Candido Dos Reis FJ, et al. Physical therapy in the management of women with chronic pelvic pain. *Int J Clin Pract*. 2008;**62**:263–9.

61. Rosenbaum TY. Pelvic floor involvement in male and female sexual dysfunction and the role of pelvic floor rehabilitation in treatment: a literature review. *J Sex Med*. 2007;**4**(1):4–13.

62. Prendergast SA WJ. Screening for musculoskeletal causes of pelvic pain. *Clin Obstet Gynecol*. 2003;**46**:773–82.

63. Hibner M, Desai N, Robertson LJ, Nour M. Pudendal neuralgia. *J Minim Invas Gynecol*. 2010;**17**(2):148–53.

64. Engeler D, Baranowski A, Borovicka J, et al. EAU guidelines on chronic pelvic pain. Paper presented at: EAU Guidelines, edition presented at the 27th EAU Annual Congress, Paris; 2012.

65. Stuge B, Sætre K, Brækken IH. The association between pelvic floor muscle function and pelvic girdle pain: a matched case control 3D ultrasound study. *Manual Ther*. 2012;**17**(2):150–6.

Pharmacological Management of Patients with Pelvic Pain

Diana T. Atashroo and Richard Cockrum

Editor's Introduction

With worsening drug epidemics in the United States, proper pharmacological management in patients with chronic pelvic pain has very significant consequences. It includes chronic management of those patients as well as perioperative management. Multiple nonnarcotic medications have been shown to be very effective in managing patients with pelvic pain. The mainstay of treatment remains nonsteroidal anti-inflammatory medications. They are effective in any type of pain but particularly in dysmenorrhea and inflammatory pain. Anticonvulsants such as gabapentin have been shown to be effective in neuropathic type of pain as well as pre- and postoperative management. Many patients with pelvic pain develop significant pelvic floor muscle spasm. They do not appear to respond well to oral muscle relaxants but usually have very good responses to vaginal suppositories with various combinations of diazepam and other medications. In patients who do not respond to muscle relaxants botulinum toxin injections to pelvic floor muscles may provide muscle relaxation and therefore pain relief. Patients with pain related to nerves may respond to gabapentin and pregabalin but also benefit from use of lidocaine patches. Narcotics pain medications should be used very cautiously and as a last resort.

Introduction

Background

Significance

An understanding of the arsenal of pharmacological interventions available to the clinician and safety is essential for any provider caring for women with chronic pelvic pain. Most gynecological societal guidelines recommend an initial thorough evaluation and acknowledge that instituting empirical therapy is reasonable given there are often multiple identifiable and nonidentifiable contributing factors [1–3]. Many chronic pelvic pain disorders alter the nervous system, resulting in neuropathic pain. An appreciation of primary and adjuvant therapies becomes even more useful in advanced pain states.

Scope

This chapter reviews the literature and best clinical practices for pharmacological management of chronic pelvic pain of benign gynecological origin. There are several common causes of pain, especially nongynecological visceral pain, that are beyond the scope of these recommendations because of inherent differences in pathophysiology. Of note, interstitial cystitis/bladder pain syndrome, endometriosis, and dysmenorrhea are commonly encountered by the gynecologist but pharmacological management will not be comprehensively reviewed here, as there are several unique targeted therapies that are described in other disorder-specific chapters.

The highest level of evidence by synthesized data either through societal guidelines or qualitative systematic reviews and quantitative meta-analyses (e.g., Cochrane Database Systematic Reviews) were used in the preparation of this chapter. Medication and disorder specific reviews within the past 15 years were included to supplement consensus statements. The Royal College of Obstetrics and Gynaecologists (2012), European Association of Urology (2014), and American College of Obstetrics and Gynecology (2020) have recently published clinical guidelines on chronic pelvic pain [1, 3]. The Society of Obstetricians and Gynaecologists of Canada (SOGC) clinical guideline on chronic pelvic pain has not been updated since 2005 [1].

Limitations of the Evidence Base

Owing to the limitation of evidence-based treatments for pelvic pain, outcomes are inferred from neuropathic pain literature from other regional and global pain syndromes [4]. These disorders include peripheral diabetic neuropathy (DN), fibromyalgia, trigeminal neuralgia, postherpetic neuralgia (PHN), and postoperative pain. Most chronic pain patients are managed with multimodal regimens as recommended by the American Pain Society; however, data are sparse regarding the most effective combinations or if combination therapies are superior to monotherapy for specific conditions [4].

Approach to Chronic Pelvic Pain Management

General Strategies

A general understanding of best practices in chronic pain management is prudent before delving into specific therapeutics. Most published algorithms are based on trial-and-error and on clinical experience. Most societal guidelines recommend a multimodal approach to maximize benefit/risk ratio; some combinations may provide synergistic benefits. Overarching themes in management reviewed in this chapter include starting with medications with greatest chance of benefit, titrating up from a low starting dose to minimize risks.

Targeted Therapy

Many pharmacological treatments have focused on specific pathologies that are common and recognizable within the modern schema for gynecological chronic pelvic pain: leiomyomata, endometriosis, adenomyosis, external genitalia pain syndromes (e.g., vulvodynia), and pelvic floor musculoskeletal and neurological disorders. Chronic pelvic pain is often an impetus in development of neuropathic pain. The etiology of neuropathic pain can be a direct result of various factors; depending on the lesion location, this can originate centrally or peripherally. Clinically, patients with this type of pain can experience different phenotypes including reflex changes to hyperalgesia, paresthesia, and dysesthesia.

Adverse Side Effects

Pharmacological management of chronic pelvic pain is not without risk of harm [5]. Throughout each section within this chapter, a brief review will be provided of clinically significant and common adverse effects with a focus on data from pelvic pain randomized controlled trials (RCTs) when available. A review

of pharmacological interactions is prudent before starting new medications, particularly for patients with polypharmacy. Many helpful web-based tools exist to this end (e.g., Lexicomp Interact online program).

Nonopioid Analgesics

Also called simple analgesics, nonopioid analgesics are among the most commonly used medications for pain in the general population owing to their easy access, low cost, generally well tolerated side effects, and suitability for long-term use. This class includes acetaminophen/paracetamol and nonsteroidal antiinflammatory drugs (NSAIDs). They all have analgesic and antipyretic properties while the latter also provides antiinflammatory effects. Most gynecological literature regarding efficacy of NSAIDs has targeted dysmenorrhea given its bioplausibility as a direct inhibitor of that pain pathway or for postprocedural pain management. There are surprisingly few placebo-controlled RCTs specifically assessing the efficacy for other etiologies of pelvic pain. In fact, there were no studies identified for the treatment of chronic noncyclic pelvic pain. In a 2012 comparative effectiveness review sponsored by the Agency for Healthcare Research (AHRQ) the authors found the literature addressing therapies for CPP in women was of poor quality and too inconclusive to guide treatment decisions [5]. Similar to other conditions, the evidence for the use of this class is otherwise derived from expert consensus, inference from studies of other pain syndromes or pathways, and common sense.

Nonsteroidal Antiinflammatory Drugs Description

NSAIDs are primarily subdivided into nonselective cyclooxygenase (COX)-1 and COX-2 enzyme inhibitors and selective COX-2 enzyme inhibitors. All of the available NSAIDs differ in the degree of the binding affinity [6]. Prostaglandins are implicated in several pathways that explain both the analgesic efficacy and also the side effect profile for NSAIDs. Unlike COX-1, COX-2 is differentially expressed and increased with inflammatory states. Endometrial tissue levels of COX-2 products are highest during menses [6]. From these findings and other basic science and clinical studies, it is hypothesized that COX-2 is implicated predominantly within the cyclic pain pathway whereas COX-1 has been more responsible for adverse side effects, especially of the gastrointestinal (GI) and cardiovascular systems. At the time of this writing, celecoxib remains the only readily available nonselective COX-2 inhibitor and requires a prescription.

Preemptive NSAID dosing has been shown to reduce overall analgesic dose requirements in postoperative pain studies and shows promise from limited basic science evidence [7]. Nearly complete prostaglandin synthesis suppression can be induced with naproxen if given before the activation of COX-1 and COX-2 pathways. The effect is dramatically less with COX-2.

Efficacy

Supporting literature is robust showing NSAIDs as a highly effective medication for management of dysmenorrhea. In a landmark 1984 systematic review, 72% of women with primary dysmenorrhea reported significant pain relief with NSAIDs alone versus 15% by placebo effect and 18% with minimal to no response [6]. However, the use of NSAIDs as they related to primary dysmenorrhea treatment will not be reviewed in this part of the chapter.

There are few trials investigating NSAIDs for the treatment of other gynecological pain conditions such as endometriosis, leiomyomas, and adenomyosis. A 2014 Cochrane review of NSAIDs used for treatment of endometriosis pain revealed only one eligible, low quality trial ($N = 24$) [8]. The reported benefit was nonsignificant (odds ratio [OR] 3.27, 95% confidence interval [CI] 0.61–17.69). There have not been any more recent RCTs for this indication. Though evidence for NSAIDs in secondary dysmenorrhea is lacking, societal guidelines agree it is a reasonable first-line analgesic because of its accessibility, affordability, familiarity to patients, and tolerability[1, 3, 9]. There is insufficient evidence evaluating NSAID use for neuropathic pain to draw conclusions on efficacy.

Comparative Effectiveness

The available literature to assess differences between NSAIDs and acetaminophen/ paracetamol is limited to dysmenorrhea trials and generally of low quality. For the purpose of this chapter, the evidence will not be reviewed here.

Adverse Side Effects and Contraindications

The only statistically significantly increased risks of adverse effects with NSAIDs included GI (e.g., nausea and indigestion) and neurological (e.g., headache, drowsiness, dizziness, and dry mouth) symptoms [10].

Overall NSAIDs were 29% more likely than placebo to result in any adverse effect, with neurological symptoms being more strongly associated than GI symptoms, OR 2.74 (95% CI 1.66–4.53) versus OR 1.58 (95% CI 1.12–2.23), respectively. This difference was not reflected in short-term follow-up studies. Robust general medicine literature clearly establishes much more serious risks for long-term use, particularly regarding cardiovascular and bleeding risks. Naproxen has been the least cardiotoxic NSAID in some studies [11].

NSAIDs should not be used in patients with significant renal dysfunction, history of GI bleeding, significant cardiovascular conditions, liver cirrhosis, and aspirin-sensitive asthma. Cautious use should be considered in the elderly, who are more susceptible to complications due to comorbidities. NSAIDs are also not recommended in patients on anticoagulation therapy, particularly coumadin, due to increased bleeding risks.

Acetaminophen/Paracetamol

The mechanism of action remains unclear for acetaminophen/paracetamol. It is thought to act similarly to NSAIDs in inhibition of the COX enzyme but only within the central nervous system (CNS) and through a different mechanism. Its lack of peripheral activity explains why it has no antiinflammatory properties. There have been well designed trials demonstrating analgesic efficacy for postoperative pain and for reducing opioid use in the immediate postoperative period [7]. Some nociceptive pain conditions such as low back pain and arthritis have evidence of small benefits over placebo as well. However, there are no RCTs assessing its efficacy for neuropathic pain or chronic pelvic pain. As it is easily accessible, has few restrictions, and is well tolerated, it is a reasonable first-line therapy and is often used in combination with NSAIDs before attempting other therapies for pelvic pain [1–3]. The primary concern with regard to adverse effects is hepatic toxicity, with the upper limit of the recommended maximum dosing at 3–4 grams per day [11]. A lower maximum threshold of 2 grams per day may be warranted for older adults and if chronic daily therapy is instituted.

Opioids

Description

Opioids include the formal class of opiates, substances derived from opium including the archetypal analgesic morphine, and synthetic compounds that bind to opioid receptors nonselectively or selectively within the CNS and peripherally. There are three subclasses of opioid receptors (mu, kappa, and delta) that are most relevant to pain physiology, and varying affinities by different opioid medications determine many of their pharmacological properties such as analgesic potency and therapeutic index. Dosing for opioids should ideally be short term with clear expectations for indication and duration using the lowest possible dose, though some patients will inevitably require chronic and escalating use. Frequent reassessment within 1–4 weeks of initiating or dose changes is indicated regarding efficacy and adverse side effects monitoring. In addition to a clearly documented pain contract delineated for the provider and patient, routine surveillance is recommended through both state-based prescription drug monitoring program databases and also urinary toxicology testing to assess for personal abuse or diversion. There are many established guidelines for prescribing opioids for chronic noncancer pain available for more thorough review; the CDC guidelines were updated in 2016 [12].

Efficacy

In a 2006 meta-analysis by Furlan et al. for opioid use in chronic noncancer pain, there was a moderate positive effect size for pain control and small positive effect size for functional outcomes when compared with placebo. Notably the number of patients who withdrew from the trials due to inadequate pain control with opioids was half the rate of placebo (15% vs. 30). Altogether 80% of trials examined nociceptive pain (e.g., arthritis, back pain), with the remainder targeting neuropathic or mixed pain (e.g., fibromyalgia, postherpetic neuropathy). Follow-up was short term, with a mean duration of 5 weeks. Medications studied including tramadol, codeine, oxycodone, morphine, and propoxyphene/dextropropoxyphene. The latter pair are no longer recommended for use due to high risk of toxicities. In a subset of trials comparing weak opioids and nonopioid analgesics there was no difference in pain control outcomes and slight but significantly worse functional outcomes for opioid use. Strong opioids (e.g., oxycodone, morphine), however, had significantly better pain control than nonopioid analgesics [13].

The CDC recommends against use of long-acting opioids for acute pain but these may be indicated for chronic pain [12]. A systematic review of 34 RCTs in chronic noncancer pain concluded there was insufficient evidence of a superior long-acting opioid or if long-acting was superior to short-acting in terms of pain or rates of adverse events [11,12].

Adverse Side Effects

CDC has recommendations for maximum doses to avoid the risk of adverse effects due to risks of respiratory depression and overdose [12]. Additionally, patients may have differential tolerance between opioids; dose reductions of at least 50% should be used for conversions. Up to two-thirds of deaths from the use of DEA Schedule II drugs involve combined opioids and benzodiazepines and thus concomitant use is ill advised [14].

The risk of chronic use after exposure to opioids has been demonstrated in some studies but a systematic review was unable to adequately address this question because of heterogeneity in study design and results [11]. It is unknown whether there are any differences in risk of abuse between various opioids. Recent retrospective evidence from state and national database studies supports that 5% of opioid-naive patients prescribed opioids for chronic pain will convert to persistent users, though several covariates are strongly predictive including age (risk during reproductive age ranging 2.2%–6.5% when stratified by decade of life) [15]. Use of opioids beyond 90 days postoperatively after minor and major procedures has similarly been demonstrated as high as 5.9% and 6.5% respectively versus 0.4% among nonsurgical controls [16]. The study authors postulated that this use consisted primarily of treatment of nonsurgical chronic pain or neuropsychiatric comorbidities. Full elucidation of this relationship and indications for which opioids may be misused is greatly needed.

Risks of adverse side effects are much more common than addiction and diversion. In systematic reviews by Moore and McQuay in 2005 and Eisenberg et al. in 2006, only nausea; vomiting; constipation; and cognitive impairments such as drowsiness, dizziness, and somnolence were more common than with placebo, ranging 15%–33% [11]. Discontinuation rates due to side effects varied as well, from 11% to 22%. Major limitations of these effect estimates are also the short duration of follow-up and fixed dosing, which do not reflect clinical use in chronic pain disorders. There are several other well recognized but less common adverse effects including hypogonadotropic amenorrhea and impaired neuropsychological performance.

Opioids with Adjuvant Mechanisms

Tramadol is a mu-opioid receptor agonist with additional effects as a weak serotonin– norepinephrine reuptake inhibitor (SNRI). Tapentadol has a stronger opioid effect than tramadol and similar to that of hydrocodone, and it only inhibits norepinephrine reuptake. The nonopioid mechanism is thought to provide additional analgesia, similar to gains seen with traditional SNRIs and tricyclic antidepressants [11]. This benefit is largely theoretical. Only small improvements in pain control and small decrements in adverse events as compared with traditional opioids have been reported in literature. Though the risks of abuse with tramadol in a large randomized controlled trial of 11,352 patients with chronic noncancer pain were similar to those for nonopioid analgesics, there are psychoneurological risks to consider [11]. Both tramadol and tapentadol can increase the risk of seizures in patients with epilepsy, and tramadol can precipitate serotonin syndrome when combined with other serotonin reuptake inhibitors. Therefore one should specifically screen for contraindications including seizures and concomitant use of psychiatric and pain medications before prescribing either medication.

Conclusion

Though opioids have a notorious reputation, there may be a role for chronic noncancer pelvic pain when reserved for acute pain flares or for short-term use while pursuing alternative therapies. A subset of patients will eventually require chronic opioid use and should be managed by a healthcare provider skilled in special challenges within this population. A goal of using the full armamentarium of pharmacological management options should be to reduce the use of opioids, especially in the setting of a national epidemic of dependence and inappropriate use for both medical and nonmedical reasons.

Antiepileptics

For several decades antiepileptics, formerly called anticonvulsants, have been used to treat a number of neurological and psychiatric disorders such as neuropathic pain and depression. In the chronic pain literature, most evidence supports treatment when pain is characterized as "lancinating or burning" [11]. Archetypal indications include PHN, DN, and fibromyalgia. The "gabapentanoids" have been the most studied compounds within this class and have the best evidence of efficacy in chronic noncancer pain as well as pelvic pain.

Gabapentanoids

Description

This subclass of antiepileptics consists of the prototypical gabapentin and its successor pregabalin, which is more lipophilic and may have improved uptake across the blood–brain barrier. Both medications act primarily in the CNS by binding the alpha-2–delta-1 subunit of voltage-gated calcium channels within inhibitory neurons, thus antagonizing excitatory neurons [11]. The complex balance of accessory excitatory and inhibitory neurons modulating nociceptive and nonnociceptive sensory transmission is implicated in the theory of central sensitization and may explain why a subset of chronic pelvic pain patients benefit from treatment with these medications. In other words, gabapentanoids may either provide analgesia from direct inhibition of increased peripheral neuropathic pain or through modulation of a more complex central process.

Owing to a common incidence of side effects, we recommend starting at a low dose and titrate up as tolerated to provide adequate analgesia (see Table 6.1 in the Appendix). These medications have few long-term serious risks if monitored appropriately, which makes them ideal candidates for management of chronic pelvic pain. However, most patients will not find substantial benefit even after escalation to therapeutic dosing, so discontinuation should be considered after a trial of 3–6 months if no effect is observed. For patients who develop bothersome side effects, weaning to either a lower dose or transitioning to an alternative therapy if there is no longer any benefit should be considered.

Efficacy

The evidence supporting the use of gabapentanoids for pelvic pain relies heavily on nongynecological literature in neuropathic pain. In a 2012 systematic review of pharmacological management noncyclic/ mixed noncyclic and cyclic pelvic pain, only one study (N = 56) was identified that compared gabapentin versus amitriptyline versus both [5]. After 2 years of follow-up, gabapentin alone (visual analog scale [VAS] pain score 1.9 ± 0.9) or in combination with amitriptyline (VAS pain score 2.3 ± 0.9) outperformed amitriptyline alone (VAS pain score 3.4 ± 0.9). There was no placebo-controlled group in that study, and at the time of this writing there is no other published evidence for efficacy of either gabapentin or amitriptyline specifically in chronic pelvic pain. A 2013 Cochrane review of antiepileptic pharmacotherapy for vulvodynia failed to identify any RCTs. While most studies reported some positive outcomes for improved pain or sexual function, there is a high rate of spontaneous resolution and fluctuation of symptoms in vulvodynia, and no studies compared the interventions with placebo [17].

Several Cochrane reviews over the past 20 years have analyzed the efficacy of antiepileptics for neuropathic pain and fibromyalgia, serving as indirect evidence used to support the use of this class in treatment of pelvic pain conditions. A 2013 Cochrane review summarized the findings of previous reports [18]. Number needed to treat (NNT) was calculated to achieve ≥50% reduction in pain for one patient. Both gabapentin and pregabalin were found to have good evidence supporting its use in diabetic neuropathy (gabapentin 600–3600 mg/day; NNT 5.8, 95% CI 4.3–9.0 and pregabalin 600 mg/day; NNT 6.3, 95% CI 4.6–10.0) and PHN (gabapentin 1800–3600 mg/day; NNT 7.5, 95% CI 5.2–14 and pregabalin 600 mg/day; NNT 4.0, 95% CI 3.1–5.5). Pregabalin was also found to be effective for central neuropathic pain (600 mg/day; NNT 5.6, 95% CI 3.5–14.0) and fibromyalgia (600 mg/day; NNT 11, 95% CI 7.1–21.0). The proportion of patients with ≥30% of pain relief is not as well correlated with clinically significant functional outcomes but nonetheless had more favorable NNTs. As gabapentin was the first of its class and had rapid uptake, becoming the most prescribed antiepileptic in the United States in less than 10 years after its initial FDA approval, there has been little incentive to conduct further studies on the majority of its use for off-label indications such as gynecological neuropathic pelvic pain [19].

Adverse Effects and Contraindications

A 2013 Cochrane review of antiepileptics for neuropathic pain summarized common adverse effects with a pooled estimate of 10% of patients discontinuing therapy for these reasons [18]. However, there was no difference in the rate of serious adverse events between gabapentanoids and placebo in RCTs, though with mostly short-term follow-up. The most common effects are neurological: somnolence, dizziness, blurry vision, and cognitive and motor impairment. Experiencing any adverse event was more common than with placebo, with both gabapentin ≥1200 mg/day (66% vs. 51%; OR 1.3, 95% CI 1.2–1.4) and pregabalin 600 mg/day (83% vs. 67%; OR 1.3, 95% CI 1.25–1.4)[18]. Rates of discontinuation due to adverse effects of pregabalin were demonstrated to have a dose–response relationship in that same Cochrane review, ranging from 7.1% for patients taking 150 mg/day to 22% for patients taking 600 mg/day compared to 6.2%–10% for placebo.

Other Antiepileptics

In a 2013 Cochrane Review of antiepileptics used for neuropathic pain and fibromyalgia, there was either inadequate or low-quality evidence for use of alternatives beyond gabapentinoid subtypes. A 2011 review specific for the management of gynecological neuropathic pain highlighted evidence against use of lamotrigine and supported topiramate as a reasonable alternative to gabapentin [20]. Side effect profiles are similar to those of gabapentanoids but rare serious events have been reported such as blood dyscrasias [18].

Antidepressants

Antidepressants have been used for the treatment of chronic pain for decades, predominantly with amitriptyline – one of the earliest synthesized tricyclic antidepressants. Other classes found in both the published literature and common use include SNRIs, and to a lesser extent, selective serotonin reuptake inhibitors (SSRIs). Dosing and monitoring guidelines for antidepressants used for the treatment of chronic pain are similar to those for gabapentanoids and are reviewed in greater detail in that section, as the body of high-quality evidence is more robust.

Tricyclic Antidepressants

Description

Though high-quality, double-blind placebo-controlled RCTs are lacking, decades of clinical experience with tricyclic antidepressants (TCAs) support the expert consensus recommendations for their use in chronic pelvic pain, particularly if neuropathic pain is within the indication for treatment. Most experts theorize that a significant benefit from TCAs is derived directly from their antidepressant effects, though these are mostly seen at higher doses than typically used for pain (>100 mg/day)[11]. However, studies investigating this relationship have failed to demonstrate a correlation between effects on mood and pain relief. Similarly, patients without depressive symptoms may still have improvement in pain scores [21]. TCAs act primarily by inhibition of the reuptake of serotonin and norepinephrine but have multiple sites of activity, including antihistamine and anticholinergic effects. While amitriptyline and nortriptyline are the best studied TCAs for this indication, others such as imipramine may be used as alternatives.

Efficacy

Studies supporting TCAs as effective medications for chronic noncancer pain have severe limitations, most notably that sample sizes were small and there was significant heterogeneity or simply lack of explanation of study design [11]. Two Cochrane reviews published in 2015 provided pooled analyses of efficacy from modernized studies of the two most commonly used TCAs: amitriptyline and nortriptyline[21, 22]. All of the 17 RCTs included for amitriptyline were no better than third-tier evidence. No data synthesis was performed because of a high risk of bias. There was no convincing benefit of amitriptyline versus active intervention shown for DN, mixed neuropathic pain, PHN, spinal cord injury, cancer-related pain, or HIV neuropathy. Only two small studies demonstrated amitriptyline improved pain over placebo and were specific to PHN. A limited analysis of the best available evidence from four studies for the first three indications suggests a significant benefit for amitriptyline over placebo (OR 2.0, 95% CI 1.5–2.8) with NNT 5.1, 95% CI 3.5–9.3, though likely overestimated [23]. This effect size is similar to that seen with gabapentanoids for the treatment of neuropathic pain. Few high-fidelity

studies were available for nortriptyline reviewed, and all proved to be short term and third-tier evidence. Nortriptyline did not perform better than active intervention (e.g., amitriptyline, gabapentin) or placebo, where most studies reported approximately one-third of participants met the prespecified goal for pain relief or improved functional outcomes regardless of which therapy was used.

An examination of the literature supporting TCA use for vulvodynia provides an excellent case study in the limitations of the available data. In a 2013 systematic review of antidepressants used for the treatment of vulvodynia, there were only 2 RCTs identified among a total of 13 studies, and both involved TCAs: oral desipramine and oral amitriptyline. Despite retrospective and prospective observational data to support efficacy of TCAs for pain control and improved sexual function in vulvodynia, there were no differences between treatment and placebo in controlled trials [24]. Base on grade A evidence, the vulvodynia expert committee recommended against the use of TCA medication for management of provoked vulvodynia [25].

Adverse Effects and Contraindications

Secondary amine TCAs (e.g., nortriptyline, desipramine) are considered to have lower rates of side effects than tertiary amine TCAs (e.g., amitriptyline, imipramine), which may be due to differential affinity for neurotransmitter inhibition. Secondary amines are more selective for norepinephrine and have fewer anticholinergic side effects. The anticholinergic effects predominant with all TCAs include dry mouth, dizziness, sedation, constipation, and weight gain. In a Cochrane review of TCA use for the treatment of neuropathic pain, 55% of participants experienced at least one adverse event as compared with 36% from placebo [21]. Importantly, there was an increased risk of serious adverse effects with TCA use in that Cochrane review: 6.6% with amitriptyline versus 1.8% with placebo including one death while using amitriptyline. Special consideration should be taken when prescribing TCAs to any elderly patient or woman with cardiovascular disease [11]. Some experts recommend performing baseline cardiac risk assessment including EKG for patients with risk factors or for age greater than 40 years [20]. There are insufficient data to estimate the rate of side effects with nortriptyline specifically from studies of neuropathic pain but most report at least two-thirds of patients will experience at least one adverse effect.

Serotonin–Norepinephrine Reuptake Inhibitors

Description

Among the antidepressant class of serotonin and nor-epinephrine inhibitors, duloxetine and venlafaxine are the best well studied for treatment of neuropathic pain and fibromyalgia. They share the same primary mechanism of action as tricyclic antidepressants, but duloxetine in particular has received FDA approval for a breadth of neuropathic pain conditions likely due to a higher quality of research standardization. Venlafaxine has evidence from animal studies for minor opioid receptor agonist activity but, like dulox-etine, acts predominantly by neurotransmitter reuptake inhibition. Similarly to TCAs, the SNRIs often exert their analgesic effects at lower doses than commonly required for their antidepressant effects [20].

Efficacy

Two Cochrane reviews in 2014 summarized available evidence for the use of duloxetine and venlafaxine for neuropathic pain and fibromyalgia. Duloxetine was investigated in 8 studies for use in diabetic neuropathy (N = 2728) and 6 studies for use in fibromyalgia (N = 2249)[26]. Notably, most studies were conducted by the manufacturer, which may explain why such a large number of participants were able to be recruited. Importantly, a clinically meaningful reduction in pain by ≥50% was assessed and decreased heterogeneity of the pooled analysis. High-quality evidence showed greater benefit for DN (NNT 5, 95% CI 4–7) than for fibromyalgia (NNT 8, 95% CI 4–21) or somatic pain symptoms related to depression (NNT 8, 95% CI 5–14). An effective dose of duloxetine to achieve significant reduction in pain was 60 mg/day, with a maximum dose of 120 mg lacking to show improved efficacy.

Only 6 of the 14 studies (total N = 460) identified for venlafaxine could be included in the Cochrane review [27]. Small sample sizes and short follow-up were primary deficiencies; no study reported on outcomes after greater than 8 weeks of treatment. Nonetheless, all studies reported positive outcomes. The largest RCT included 245 participants and demonstrated a significantly greater proportion of patients achieving ≥50% reduction in pain with ven-lafaxine (56% vs. 34% placebo, NNT 4.5).

Adverse Effects

SNRIs are generally better tolerated than TCAs because of their lack of nonselective effects. A 2017 Cochrane review of venlafaxine used for the treatment of neuropathic pain showed significantly greater rates of adverse effects with treatment but also high rates with placebo, 89% versus 75% respectively [26]. Other, non-placebo-controlled studies, reported rates as low as 44%. The most common side effect of SNRIs is nausea, which may be limited by titration from a low starting dose and taking the medication with food [11]. Other adverse effects include dizziness, somnolence, dry mouth, and sweating.

Selective Serotonin Reuptake Inhibitors

A 1997 systematic review failed to show any benefit of SSRIs for chronic pain management. Alternative therapies have been shown clearly superior in classic syndromes of neuropathic pain. Limited data support use in fibromyalgia, though other antidepressants – particularly TCAs – are likely more efficacious [11]. Nonetheless, 47% of patients treated with SSRIs in the review reported some degree of improvement in somatic symptoms, predominantly pain.

Muscle Relaxers

Description and Efficacy

Muscle relaxers include a heterogeneous group of medications that act primarily as antispasmodics. One review of pharmacotherapy for chronic noncancer pain subclassifies them by FDA-approved indication either for spasticity (e.g., baclofen, dantrolene, tizanidine) or musculoskeletal conditions (e.g., carisoprodol, cyclobenzaprine, metaxalone, methocarbamol, and orphenadrine)[11]. No studies demonstrated superiority among the class of muscle relaxers. Most evidence of efficacy in chronic noncancer pain is derived from use in fibromyalgia, which often has additional spasticity symptoms separate from central or neuropathic pain. A 2005 meta-analysis found 5 placebo-controlled RCTs for the treatment of fibromyalgia with cyclobenzaprine with a pooled OR 0.21 (95% CI 0.09–0.34) and NNT 4.8 (95% CI 3.0–11)[28]. A significant component of therapeutic benefit from muscle relaxers is likely from its sedative effects and improvement in sleep dysfunction, as evidenced in that same review. Pain and sleep had small improvements, and while there were small initial improvements in fatigue or tender points at 4 weeks, the benefit did not persist. This finding is consistent with the manufacturer prescribing guidance for short-term acute muscle spasm. Another possible mechanism for efficacy for cyclobenzaprine in particular is that its chemical structure is similar to that of tricyclic antidepressants. Accordingly, it carries risks of serotonin syndrome when combined with other psychoactive drugs. Tizanidine is a centrally acting alpha-2 receptor inhibitor, and in addition to sedation commonly seen with that class, it carries risks for hypotension because of its concomitant vasodilatory effect. A systematic review was unable to assess risks of abuse with muscle relaxers, which has been a concern because of the sedative effects. Most reports of abuse have involved carisoprodol, though baclofen is also associated with risks of withdrawal [11].

There are no high-quality RCTs assessing long-term outcomes. Patients with chronic pelvic pain who may benefit most from treatment would likely have concomitant myofascial pain involving the pelvic floor, abdomen, or lower back and significant sleep dysfunction. The evidence to support the use of muscle relaxers is limited; however, they might be beneficial as adjunctive multimodal therapy versus maintenance therapy.

Off-Label Medications

Vaginal Suppositories: Benzodiazepines and Belladonna

Description

Benzodiazepines are known to have antispasmodic and anxiolytic properties. Related to chronic pelvic pain, experts suggest musculoskeletal pain disorders should also be part of the initial workup for chronic pain conditions [29]. High-tone pelvic floor dysfunction is often associated with other pain conditions such as interstitial cystitis/bladder pain syndrome and vestibulodynia. Vaginally and rectally placed muscle relaxants are thought to relax the rectum, bladder, and vagina. Vaginal diazepam, a benzodiazepine derivative, has been reported for off-label use to treat pelvic floor hypertonicity and urogenital pain. The usual prescribed dose is 5–10 mg tablets or compounded suppositories or creams that are used vaginally up to two or three times daily. Similar to gabapentin, it acts on the inhibitory GABA receptors. Anecdotally, vaginal use is thought to be effective without the potential side effects of their oral counterparts. however, this is an assumption that is not grounded in strong data. Albeit, the neurobiology and pharmacology do not support its use, there is a potential placebo benefit that should be considered.

Efficacy

High-fidelity studies are limited in this area due to low sample sizes with conflicting results. Data are also limited in quality and quantity to definitively conclude superior efficacy and safety of one agent versus another for musculoskeletal conditions. There are only two placebo-controlled RCTs looking at the clinical effects of vaginal diazepam on pain reduction. One placebo-controlled RCT showed that 10 mg of vaginal diazepam used nightly for 4 weeks in 21 patients with high-dose pelvic floor dysfunction did not show any significant improvement in EMG tone, pain, or sexual functioning indices [30]. Of note, this study also limited patients to only medical therapy. A second placebo-controlled RCT also failed to show improvement of VAS scores in women with pelvic pain and levator spasms compared to placebo (50 vs. 39 mm, $p = 0.36$) [31]. Efficacious therapy was elucidated in one retrospective study with no placebo arm, where clinical improvement in sexual pain scores as well as PFM tone based on resting ($p < 0.001$), squeezing ($p = 0.014$), and relaxation ($p = 0.003$) perineometry readings were seen in 25 of 26 women treated with 10 mg of vaginal diazepam daily [32]. Its worthwhile to note that this cohort also received physical therapy and trigger points, further confounding the strength of these findings.

Belladonna is a plant derivative with muscarinic antagonist properties. Belladonna 16.2 mg, when combined with opium 30 mg (B&O) as a rectal suppository, can also be used clinically as an off-label alternative for pelvic floor dysfunction similarly to diazepam. Unfortunately, there is no evidence to support its use in patients with pelvic pain beyond the urological literature. For perioperative pain management postprostatectomy and ureteral stent placement, B&O rectal suppositories are shown to decrease urinary pain and narcotic use [33]. However, in the gynecology literature, the evidence is limited to one RCT. When compared to placebo for pain reduction post vaginal surgery, no benefit was elucidated in postoperative pain scores, narcotic use, nausea, vomiting, or patient satisfaction [34].

Adverse Effects

In the musculoskeletal literature, benzodiazepines' adverse events are linked to dizziness (17%), drowsiness (33%), and dry mouth [35]. However, there is a wide disparity regarding the adverse event rates among studies of diazepam, making reliable conclusions about adverse event rates inconclusive.

One small (level VI evidence) prospective study looking at the safety profile and found even with daily use of dosages 2–10 mg of vaginal diazepam, no supratherapeutic serum levels were noted after one month of use (mean 0.29, normal = 0.02–1.0 µg/mL), with only 33% patients reporting dizziness. Improvements were seen in levator (mean VAS 3.8/10 to 1.8/10) and vulvar pain (VAS mean 5.9/10 to 2.2/10) levels post diazepam use [36].

The overall safety profile of B & O suppositories is favorable, with common adverse events including urinary retention (51%) and constipation, but lacked statistical significant between the groups. Limitation of ubiquitous use includes their high cost of $32 per suppository [34]. The challenge with the presented treatments is the lack of validated use in the chronic pain subpopulation. The challenge for clinicians is to weigh the risks/benefits in spite of the lack of consensus criteria on the appropriate use of these medications as well as on how to properly diagnose pelvic floor dysfunction.

Topical and Transdermal Agents

Topical agents (e.g., creams, gels, patches) are formulated for local delivery to the skin. Because of their pharmacodynamics, these agents have been investigated for treatment of localized neuropathic pain conditions [37]. Compared to systemic neuropathic pain agents, they offer site specific therapy, while minimizing drug–drug interactions, and potential systemic side effects associated with oral medications. Current data suggest that the elderly population and poly-medicated patients with neuropathic pain are two subgroups that could have the most relevant benefit from the use of topically delivered agents.

Select localized neuropathic pain disorders include vulvodynia, PHN, and musculoskeletal conditions such as osteoarthritis, rheumatoid arthritis, fibromyalgia, and spinal conditions. We will be reviewing the available evidence on the use of topical agents for some of these conditions specific to their efficacy in the treatment of localized neuropathic pain. The only licensed topical agents for neuropathic pain are a 5% lidocaine plaster for neuropathic pain and capsaicin 8% with and without topical patch for PHN and HIV neuropathy [38]. Mixtures of topical agents have been used based either on previous knowledge about the potential efficacy and mechanisms of action or more arbitrarily.

Capsaicin Description

Capsaicin is an analog of chili peppers and has shown to be useful for neuropathic pain. Topical capsaicin targets vanilloid receptors (VR1) that leads to a depletion of substance P, which is associated with pain and inflammation. Repeat local application of this agent results in a functional block of nerve terminals responsive to capsaicin in the epidermis and dermis, resulting in long-lasting desensitization of nerve endings. Capsaicin is available as a topical analgesic cream (0.025%–0.075%) or high concentration (8%) patch formulation.

Efficacy

A 2017 Cochrane review analyzed the efficacy of high concentration (8%) capsaicin for a heterogeneous group of peripheral neuropathic pain patients, showing that 10% of patient reported pain improvement at 8 and 12 weeks with NNT 8.8 (95% CI 5.3–26) compared to placebo with NNT 7.0 (95% CI 4.6–1.5) [39]. There was no difference in adverse events between the studies. A low concentration of the agent (<1%) did not show meaningful results over placebo. This evidence was low to moderate quality, as the benefiting group cohort wasn't large, but did show significant improvements in sleep, fatigue, depression, and quality of life [39].

Vulvodynia is also characterized by burning and hyperalgesia in the location of the vulvar vestibule. An increase expression of VR1 with immunostaining was seen in women with this condition [40]. One prospective study of 32 patients and one retrospective study of 52 patients did look at topical capsaicin for the treatment of provoked vulvodynia (PVD). In both studies, topical lidocaine was placed on the treatment area before to prevent contact irritation. Using concentrations of 0.025% and 0.05% with treatment protocols from 3 to 6 months, both studies did show improvement in pain scores and dyspareunia [41, 42] However, given the uncontrolled nature of these studies, experts do not recommend capsaicin as first-line therapy for PVD but as a second- line alternative (grade C evidence)[25].

Adverse Effects

The safety profile of topical capsaicin is favorable given its rapid elimination profile and limited systemic absorption. After 60- and 90-minute application, the volume of distribution of this agent is quite high, with a low plasma concentration. The predominant adverse event was localized skin sensitivity such as a burning itching and erythema secondary to the release of substance P. These effects are quickly reversed, notable for 1.64 hour elimination half-life with removal of the dermal product [43]. Despite the safety profile, a recent International Association for the Study of Pain (IASP) neuropathic pain (NeuPSIG) update recommend these agents at second-line treatment options for local neuropathic pain.

Lidocaine

Description

Lidocaine is a local anesthetic that is formulated as a spray, cream, plaster (i.e., patch). Standard concentration varies from 2% to 5% for commercially available products. Topical lidocaine exerts its anesthetic relief with nonselective blockade of sodium channels on sensory afferents in peripheral tissue at the site of application [44]. There is also some suggestion of an additive mechanical barrier effect on placement site localized pain reduction. It has been studied most extensively in patients with localized neuropathic pain. Currently, it is FDA approved as first- and second-line therapy for PHN and DN [45].

Efficacy

A 2014 Cochrane review identified 12 studies (508 participants) that were eligible for qualitative analysis comparing topical lidocaine (5% patch, gel, cream, and 8% spray) versus placebo [46]. Half of the study enrollments included patients with PHN and the remaining included patients with mixed neuropathic conditions. Most participants had pain durations of at least 3 months and treatment periods varied from 1 to 4 weeks. Study designs varied but all were considered second and third tier data quality. Seven of the studies included multiple doses, and the rest used a single application. Of note, many of the studies did allow concomitant analgesic medication, which likely led to some bias on effects of topical monotherapy. A 30% reduction of pain over baseline was defined as moderate relief, with at least 50% defined as substantial. In all but two studies reviewed, lidocaine was better than placebo for some measure of pain relief. The trend noted among the data was that time to significant pain relief was short (ranging 15 minutes to 4 hours) and persisted for a median of 4–5 hours. The strength of any finding is subject to inherent study biases including small treatment groups; unclear blinding methods; and short duration of treatment, ranging from a single dose to 4 weeks. The Cochrane review did not include any long-term data on topical lidocaine efficacy. There are open label and observational retrospective studies that look at extensive use of 5% lidocaine and do show consistent efficacy, patient satisfaction, and safety profiles from a 12-month up to 4-year time period, which even suggests reduction in use of other coanalgesics for neuropathic pain [tricyclic antidepressants 14.9% ($p < 0.001$), antiepileptics 20.8% ($p < 0.0001$, and SSRIs (4.9%, $p = 0.05$)] and is particularly significant for the refractory neuropathy pain population [47].

Regarding gynecological conditions, the data on topical lidocaine are lacking. There was a single placebo-controlled RCT that looked at the use of 5% lidocaine specifically for 133 patients with PVD [48]. There was no significant difference in tampon test scores between the groups or sexual satisfaction within the lidocaine-treated group after 12 weeks of treatment. Other, nonrandomized, studies showed around 50% improvement in dyspareunia sustained at 6-month follow-up [49]. Based on available evidence, expert opinion is not to use for long-term management of PVD symptoms [25].

Adverse Effects

The available data suggest topical lidocaine is well tolerated in patients with localized neuropathic pain. Based on the Cochrane pooled data analysis, minimal side effects are reported, which included localized skin reactions or itching, numbness, burning, tingling (e.g., cream) that did not differ between lidocaine and placebo groups (RR 1.24, 95% CI 0.34–4.55). The combined withdrawal rate among the studies was 10/147 (6.8%) with topical lidocaine and 18/146 (12% placebo) due to lack of efficacy and no adverse events.

Conclusion

The weakness of the evidence is lack of NNT, which might not have been inherently possible based on available study designs. However, the available NNT data do suggest that 5% lidocaine plaster as an add-on therapy reduced pain and allodynia with NNT of 4.4 (2.5–17.5). This observation is clinically relevant, as current guidelines do not account for recommendations after failed monotherapy, in which topical therapies could have relevant adjuvant pain advantages.

Topical Tricyclics and Analogs

Description

As described earlier, dose-dependent anticholinergic effects of oral TCAs often limit treatment compliance. In animal studies, topical formulations of these agents have been shown to have peripheral antinociceptive and antiinflammatory effects in rat models of neuropathic and inflammatory pain [50].

Efficacy

Available evidence for efficacy of topical TCAs in the treatment of neuropathic pain consists of controlled clinical trials, uncontrolled trials, and case reports. Only one prospective study looked at the efficacy of amitriptyline cream in the management of dyspareunia related to VD. Thompson and Brooks reviewed the available evidence on the use of amitriptyline for neuropathic pain. There are five RCTs that compared amitriptyline to placebo. All studies included patients with neuropathic pain of various etiologies. Amitriptyline concentrations ranged from 1% to 5% and treatment length varied from 2 days to 6 weeks. Amitriptyline concentrations were compared solo versus lidocaine or in combination with ketamine (see Appendix, Table 6.2). In summary, topical amitriptyline of varying concentrations did not show any significant improvement in pain scores by itself or when combined with other agents versus placebo. Only lidocaine reduced pain, albeit without statistical significance compared to placebo. Other level B and C evidence studies did seem to show benefit [51].

Another RCT looked at 200 patients with chronic neuropathic pain and the effects of doxepin 3.3% and capsaicin 0.025%, alone or in combination, and placebo applied to affected areas daily for 4 weeks [52].

Improvement in pain scores was seen in the three treatment groups with more rapid onset that is, 1 versus 2 weeks with the doxepin/capsaicin versus capsaicin or doxepin singularly. Capsaicin more greatly reduced sensitivity from baseline after the first week compared to other cohorts 1.2 (95% CI, 0.1–2.3), especially after 1 week of use. Reduction of shooting and burning pain was seen only in the capsaicin and combination group, 0.75 versus 0.73 ($p < 0.001$).

There are only uncontrolled studies that looked at tricyclics for treatment of vulvar pain. A 2012 prospective study of 150 patients using 2% amitriptyline for dyspareunia related PVD of at least 5 years' duration [53]. Daily use of the cream to affected areas resulted in a 56% ($N = 84/150$) positive response, with 15 patients reporting resolution of pain after 12 months. Of note, 10% of cohorts ceased treatment because of local sensitivity. These positive results are similar to those of other, nonrandomized, studies; however, small sample size, absence of control groups, and lack of validated pain reporting limit the clinical significance of the data.

Adverse Effects

Topical tricyclics are generally well tolerated compared to their oral counterparts. Among studies, temporal skin irritation was most commonly reported and the reason for discontinuing therapy. The most common deleterious side effect in the doxepin study was burning with application in 27 of 33 (61%) of the doxepin group, 4 of 41 (17%) of the doxepin/capsaicin group, and 81% of the capsaicin patients, indicating that capsaicin is likely the greater contributing factor in side effects. Other small side effects included drowsiness, skin rash, headaches, and itching.

Conclusion

There is a mechanistic rationale in the use of topical amitriptyline in treating neuropathic pain. Controlled studies for the use of topical TCAs for pelvic pain conditions are lacking. In summary, data from controlled studies on neuropathic pain do not support the use of topical amitriptyline for neuropathic pain, while a single trial on doxepin plus or minus capsaicin suggested some benefit. Further studies with blinded control groups, using various strengths of amitriptyline topical preparations, are needed to guide clinical recommendations on the optimal concentration of individual versus combined agents.

Topical Nonsteroidal Antiinflammatory Drugs

Description

Similar to their oral counterparts, topical NSAIDs also have analgesic and antiinflammmatory properties with less risks of systemic side effects. A 2017 Cochrane review looked at eight moderate to high-quality studies using NSAIDs (ketorolac and diclofenac) for chronic musculoskeletal pain(OA and knee pain) [54]. Only three studies in the analysis used topical NSAIDs (ketorolac and diclofenac) for chronic musculoskeletal pain (OA and knee pain) versus acute conditions. Unlike for acute pain, the evidence for topical NSAIDS in chronic pain conditions was not seen but safety profiles were favorable.

Ahmed et al. challenged the value of 1.5% diclofenac for neuropathic conditions such as PHN and chronic region pain syndrome (CRPS). Daily use of 1.5% diclofenac three times versus placebo in 28 patients were followed for 2 weeks of therapy. The treatment group showed lower overall visual pain score compared with the placebo group (4.9 vs. 5.6, $p = 0.04$) as well as decreased burning pain (2.9 vs. 4.3 difference, 1.4; $p = 0.01$). The study failed to show significant changes in quality of pain (constant, shooting, hypersensitivity) over the painful areas or functional statues (SF-36) [55]. Unlike the Cochrane review, no complications of treatment were seen. Inherent weakness in this study was it underpowered state and lack of generalizability to other chronic pain conditions.

Adverse Effects

Localized sensitivity and pain can occur with application, which is an inherent albeit uncommon disadvantage of use similar to that for other topical analgesic formulations described in this chapter. Local reactions were seen in the topical diclofenac (NNH 16) but not the ketorolac group.

Cannabinoids

Description

Preclinical and clinical studies have suggested that cannabis extract and synthetic cannabinoids containing only tetrahydrocannabinol (THC) and combination with cannabidiol (CBD), may be useful to treat diverse diseases including acute and chronic pain conditions. It exists in a variety of forms including sublingual, topical, and oral that can be smoked, inhaled, or ingested.

The biological pain effects of cannabinoids are thought to work on CB1 and CB2 receptors harbored in pain circuits within the spinal, peripheral, and central centers that modulate nociception and inflammation. Pain models have shown that cannabinoid receptors (CBR) agonists have antinociceptive and antihyperalgesic effects, even showing synergistic activity within the endogenous opioid system, further potentiating their analgesic affects.

Guidelines from national and international pain societies are not unified in their recommendations of use. There is no consensus on the role of these agents in treating neuropathic pain that is refractory to first-line recommendations. The Canadian Pain Society advocates for the use of selective cannabinoids as a third-line option for NP whereas the Special Interest Group on NP of the IASP weakly recommend its use.

While there are no available data linking efficacy in pelvic pain specifically, histological studies have shown cannabinoid nerve fibers in pain conditions such as painful bladder syndrome and expression of CB1 receptor in animal endometriosis models [56]. We can extrapolate the analgesic outcomes from other central/peripheral neuropathic pain conditions to gynecological pain pathologies. In the literature, there are a variety of heterogeneous studies looking at selective cannabinoids versus placebo or adjunctive treatment which will be reviewed.

Efficacy

Meng and colleagues reviewed 11 RCTs including 1219 patients, comparing selective cannabinoids (dranabinol, nabilone, and nabiximols) with traditional treatments (e.g., pharmacotherapy, physical therapy, or a combination) or placebo in patients with chronic neuropathic pain. Neuropathic pain was defined based on clinical criteria or validated screening tools. In patients with multiple sclerosis, dronabinol and nabilone were superior to placebo in pain improvement based on validated pain score resulting in at least 30% reduction of pain [57]. However, combination nabilone with gabapentin proved to be superior to placebo in regard to VAS and patient global assessment of change after 9 weeks of treatment. These pain benefits were not corroborated with nabilione vs control group with amitriptyline in fibromyalgia patients (h= 29/32) after 2 weeks of therapy. Similar when comparing 96 patients with chronic neuropathic pain, nabilione failed to show better pain relief vs dihydrocodeine with slightly more side effects specific to nausea/vomiting. The most common adverse effects in these trials included dizziness/lightheadedness, somnolence, and dry mouth.

A European double-blind placebo-controlled RCT looked at 125 patients with peripheral neuropathy treated with oromucosal sativex. Compared to the placebo group, the treatment group showed improvement in numerical rating scale (NRS) pain scores 22% vs. 8% ($p < 0.001$; 95% CI: −2.10, −0.74) and mechanical allodynia 20% vs 5% in placebo that was sustained for 5 weeks. Adverse effect were present in > 90% of sativex group of which GI and CNS complaints predominated that resulted in 18% of patient withdrawing from the study. There did not seem to be a correlation with dose and severity of side effects. Of note, 63% of the treatment group were concurrently on neuromodulator or opioid agents, which suggested an additive analgesic effect to multimodal therapy.

Inherent weakness included varied treatment duration from 2 to 15 weeks, making it difficult to establish long-term clinical significance. Although there was heterogeneity among the studies, meta-regression analysis did not show analgesic differences between selective cannabinoids based on central or peripheral pain. Secondary outcome showed an improvement in quality of life (QoL) outcomes and patient satisfaction, including better sleep quality despite short treatment duration.

Adverse Effects

A 2015 prospective cohort study out of Canada was designed to look at the long-term adverse events of cannabis (12% THC) users among noncancer patients versus nonusers for a 1-year period. There was no statistical difference in serious side effect (adjusted incidence rate ratio = 1.08, 95% CI: 0.57−2.04). Medical cannabis users were more likely to have nonserious side effects, the most common being GI disorder (17%) and nervous system disorders (16%). There was also no difference in

pulmonary and neurocognitive function and standard hematology, biochemistry, renal, liver, and endocrine function [58].

In summary, patients who did receive selective cannabinoids had significant albeit small improvement in numerical pain scores compared to controls. However, given the variability of the studies, validated outcome reporting, etiology of neuropathic pain, and dose of the selective cannabinoids, these agents should be limited to adjunctive use as part of the multimodal approach to chronic pain therapy or for those patients who are recalcitrant to first- and second-line therapies (GRADE [Grading of Recommendations Assessment, Development and Evaluation] weak recommendation; moderate quality evidence). When counseling patients, attention should focus on risk and benefit ratio given overall small increase analgesic benefit in the setting of nonstandardized dosages and duration of treatment. Ultimately, future well-designed studies are needed to better guide clinicians prior to routine prescribing.

Five Things You Need to Know

- There is no universally proposed treatment approach to guide pharmacological management of patient with neuropathic pain, although national societies have recommended guidelines for certain pain conditions. We have extrapolated the available nongynecological pain data to a broad range of pelvic pain conditions. Most societal guidelines recommend a multimodal approach to maximize the benefit/risk ratio; some combinations may provide synergistic benefits.

- Opioids have a role for chronic noncancer pelvic pain when reserved for acute pain flares or for short-term use while pursuing alternative therapies.

- Gabapentinoids and antidepressants have benefit for treatment of neuropathic pain, though tricyclic antidepressants have not been shown to be helpful for vulvodynia.

- Muscle relaxants can be beneficial adjunctive therapy for chronic pelvic pain in patients with concomitant myofascial pain involving the pelvic floor, abdomen, or lower back and significant sleep dysfunction.

- Topical/transdermal analgesic agents might have some benefit for neuropathic pain with limited evidence, but overall low side effect profile.

Appendix

Table 6.1 Summary of nonhormonal therapies

Drug	Efficacy	Side effects	Comments
Nonopioid Analgesics Nonselective- NSAIDs • Ibuprofen (400–800 mg 1–4×/d; max: 2400 mg/day) • Naproxen (500 mg 1–2×/day; max: 1000 mg/day) • Diclofenac 50 mg q 8 hours (max 150 mg) • Salsalate 1000 mg q 8 hours or 1500 mg q 12 hours; max: 30,000 mg/day • Etodolac 300 mg q 8 hours, or 500 mg q 12 hours; max: 1000 mg/day) • Others (see references)	Highly effective for dysmenorrhea (NNT 3) but limited to no evidence in other pain disorders. Limited data suggest naproxen outperforms COX-2 inhibitors for dysmenorrhea.	GI upset, peptic ulcers, GI bleeding, risk of severe bleeding generally, renal dysfunction Avoid use if coronary artery disease Risk of hepatic toxicity	Naproxen sodium is absorbed faster and may better treat acute pain than naproxen. Naproxen has safest cardiovascular profile. Consider max 2 g/day in chronic treatment or elderly.
COX-2 Selective NSAID • Celecoxib (100–200 mg 1–2×/day; max: 400 mg/day)			
Other • Acetaminophen/ Paracetamol (650–1000 mg, 4–6×/day; max: 3–4 g/day)			
Opioid Analgesics Traditional Opioids • Morphine, SR, 15 mg bid and increase as needed • Oxycodone, SR, 5–10 mg qd to bidHydrocodone (combined with acetaminophen) Opioids with Adjuvant Effects • Tramadol: 25 mg bid or tid, titrate to max of 100 mg qid • Tapentadol: 50–100 mg q 4–6 hours; max: 700 mg/day	Moderate effect on pain control and small effect on functional outcomes. Not recommended for chronic noncancer pain but may be indicated for acute pain flares.	Nausea and vomiting, constipation, sedation, risks of abuse/ addiction/ diversion	Short acting use first to determine dosing and side effects. Maximum of 50 MME/day, ≥ 90 MME/day are recommended against due to risks of respiratory depression and overdose Consider constipation prophylaxis for at risk patients. Recommend consultation with pain specialist beyond treating postoperative or acute pain.
Antiepileptics Gabapentanoids • Gabapentin 300–1200 mg, 1–3×/day max: 3600 mg/day	Effective for non–gynecological neuropathic pain conditions (NNT 5.6–7.5) and fibromyalgia (NNT 11). Only related study of noncyclic pelvic pain favored gabapentin over amitriptyline.	Rash, dizziness, somnolence, nausea, constipation, blurred vision, mood changes	Start gabapentin or pregabalin at lowest dose and titrate up by that amount weekly. May start at 100 mg for elderly. Discontinue if no benefit within 12 weeks.

Medication/Dose	Evidence/Indication	Side effects	Notes
Pregabalin 75–300 mg, 1–2x/day max: 600 mg/day	No other antiepileptics have proven efficacy for pelvic pain.		
Others • Carbamazepine • Topiramate • Lamigotrine			
Antidepressants Tricyclic (TCAs) • Amitriptyline (10–150 mg, 1–2x/d; max: 150 mg) • Nortriptyline (10–150 mg, 1–2x/d; max: 150 mg) • Desipramine (12.5–150 mg 1–2x/day; max: 300 mg/day)	Limited studies of TCAs report some pain relief (NNT 5) but Cochrane reviews failed to show conclusive benefit for any indication besides postherpetic neuralgia. Recommend against TCAs for vulvodynia. Effective for diabetic neuropathic pain (NNT 5) and fibromyalgia (NNT 8). Have not been assessed for pelvic pain specifically.	Anticholinergic effects (dry mouth, sedation, dizziness, constipation). Risks of syncope, arrhythmias.	Start TCAs at 10–25 mg nightly and increase by that dose weekly. May split dosing in half if better tolerated. Discontinue if no benefit after 12 weeks. Risk of seizures in patients with epilepsy and tramadol can precipitate serotonin syndrome when combined with other SSRIs
SNRIs • Duloxetine (30–60 mg, 1–2x/day; max: 120 mg/day) • Venlafaxine (37.5–225 mg, once daily; max: 225 mg/day) SSRIs	SSRIs are not recommended for the treatment of pelvic pain.	Nausea/ GI upset, sedation, dizziness, night sweats. Risks of serotonin syndrome. Similar to those with SNRIs	Start SNRIs at lowest dose and increase by that dose weekly. Studies of duloxetine have not shown much benefit for >60 mg/day. Discontinue if no benefit after 12 weeks. Do not exceed 50 mg if on SSRI or SNRI Relatively contraindicated in elderly or cardiovascular disease
Muscle Relaxers Cyclobenzaprine (5–10 mg 1–3x/day; max: 30 mg/day) Baclofen (5–20 mg 1–3x/day; max: 60 mg/day, usually ≤30) Tizanidine (2–4 mg 1–3x/day; max 12 mg/day)	Evidence limited to fibromyalgia, low back pain, and mostly only with cyclobenzaprine. All agents within class were studied primarily for adjuvant treatment of acute pain.	Well tolerated. Shares chemical structure and side effects with TCAs. Central alpha-2 agonist with risks of hypotension, sedation	Most benefit noted from improving sleep dysfunction. Start at lowest dose 1–3x/day. Titrate weekly if desired but unclear if additional benefit. Recommend tapering down over 1–4 weeks if discontinuing.
Topicals Capsaicin cream 0.025% 4 times per day over painful area Lidocaine 5% patch (max: 3 patches)	Good evidence for NP. Weak evidence for VD. Good evidence for DN, weak evidence for VD.	Localized skin reaction	
Suppositories Vaginal Valium: 5–10 mg, qd–tid Rectal belladonna/opium 16.2/30 mg: qd–bid	Weak evidence for pelvic floor muscle dysfunction, sexual pain.	Minimal side effects Constipation	Belladonna is expensive.

bid, twice daily; COX, cyclooxygenase; GI, gastrointestinal; MME, morphine milligram equivalents; NNT, number needed to treat; NP, neuropathic pain; NSAID, nonsteroidal antiinflammatory drug; qd, daily; SNRI, serotonin–norepinephrine reuptake inhibitor; SR, sustained release; SSRI, selective serotonin reuptake inhibitor; VD, vulvodynia.

Table 6.2 Review of topical analgesics

Author	Subject no.	Study design	Topical treatment	Study length	Outcomes	Adverse events	Limitation of study
Lynch et al. (2003)	20 • Post-herpetic neuralgia • Diabetic neuropathy • Posttraumatic neuropathic pain	Double-blinded RCT	• 1% Amitriptyline • 0.5% Ketamine • 1% Amitriptyline/ 0.5% ketamine5 mL qid × 4 days	2 days	No statistically significant MPQ and VAS score	Rash Burning skin	Short study length, low treatment concentrations
Lynch et al (2005)	92 • Diabetic neuropathy • Postherpetic neuralgia • Postsurgical neuropathy	Double-blinded RCT, PCT	• 2% Amitriptyline • 2% Amitriptyline + 1% ketamine4 mL to site tid	3 weeks	No statistically significant decrease in MPQ or VAS score	Skin irritation Sedation (combo group)	Short study length, heterogenous population, low treatment concentration
Ho et al. (2008)	35 • Postsurgical pain • Diabetic neuropathy • Postherpetic neuropathy	Double-blinded RCT, PCT, crossover	• 5% Amitriptyline 5% Lidocaine3–5 mL bid for 1 week then washout 1 week	6 weeks	No statistical significance with amitriptyline Pain improvement with lidocaine vs. placebo ($p < 0.005$)	Itching, numbness, burning, blurred vision	Small study, Heterogeneous population, low baseline pain
Barton et al. (2011)	208 • Chemotherapy-induced peripheral neuropathy	Double-blinded RCT	• 40 mg amitriptyline + 20 mg ketamine + 10 mg baclofen in 1.31 g PLO gel • 1 teaspoon twice daily	4 weeks	Improvement in sensory pain and motor function, but not statistically significant	None	Unclear singular benefit of amitriptyline due to multi-combination medication
Gewandter et al. (2014)	462 • Chemotherapy-induced peripheral neuropathy	Double-blinded RCT	• 4% Ketamine + 4% amitriptyline up to 4 g bid	6 weeks	No difference in pain states	No difference between treatment and placebo	Chemotherapy treatment variability
McCleane et al. (2000)	200 • Chronic neuropathic pain	Double-blinded RCT	• 3.3% Doxepin • 0.025% Capsaicin • 3.3% Doxepin/ 0.025% Capsaicin Grain of rice tid application	4 weeks	Improvement in pain scores (VAS) in all treatment groups Shooting pain improvement with doxepin (0.75, 0–1.5) and combination (0.73, 0.28–1.18) Increased burning pain with doxepin 2.1 (1.62–2.58)	Drowsiness, skin rash, headache, itch, burning	Lack of validated pain scores

Study	N	Condition	Study type	Treatment	Duration	Outcome	Side effects	Limitations
Lynch et al. (2005)	21	• Peripheral neuropathic pain	Prospective	2% Amitriptyline + 1% ketamine	6 months	89% of subjects rated their satisfaction as 3/5 or greater and 2 subjects (10%) were pain free minimal systemic absorption	Drowsiness, dry mouth, rapid heart rate, heart palpitations	Lack of randomization or placebo group
Uzarga et al. (2012)	16	• Neuropathic pain from radiation dermatitis	Prospective	• 2% Amitriptyline + 1% ketamine + 5% lidocaine tid for at least 2 weeks	Up to 6 weeks	Reduce short-term pain intensity, sharpness, burning, sensitivity, itchiness, unpleasantness, deepness, and surfaceness ($p < 0.05$) Significant reduce burning pain on long-term basis ($p < 0.05$)	Fatigue, irritation	Lack of randomization
Pagano et al. (2012)	150	• Entry dyspareunia • Provoked vestibulodynia (102 patients) • Provoked and unprovoked vestibulodynia [48 patients]	Prospective	2% Amitriptyline	12 months	56% improved response with treatment, 10% pain free	None	Lack of randomization, low treatment concentration

DN, diabetic neuropathy; MPS, McGill pain questionnaire; PCT, placebo-controlled trial; PHN, postherpetic neuropathy; PSN, postsurgical neuropathy; RCT, randomized controlled trial; VAS, visual analog scale.

References

1. Jarrell JF, Vilos GA, Allaire C, Burgess S, Fortin C, Gerwin R, et al. Consensus guidelines for the management of chronic pelvic pain. *J Obstet Gynaecol Can JOGC J Obstet Gynecol Can JOGC*. 2005;**27**(9):869–910.

2. Fall M, Baranowski AP, Elneil S, Engeler D, Hughes J, Messelink EJ, et al. EAU guidelines on chronic pelvic pain. *Eur Urol*. 2010;**57**(1):35–48.

3. Royal College of Obstetricians and Gynecologists. The initial management of chronic pelvic pain. Guideline No. 41. 2nd ed.; 2012.

4. American Pain Society. Pain: Current understanding of assessment, management and treatments. 1st ed; 2001.

5. Yunker A, Sathe NA, Reynolds WS, Likis FE, Andrews J. Systematic review of therapies for noncyclic chronic pelvic pain in women. *Obstet Gynecol Surv*. 2012;**67**(7):417–25.

6. Oladosu FA, Tu FF, Hellman KM. Nonsteroidal antiinflammatory drug resistance in dysmenorrhea: epidemiology, causes, and treatment. *Am J Obstet Gynecol*. 2018;**218**(4):390–400.

7. Wong M, Morris S, Wang K, Simpson K. Managing postoperative pain after minimally invasive gynecologic surgery in the era of the opioid epidemic. *J Minim Invasive Gynecol*. 2018;**25**(7):1165–78.

8. Brown J, Farquhar C. Endometriosis: an overview of Cochrane Reviews. *Cochrane Database Syst Rev*. 2014 Mar 10;(3):CD009590.

9. ACOG (American College of Obstetricians and Gynecologists).Practice bulletin no. 114: management of endometriosis. *Obstet Gynecol*. 2010;**116**(1):223–36.

10. Marjoribanks J, Ayeleke RO, Farquhar C, Proctor M. Nonsteroidal anti-inflammatory drugs for dysmenorrhoea. *Cochrane Database Syst Rev*. 2015 Jul A**30**;(7):CD001751.

11. Kroenke K, Krebs EE, Bair MJ. Pharmacotherapy of chronic pain: a synthesis of recommendations from systematic reviews. *Gen Hosp Psychiatry*. 2009;**31**(3):206–19.

12. Dowell D, Haegerich TM, Chou R. CDC guideline for prescribing opioids for chronic Pain–United States, 2016. *JAMA*. 2016;**315**(15):1624–45.

13. Furlan AD, Sandoval JA, Mailis-Gagnon A, Tunks E. Opioids for chronic noncancer pain: a meta-analysis of effectiveness and side effects. *CMAJ Can Med Assoc J J Assoc Medicale Can*. 2006;**174**(11):1589–94.

14. Lamvu G, Feranec J, Blanton E. Perioperative pain management: an update for obstetrician-gynecologists. *Am J Obstet Gynecol*. 2018;**218**(2):193–9.

15. Deyo RA, Hallvik SE, Hildebran C, Marino M, Dexter E, Irvine JM, et al. Association between initial opioid prescribing patterns and subsequent long-term use among opioid-naïve patients: a statewide retrospective cohort Study. *J Gen Intern Med*. 2017;**32**(1):21–7.

16. Brummett CM, Waljee JF, Goesling J, Moser S, Lin P, Englesbe MJ, et al. New persistent opioid use after minor and major surgical procedures in US adults. *JAMA Surg*. 2017;**152**(6):e170504.

17. Leo RJ. A systematic review of the utility of anticonvulsant pharmacotherapy in the treatment of vulvodynia pain. *J Sex Med*. 2013;**10**(8):2000–8.

18. Wiffen PJ, Derry S, Moore RA, Aldington D, Cole P, Rice ASC, et al. Antiepileptic drugs for neuropathic pain and fibromyalgia: an overview of Cochrane reviews. *Cochrane Database Syst Rev*. 2013 Nov 11;(11):CD010567.

19. Wallach JD, Ross JS. Gabapentin approvals, off-label use, and lessons for postmarketing evaluation efforts. *JAMA*. 2018;**319**(8):776–8.

20. Tu FF, Hellman KM, Backonja MM. Gynecologic management of neuropathic pain. *Am J Obstet Gynecol*. 2011;**205**(5):435–43.

21. Moore RA, Derry S, Aldington D, Cole P, Wiffen PJ. Amitriptyline for neuropathic pain in adults. *Cochrane Database Syst Rev*. 2015 Jul 6;(7):CD008242.

22. Derry S, Wiffen PJ, Aldington D, Moore RA. Nortriptyline for neuropathic pain in adults. *Cochrane Database Syst Rev*. 2015 Jan 8;1:CD011209.

23. Leo RJ. A systematic review of the utility of anticonvulsant pharmacotherapy in the treatment of vulvodynia pain. *J Sex Med*. 2013;**10**(8):2000–8.

24. Leo RJ, Dewani S. A systematic review of the utility of antidepressant pharmacotherapy in the treatment of vulvodynia pain. *J Sex Med*. 2013;**10**(10):2497–505.

25. Goldstein AT, Pukall CF, Brown C, Bergeron S, Stein A, Kellogg-Spadt S. Vulvodynia: assessment and treatment. *J Sex Med*. 2016;**13**(4):572–90.

26. Gallagher HC, Gallagher RM, Butler M, Buggy DJ, Henman MC. Venlafaxine for neuropathic pain in adults. *Cochrane Database Syst Rev*. 2015 Aug 23; (8):CD011091.

27. Lunn MPT, Hughes RAC, Wiffen PJ. Duloxetine for treating painful neuropathy, chronic pain or fibromyalgia. *Cochrane Database Syst Rev*. 2014 Jan 3;(1):CD007115.

28. Tofferi JK, Jackson JL, O'Malley PG. Treatment of fibromyalgia with cyclobenzaprine: a meta-analysis. *Arthritis Rheum*. 2004;**51**(1):9–13.

29. Howard FM. Chronic pelvic pain. *Obstet Gynecol*. 2003;**101**(3):594–611.

30. Crisp CC, Vaccaro CM, Estanol MV, Oakley SH, Kleeman SD, Fellner AN, et al. Intra-vaginal diazepam for high-tone pelvic floor dysfunction: a randomized placebo-controlled trial. *Int Urogynecol J.* 2013;**24**(11):1915–23.

31. Holland MA, Joyce JS, Brennaman LM, Drobnis EZ, Starr JA, Foster RT. Intravaginal diazepam for the treatment of pelvic floor hypertonic disorder: a double-blind, randomized, placebo-controlled trial. *Female Pelvic Med Reconstr Surg.* 2019;**25**(1):76–81.

32. Rogalski MJ, Kellogg-Spadt S, Hoffmann AR, Fariello JY, Whitmore KE. Retrospective chart review of vaginal diazepam suppository use in high-tone pelvic floor dysfunction. *Int Urogynecol J.* 2010;**21**(7):895–9.

33. Lee FC, Holt SK, Hsi RS, Haynes BM, Harper JD. Preoperative belladonna and opium suppository for ureteral stent pain: a randomized, double-blinded, placebo-controlled study. *Urology.* 2017;**100**:27–32.

34. Butler K, Yi J, Wasson M, Klauschie J, Ryan D, Hentz J, et al. Randomized controlled trial of postoperative belladonna and opium rectal suppositories in vaginal surgery. *Am J Obstet Gynecol.* 2017;**216**(5):491.e1–e6.

35. Nibbelink DW, Strickland SC, McLean LF, et al. Cyclobenzaprine, diazepam and placebo in the treatment of skeletal muscle spasm of local origin. *Clin Ther.* 1978;**1**(6):409–24.

36. Carrico DJ, Peters KM. Vaginal diazepam use with urogenital pain/pelvic floor dysfunction: serum diazepam levels and efficacy data. *Urol Nurs.* 2011;**31**(5):279–84, 299.

37. Sommer C, Cruccu G. Topical treatment of peripheral neuropathic pain: applying the evidence. *J Pain Symptom Manage.* 2017;**53**(3):614–29.

38. Attal N, Cruccu G, Baron R, Haanpää M, Hansson P, Jensen TS, et al. EFNS guidelines on the pharmacological treatment of neuropathic pain: 2010 revision. *Eur J Neurol.* 2010;**17**(9):1113–e88.

39. Derry S, Rice AS, Cole P, Tan T, Moore RA. Topical capsaicin (high concentration) for chronic neuropathic pain in adults. *Cochrane Database Syst Rev.* 2017 Jan 13;(1):CD007393.

40. Tympanidis P, Casula MA, Yiangou Y, Terenghi G, Dowd P, Anand P. Increased vanilloid receptor VR1 innervation in vulvodynia. *Eur J Pain Lond Engl.* 2004;**8**(2):129–33.

41. Murina F, Radici G, Bianco V. Capsaicin and the treatment of vulvar vestibulitis syndrome: a valuable alternative? *Medscape Gen Med.* 2004;**6**(4):48.

42. Steinberg AC, Oyama IA, Rejba AE, Kellogg-Spadt S, Whitmore KE. Capsaicin for the treatment of vulvar vestibulitis. *Am J Obstet Gynecol.* 2005;**192**(5):1549–53.

43. Babbar S, Marier J-F, Mouksassi M-S, Beliveau M, Vanhove GF, Chanda S, et al. Pharmacokinetic analysis of capsaicin after topical administration of a high-concentration capsaicin patch to patients with peripheral neuropathic pain. *Ther Drug Monit.* 2009;**31**(4):502–10.

44. Cline AE, Turrentine JE. Compounded topical analgesics for chronic pain. *Dermat Contact Atopic Occup Drug.* 2016;**27**(5):263–71.

45. Pickering G, Martin E, Tiberghien F, Delorme C, Mick G. Localized neuropathic pain: an expert consensus on local treatments. *Drug Des Dev Ther.* 2017;**11**:2709–18.

46. Derry S, Wiffen PJ, Moore RA, Quinlan J. Topical lidocaine for neuropathic pain in adults. *Cochrane Database Syst Rev.* 2014 Jul 24;(7):CD010958.

47. Binder A, Rogers P, Hans G, Baron R. Impact of topical 5% lidocaine-medicated plasters on sleep and quality of life in patients with postherpetic neuralgia. *Pain Manag.* 2016;**6**(3):229–39.

48. Zolnoun DA, Hartmann KE, Steege JF. Overnight 5% lidocaine ointment for treatment of vulvar vestibulitis. *Obstet Gynecol.* 2003;**102**(1):84–7.

49. Zolnoun DA, Hartmann KE, Steege JF. Overnight 5% lidocaine ointment for treatment of vulvar vestibulitis. *Obstet Gynecol.* 2003;**102**(1):84–7.

50. Moore RA, Derry S, Aldington D, Cole P, Wiffen PJ. Amitriptyline for neuropathic pain in adults. *Cochrane Database Syst Rev.* 2015 Jul 6;(7):CD008242.

51. Thompson DF, Brooks KG. Systematic review of topical amitriptyline for the treatment of neuropathic pain. *J Clin Pharm Ther.* 2015;**40**(5):496–503.

52. McCleane G. Topical application of doxepin hydrochloride, capsaicin and a combination of both produces analgesia in chronic human neuropathic pain: a randomized, double-blind, placebo-controlled study. *Br J Clin Pharmacol.* 2000;**49**(6):574–9.

53. Pagano R, Wong S. Use of amitriptyline cream in the management of entry dyspareunia due to provoked vestibulodynia. *J Low Genit Tract Dis.* 2012;**16**(4):394–7.

54. Derry S, Wiffen PJ, Kalso EA, Bell RF, Aldington D, Phillips T, et al. Topical analgesics for acute and chronic pain in adults: an overview of Cochrane Reviews. *Cochrane Database Syst Rev.* 2017 May 12;5:CD008609.

55. Ahmed SU, Zhang Y, Chen L, Cohen A, St Hillary K, Vo T, et al. Effect of 1.5% topical diclofenac on clinical neuropathic pain. *Anesthesiology.* 2015;**123**(1):191–8.

56. Dmitrieva N, Nagabukuro H, Resuehr D, Zhang G, McAllister SL, McGinty KA, et al. Endocannabinoid involvement in endometriosis. *Pain.* 2010;**151** (3):703–10.

57. Meng H, Johnston B, Englesakis M, Moulin DE, Bhatia A. Selective cannabinoids for chronic neuropathic pain: a systematic review and meta-analysis. *Anesth Analg.* 2017;**125**(5):1638–52.

58. Ware MA, Wang T, Shapiro S, Collet J-P, COMPASS study team. Cannabis for the Management of Pain: Assessment of Safety Study (COMPASS). *J Pain Off J Am Pain Soc.* 2015;**16**(12):1233–42.

Evidence for Surgery for Pelvic Pain

Nita Desai and Anna Reinert

Editor's Introduction

Among the physicians who see patients for pelvic pain some feel that the only proper treatment is surgery and others that nonsurgical treatment should be the mainstay of therapy. The truth of course lies in the middle, and the most effective providers are not only excellent surgeons but also recognize the importance of physical therapy, pharmacological treatments, and psychological counseling. One of the problems with assessing the effectiveness of surgery and comparing outcomes between the providers is that there are different skill levels, and what one provider calls complete resection of endometriosis or adhesiolysis another may deem as incomplete. In the hands of good and qualified surgeons some procedures unequivocally are beneficial for patients. Resection of endometriosis has clearly been shown to be beneficial provided other causes of pain are also treated. In our practice patients with complete adhesiolysis also seem to have good improvement of pain. It is true that pain may return with time but patients may have few good years, after which they may be candidates for a repeat procedure. Hysterectomy for pain is of course controversial, especially in younger or nulligravid patients. Nevertheless, evidence shows that the majority of patients with pelvic pain, especially those with endometriosis, adenomyosis, or dysmenorrhea, will experience pain improvement after hysterectomy. Proper counseling, documentation, and obtaining consent are of utmost importance.

Introduction

As illustrated throughout this book, female pelvic pain may be caused by a wide variety of conditions and is often multifactorial. Surgery serves an important role in the treatment of many of these conditions and is best addressed specifically rather than generally. This chapter aims to address the use of each procedure by specific indication or diagnosis. For many procedures, there may be only limited data by which to judge the efficacy of the surgery for treatment of pelvic pain.

Among women with chronic pelvic pain of unknown etiology, certain procedures may help identify or confirm a cause of their pain, as in the case of laparoscopy identifying endometriosis or adhesions, or hysterectomy identifying adenomyosis. While rarely addressed within clinical studies, there may be psychological benefits to patients from identifying a cause of their chronic pain.

Any decision about surgery involves counseling the patient about risks, benefits, alternatives, indications, and contraindications of performing surgery. Risks of not performing surgery should also be discussed, including the risk of delaying diagnosis and treatment for the cause(s) of the patient's pain. Surgical risk is influenced by patient factors such as obesity or other medical comorbidities, as well as by surgeon factors such as experience with the proposed procedure, surgical volume, comfort managing complications, and availability of surgical assistance for management of a complication.

Laparoscopy for the Evaluation of Acute Pelvic Pain

While the primary focus of this chapter is chronic pelvic pain, a manual on management of pelvic pain merits discussion of acute pelvic pain: both isolated and superimposed upon chronic pelvic pain. A woman of reproductive age presenting with acute pelvic or lower abdominal pain represents a broad differential diagnosis, as pain may include gynecological, urological, musculoskeletal, gastrointestinal, vascular, or metabolic disorder etiologies [1, 2]. Initial assessment should include testing for pregnancy, as ectopic pregnancy may be a life-threatening cause of acute pain in women. Additional causes of acute pelvic pain requiring urgent assessment and management include acute appendicitis, pelvic inflammatory disease, obstructive renal stones, and/or ovarian torsion. Ovarian cyst, cyst rupture, or ovulation pain may also result in acute pelvic pain, but rarely requires surgical management unless ovarian torsion is present, significant and ongoing blood loss from a hemorrhagic cyst is suspected, or imaging suggests dermoid cyst rupture. Surgical management of symptomatic, presumed benign ovarian cysts should be through a laparoscopic approach, with a goal of fertility preservation [3]. Presentation of complicated myomas may be varied, with myomectomy indicated for cases of torsion versus expectant management for other instances of acute myoma degeneration.

Imaging is crucial in the evaluation of acute female pelvic pain; abdominal ultrasound can accurately identify most gynecological pathologies requiring emergent intervention, and further characterization may be provided through the use of transvaginal ultrasound, computed tomography, or magnetic resonance imaging [4]. Absence of Doppler flow on imaging is diagnostic for torsion of an ovary or of a pedunculated myoma.

A benefit to diagnostic laparoscopy in the evaluation of acute female pelvic pain is the ability to diagnose and institute appropriate care for disease of the appendix or female reproductive tract. A Cochrane review looked at the use of laparoscopy among women of childbearing age presenting with acute lower abdominal pain and/or suspected appendicitis; they concluded that the use of laparoscopy was more likely to result in a specific diagnosis before discharge when compared to open appendectomy (odds ratio [OR] 4.10) or to a 'wait and see" strategy (OR 6.07), without a change in adverse events (OR 0.46 compared to open appendectomy, OR 0.87 compared to "wait and see"). The rate of normal appendix removal with laparoscopy was lower compared to open appendectomy (OR 0.13), but higher compared a "wait and see" strategy (OR 5.14) [5]. Early laparoscopy (within 18 hours of admission) for nonspecific abdominal pain has also been shown to result in a greater improvement in well-being scores at 6 weeks follow-up compared to a close-observation approach (149 points from baseline of 134 points vs. 143 points from baseline of 132 points using a 177-point scale) [6]. In a review of 2365 patients with acute and chronic pelvic pain, laparoscopy was used to evaluate 736 (31.1% of) patients with acute pelvic pain, and yielded a diagnosis in 681 (92.5% of) cases,

with salpingo-oophoritis and pelvic adhesions each diagnosed among 168 (22.8% of) patients [41].

For patients with chronic pelvic pain, assessment of an acute pain flare should take into consideration the patient's underlying chronic pain diagnoses, but also consider the possibility of a superimposed acute abdominopelvic process [7]. In our clinical experience, acute pelvic pain flares are often related to worsening pelvic floor muscle spasm in women with this spastic pelvic floor syndrome and may respond to treatment with muscle relaxant medications. Ultrasound imaging for women with unilateral exacerbation of pelvic pain may demonstrate a new ovarian cyst; for women with a known ovarian cyst, adnexal torsion should be considered as a cause of worsening pain and evaluated appropriately. In our experience, laparoscopy is rarely indicated for evaluation of an acute flare of chronic pelvic pain. Evidence for laparoscopy for evaluation of acute pelvic pain: Level II-2.

Laparoscopy for the Evaluation of Chronic Pelvic Pain

Laparoscopy can be instrumental in diagnosing and managing chronic pelvic pain arising from endometriosis, adnexal masses, adhesions, or peritoneal cysts. Appropriate patient selection for laparoscopy is crucial to avoid delaying diagnosis and treatment among women with chronic pain causes amenable to laparoscopic treatment, while not subjecting to unnecessary surgical risks women whose chronic pelvic pain likely arises from other causes, or whose pain may be adequately controlled with medical management. There are no clinical guidelines or quality evidence to guide the timing of laparoscopy for evaluation and treatment of women with unknown cause of chronic pelvic pain, and most authors agree that this decision should be made collaboratively between a patient and her physician [7]. A study of 370 women with chronic pelvic pain evaluated in a specialty clinic showed similar improvements in pain and depression scores at one year among women recommended to undergo surgery compared to those recommended to undergo nonsurgical treatment [8].

In our practice, the initial evaluation of a patient often leads us to suspect multifactorial causes of their chronic pelvic pain. If abdominopelvic visceral causes are suspected in additional to musculoskeletal causes, we usually recommend early laparoscopic evaluation and treatment prior to referral to pelvic physical therapy for treatment of spastic pelvic floor syndrome. We find this approach more effective than delaying surgery and subsequently interrupting a patient's pelvic physical therapy course for several weeks to allow for surgical recovery.

Conscious laparoscopic pain mapping was historically advanced as a useful tool in the evaluation of chronic pelvic pain, and despite difficulties in study design, small case series demonstrated high success of this approach in identifying visceral sources of pain [9]. More recent literature on this procedure suggests that it may be helpful in establishing a diagnosis in only a small portion of patients (27%) [10], and there is presently inadequate evidence to support its routine use in treatment of chronic pelvic pain [11].

Large studies have shown varied outcomes for laparoscopic evaluation of chronic female pelvic pain, with negative or nondiagnostic findings reported in 15% to 35% of cases [12–14, 15]. Reasons for this variability in findings may relate to patient selection factors, as well as variability in the use of peritoneal biopsies for histological diagnosis confirmation. Studies comparing visual identification of endometriosis by the surgeon with histological diagnosis confirmation have shown poor specificity of visual identification (77%–79.23%) [16–1875]. Sensitivity of visually identified endometriosis is reported to be better than specificity, 94% per one meta-analysis [18]; however, within our practice, routine biopsy of normal-appearing peritoneum in laparoscopy for patients with symptoms suggestive of endometriosis has yielded a histological diagnosis of endometriosis in up to 39% of patients, suggesting poor sensitivity of visual identification. For these reasons, within our practice we often routinely obtain peritoneal biopsies from the anterior and posterior cul de sac and right and left ovarian fossae on patients undergoing laparoscopy for chronic pelvic pain of unknown cause with intraoperative findings of normal anatomy and no clear endometriosis or adhesive disease.

Negative laparoscopy may still benefit patients, resulting in a lasting reduction in pain scores. A study of 71 patients undergoing laparoscopy for evaluation of chronic pelvic pain included 34 women with no pathology at time of surgery (47.9%); the entire cohort demonstrated reduction in visual analog scale (VAS) usual pain and VAS worst pain scores from presurgery baseline to 6 months postsurgery

[19]. Subgroup analysis of women with no surgical findings of pathology was not performed. Evidence for laparoscopy for evaluation of chronic pelvic pain: Level II-2.

Laparoscopic Surgery for Treatment of Endometriosis

The goal of laparoscopic surgery for endometriosis is to remove or destroy all visible endometriotic lesions and to restore normal anatomy. There is strong evidence that excision or ablation of minimal to moderate endometriosis results in an improvement in chronic pelvic pain. A Cochrane review looked at seven studies comparing operative laparoscopy to diagnostic laparoscopy for management of endometriosis, and found that excision or ablation was associated with decreased pain score at 6 months (OR 6.58, $p = 0.00001$) and 12 months (OR 10.00, $p = 0.001$) [20]. A single randomized controlled trial (RCT) from the meta-analysis included data from 3 months postsurgery comparing laparoscopic ablation to diagnostic laparoscopy and found no difference in pain scores at that time point (OR 1.37, $p = 0.53$), which may be attributable to placebo effect from surgery within the diagnostic laparoscopy group. The Cochrane meta-analysis included only a limited number of patients with severe endometriosis, and therefore recommends that conclusions regarding surgery for treatment of severe endometriosis "should be made with caution." Regarding duration of pain reduction after local surgical treatment of endometriosis, a retrospective study of 850 women showed a surgery-free percentage of 79.4% at 2 years, 53.5% at 5 years, and 44.6% at 7 years [21].

There is insufficient evidence to recommend a surgical approach of excision versus one of ablation of endometriosis lesions, with similar outcomes for overall pain, pelvic pain, dyspareunia, and dyschezia when the two approaches are compared within meta-analysis [20], and limited studies comparing the two approaches directly [22]. An RCT of 103 patients with superficial endometriosis showed similar VAS score outcomes at 1 year postsurgery between patients who had undergone ablation versus excision approaches, but did not address treatment of deep infiltrating endometriosis [23]. An RCT of 24 patients with mild endometriosis compared ablation versus excision and found similar outcomes at 6 months postsurgery [24]. In our practice, we prefer an excisional approach, which allows for histopathological confirmation of endometriosis; and exception is diaphragmatic endometriosis lesions, which we treat with argon beam ablation. Evidence for excision or ablation of mild to moderate endometriosis: Level I.

Treatment of Deep Infiltrating Endometriosis

Deep infiltrating endometriosis (DIE), defined as lesions penetrating more than 5 mm into the affected tissue, is a severe form of endometriosis that manifests as retroperitoneal nodules associated with severe pelvic pain as well as organ-specific symptoms when localized to the urinary or gastrointestinal tracts. Preoperative imaging with ultrasound and magnetic resonance imaging can help identify lesions prior to surgery; additionally, organ-specific symptoms can be evaluated through cystoscopy and colonoscopy prior to a laparoscopic procedure and allow for appropriate multidisciplinary surgical planning [25]. Complete surgical excision of DIE is considered definitive treatment, as symptoms may not respond to medical management and often recur after the medication is discontinued. Best surgical practice is controversial, as complete surgical excision entails greater risk of complications and morbidity, and literature comparing complete versus incomplete excision of DIE is limited.

A retrospective cohort study of 93 women undergoing surgical treatment of DIE looked at postoperative outcomes with complete and incomplete excision, but involved a heterogeneous cohort including 46 rectovaginal septum lesions and 5 uterosacral ligament lesions that were completely excised as well as diverse genitourinary and gastrointestinal lesions that were both partially and completely excised, and included 3–36-month postoperative follow-up [26]. Patients with complete excision had a greater reduction in VAS postoperative pain scores, which was not improved by postoperative gonadotropin-releasing hormone (GnRH) agonist use (6.9 vs. 5.5, $p = 0.317$); patients with incomplete excision had less reduction in VAS postoperative pain scores and GnRH significantly improved these scores (1.2 vs. 4.5, $p = 0.003$). Recurrence rate was not significantly reduced by use of GnRH agonists and was higher for the incomplete excision group versus the complete excision group (0–10% vs. 29.4–41.2%).

A retrospective cohort study of 132 patients with histologically proven DIE surveyed at a mean of 3.3 years postsurgery analyzed patients according to a proposed surgical classification based on anatomical location: uterosacral, vaginal, bladder, or intestinal [27]. For 78 patients with uterosacral lesions and 25 patients with vaginal lesions included in the study, complete surgical excision resulted in significant improvements in dysmenorrhea (delta 4.36 and 5.17, $p = 0.0001$), deep dyspareunia (delta 4.30 and 4.41, $p = 0.0001$), painful defecation during menstruation (delta 3.72, $p = 0.0001$ and delta 5.17, $p = 0.0007$), and noncyclic chronic pelvic pain scores (delta 4.11, $p = 0.0001$ and delta 6.00, $p = 0.0171$). These results strongly support the efficacy of complete excision of posterior DIE lesions for management of pain symptoms.

Recurrence of DIE lesions remains a risk even with complete lesion excision at time of primary surgery. A recent meta-analysis identified elevated body mass index (BMI) and younger age at primary surgery as risk factors for DIE recurrence [28]. Evidence for resection of DIE: Level II-2.

Treatment of Intestinal Deep Infiltrating Endometriosis

In patients with intestinal DIE, treatment may involve a conservative nodulectomy approach of lesion shaving or discoid resection, versus a radical approach of segmental bowel resection with colorectal anastomosis. Segmental bowel resection is appropriate when lesions exceed 3 cm size or involve >50% of the bowel circumference [29]. Nodulectomy may be safely performed in multicentric disease if lesions are separated by at least 5 cm of healthy bowel [30]. A retrospective comparative study of 77 women undergoing surgical treatment of DIE of the rectum showed a recurrence rate at 5 years postsurgery of 8.7% for those undergoing rectal shaving compared with colorectal resection; the authors concluded that for colorectal resection be performed in lieu of rectal shaving, the number needed to treat is 11 patients to prevent one patient recurrence [31]. Given postoperative complications including anal incontinence and lower quality of life scores with colorectal resection, conservative treatment is preferred in appropriate candidates [32]. Preoperative imaging and multidisciplinary consultation is appropriate for patients with intestinal DIE. Evidence for discoid bowel resection of DIE: Level II-2.

Treatment of Urinary Tract Deep Infiltrating Endometriosis

In patients with urinary tract DIE, treatment may involve resection of bladder endometriosis nodules with full or partial thickness bladder cystectomy, advanced ureterolysis, and segmental ureteral resection with end-to-end anastomosis or ureteroneocystotomy. Literature on this topic is limited to retrospective noncomparative studies, so there is a lack of evidence-based practice guidelines. A retrospective study of 81 women treated for urinary tract DIE including 42 cases of ureteral endometriosis and 50 cases of bladder endometriosis looked at outcomes and postoperative complications through 5 years postsurgery [30]. Ureterolysis was preferred over segmental ureter resection, unless there was evidence of ureteral muscularis infiltration; end-to-end reanastamosis was preferred over ureteroneocystotomy unless ureteral stenosis exceed 2–3 cm or was located adjacent to the vesicoureteral junction. Of the 42 patients treated for ureteral nodules, 28% experienced postoperative complications: seven presented with complications requiring reintervention, five had complications requiring medical management. Among the 50 patients treated for bladder endometriosis, four (8%) experienced postoperative complications, all requiring reintervention. None of the patients in the study had recurrence of urinary tract endometriosis at 5-year follow-up. Evidence for resection of urinary DIE: Level II-2.

Laparoscopic Appendectomy

Incidental appendectomy at time of laparoscopy has been explored as a treatment option for women with both known and unknown causes of pelvic pain. Elective coincidental appendectomy performed for a normal-appearing appendix at the time of another surgical procedure may be considered for purposes of reducing risk of subsequent appendicitis and simplifying the differential diagnosis for an acute pain flare in a patient with chronic pelvic pain [33]. There is no evidence from RCTs to guide whether the increase in cost and surgical morbidity from elective coincidental appendectomy outweigh the cost and risk from patients developing future appendicitis. Studies suggest benefit to removal of a normal or abnormal-appearing appendix during laparoscopy or laparotomy for chronic abdominopelvic pain. A retrospective study reported 63 cases of appendectomy performed for abnormal-appearing appendix at the time of laparoscopy for chronic female pelvic pain: all patients reported pain in the right lower quadrant pain before surgery [34]. Pathology was present in 92% of appendiceal specimens, and 89% of patients reported complete and permanent relief of pain at 1-year postoperative follow-up. A retrospective cohort study of women undergoing laparoscopic surgery for chronic pelvic pain without identifiable intraoperative pathology (including normal-appearing appendix) showed improved postoperative pain score in women undergoing appendectomy ($n = 19$) compared to those who did not ($n = 76$) [35]. Women who underwent appendectomy were more likely to have reported right-sided pain preoperatively (58% vs. 22%, $p = 0.002$); only 2 of 19 patients had pathology noted at the appendix (mild acute and chronic appendicitis). At 6 weeks postsurgery, improvement in pain was reported by 93% of appendectomy group patients versus 16% of nonappendectomy group patients (OR 69.9, $p < 0.001$); when surveyed at an average of 4.2 years postsurgery, only 38% of patients responded, but results indicated greater improvement in Pain Disability Index Scores following surgery among appendectomy patients. Among women with DIE, there is an increased risk of appendiceal endometriosis compared to women with superficial endometriosis (39.0% vs. 11.6%, OR 2.7, $p < 0.001$) [36].

Overall, evidence supports consideration of appendectomy at time of gynecological laparoscopy among women with chronic pelvic pain and should be especially considered if patients have preoperative right lower quadrant pain and/or an abnormal appearing appendix at time of laparoscopy. Among patients with endometriosis, appendiceal endometriosis is present in more than one third of patients with DIE and should be especially considered in this population. Evidence for appendectomy for chronic right lower quadrant pain: Level II-2.

Laparoscopy for Adhesiolysis

Although intraabdominal adhesions are considered a common cause for abdominopelvic pain, with 47% of adhesions shown to be a source of pain at the time of conscious laparoscopy [37], the efficacy of adhesiolysis remains controversial. A meta-analysis from 2015 looked at 25 studies with a total of 1281 patients, including three RCTs and 22 case-control studies, many of which were judged to be at high risk of bias

[38]. Results of the three RCTs were highly varied, with one study showing benefit, one study showing benefit only within a subgroup of patients with dense and vascularized adhesions, and one showing no benefit for adhesiolysis. The majority of studies showed improvement in pain in more than 50% of patients. The authors of the review concluded that there was inadequate evidence to definitively conclude that adhesiolysis is effective in the treatment of chronic abdominal pain. Subsequent studies of adhesiolysis efficacy have shown variable results. An RCT of 100 patients randomized to laparoscopic adhesiolysis versus diagnostic laparoscopy showed poorer outcomes with adhesiolysis at 12-year follow-up, including lower risk of being pain free (relative risk [RR] = 1.3, $p = 0.033$), and higher risk of repeat surgery for persistent abdominal pain (RR = 1.67, $p = 0.042$) [39]. An RCT of 50 women with chronic pelvic pain randomized to laparoscopic adhesiolysis versus diagnostic laparoscopy showed improvement in VAS scores at 6 months postsurgery among the adhesiolysis group (-17.5 vs. -1.5, $p = 0.048$) [40]. Within our practice, adhesiolysis is performed when adhesions are noted at the time of surgery; clinical experience has shown us that patients often report improved pain following adhesiolysis, and that patients undergoing future surgery for recurrent pain typically have decreased adhesive disease burden compared to their primary surgery. Evidence of adhesiolysis for chronic pelvic pain: Level II-2.

Laparoscopic Ovarian Cystectomy

Most benign ovarian cysts are functional and asymptomatic, but may cause pain from large size, ovarian, torsion, or hemorrhage. Reasons for surgical management of an ovarian cyst include persistence over several menstrual cycles or increasing size on serial imaging. A laparoscopic approach is considered the gold standard for management of benign ovarian masses, with cystectomy favored over cyst aspiration or oophorectomy for purposes of fertility preservation in premenopausal women who have not yet completed child bearing [3]. For endometrioma cysts, ovarian cystectomy is recommended. A Cochrane review compared laparoscopic excision of the endometrioma cyst wall to laparoscopic drainage and ablation of the endometrioma and found excision to be associated with a reduced rate of dysmenorrhea (OR 0.15), dyspareunia (OR 0.08), nonmenstrual pelvic pain (OR 0.10), and recurrence of the endometrioma

(OR 0.41) [41]. For ovarian mature cystic teratomas (dermoid cysts), a laparoscopic approach is preferred over laparotomy despite being associated with a longer operative time and higher risk of intraabdominal cyst rupture; cystectomy should be attempted in a young patient for purposes of fertility preservation, unless she requests oophorectomy [42]. Evidence for ovarian cystectomy with cyst wall excision for management of endometrioma: Level I.

Oophorectomy

Ovarian preservation is recommended for women under age 65 who are undergoing hysterectomy for benign indications, owing to decreased life expectancy associated with ovary removal [43]. Bilateral oophorectomy at time of hysterectomy is associated with having as many or more symptoms at problematic–severe levels at two years postsurgery compared to presurgery in a prospective cohort study of 1299 women undergoing hysterectomy for benign indications (OR 2.01, $p = 0.02$) [44]. A case-control study of 4931 women undergoing ovary-sparing hysterectomy compared to 4931 age-matched women who did not have hysterectomy showed the incidence of subsequent oophorectomy by 30-year follow-up to be 9.2% versus 7.3% for controls (hazard ratio [HR] = 1.20, $p = 0.03$) [45], suggesting that indications for hysterectomy may also raise the risk of subsequent oophorectomy, but that most patients with ovarian conservation at time of hysterectomy will not require subsequent surgery for oophorectomy.

Among patients with endometriosis, oophorectomy at time of hysterectomy is controversial. A retrospective study of 138 women undergoing hysterectomy for endometriosis compared rates of recurrent symptoms and reoperation among women with and without ovarian preservation: ovarian preservation was associated with 62% risk of recurrent symptoms compared with 10% among castrated patients (RR 6.1), and 31% risk of reoperation versus 3.7% (RR 8.1) [46]. A more recent study showed that among women with endometriosis undergoing surgical management, 77% of those who underwent hysterectomy with ovarian preservation had not undergone reoperation at 7-year follow-up, compared to 91.7% of those who underwent hysterectomy without ovarian preservation; this study showed that among the subgroup of women age 30–39, those undergoing hysterectomy with ovarian preservation had a reoperation risks similar to those of women who underwent hysterectomy without ovarian preservation (surgery-free percentage of 89.6% vs. 85.7%) [21]. The authors concluded that for women under age 40, bilateral oophorectomy did not substantially reduce the risk of reoperation, and therefore hysterectomy with ovarian preservation is preferable for these women. On the basis of these studies, ACOG recommends that in patients with normal ovaries undergoing hysterectomy, ovarian conservation with removal of endometriotic lesions should be considered. In our practice, we recommend ovarian preservation for women under age 40 undergoing hysterectomy for treatment of endometriosis, as the benefits of ovarian conservation outweigh the risk of disease recurrence.

When oophorectomy is performed for reasons of pain, proper surgical technique can help lower the risk of ovarian remnant syndrome, a cause of chronic pelvic pain that is discussed in a separate chapter. In our practice, retroperitoneal dissection is performed lateral to the infundibulopelvic ligament, to dissect the ovary, infundibulopelvic ligament, and obliterated broad ligament off of the pelvic sidewall and to identify and lateralize the ureter prior to transecting the infundibulopelvic ligament with a margin of vessel proximal to the ovary. Obliterated broad ligament and surrounding tissues are removed with the ovary. Evidence for oophorectomy for management of chronic pelvic pain from endometriosis: Level II-2.

Hysterectomy

Hysterectomy, both with and without ovarian conservation, is commonly performed for management of chronic pelvic pain, and is generally considered effective for appropriately selected patients. Of the 600,000 hysterectomies performed each year in the United States, approximately 12% have chronic pelvic pain as the primary indication [47]. A 2-year prospective study of 1299 women undergoing hysterectomy showed 63.1% of patients reporting pelvic pain prior to surgery, but only 7.8% reporting this symptom at 2 years postsurgery [44]. These findings are similar to those of prior studies demonstrating resolution of chronic pelvic pain among 74% of women for whom this was the primary indication for hysterectomy [48].

For patients with endometriosis, there is considerable evidence for the efficacy of hysterectomy for management of pelvic pain; however, the literature is not specific about different varieties of preoperative pelvic pain among patients undergoing hysterectomy, making it challenging to identify risk factors for poor

response to hysterectomy [49]. Supracervical hysterectomy among patients with endometriosis may be associated with continued or recurrent pain and severe adhesions at time of trachelectomy for persistent symptoms, as well as risk of implantation of tissue at the incision through which the specimen is removed or dissemination from morcellation for tissue removal. Complete removal of endometriosis tissue at time of hysterectomy is recommended to avoid residual pain. Women with endometriosis should be counseled that even with hysterectomy, they remain at risk for continued symptoms or recurrence of endometriosis and chronic pelvic pain, which may occur in up to 62% among women with ovarian conservation [50]. A retrospective study of 120 women with endometriosis showed that among 47 women undergoing hysterectomy with ovarian preservation, 95.7% were surgery free at 2 years, and 77.0% at 7 years; among 50 women undergoing hysterectomy with bilateral salpingo-oophorectomy (BSO), 96.0% were surgery free at 2 years, and 9.17% at 7 years [21]. Evidence for hysterectomy for endometriosis: Level II.

For women with pain arising from pelvic congestion syndrome, hysterectomy with BSO results in significant improvement in pain: a prospective non-randomized study of 36 patients showed complete pain resolution in 67% at 1 year, and only one woman (3%) had no improvement in her chronic daily pain after the procedure [51]. An RCT of 164 women with pelvic congestion syndrome stratified by preoperative stress score showed 39.5%–46.5% improvement in VAS score at 12 months postsurgery for 27 women undergoing hysterectomy with BSO followed by hormone replacement therapy, and 33.4%–34.6% improvement in VAS score at 12 months postsurgery for 27 women undergoing hysterectomy with unilateral salpingo-oophorectomy (USO) [52]. Evidence for hysterectomy for pelvic congestion syndrome: Level I.

The value of hysterectomy for patients without endometriosis or other identified extrauterine cause of pelvic pain has been demonstrated: a retrospective study of 99 premenopausal patients undergoing hysterectomy with no evidence of extrauterine pathology showed significant symptom improvement in 77.8% of patients at an average of 21.6-month postoperative follow-up [53]. Among these patients, no pathological alteration of the uterus was noted in 65.7% of patients (34.3% had leiomyomata and/or adenomyosis identified on pathology). While the majority of patients with pelvic pain demonstrate a positive response to hysterectomy, regardless of pelvic pain etiology, authors have called for greater research to identify risk factors for continued pain after hysterectomy and full preoperative evaluation of nonreproductive causes of pain [54]. A prospective cohort study of 1249 women undergoing hysterectomy for benign indications showed that women with both preoperative pelvic pain and depression were at a three to five times increased risk of continued impairment in quality of life at 2 years following hysterectomy, including OR 4.91 for continued pelvic pain and OR 2.41 for dyspareunia [55]. Evidence for hysterectomy for management of chronic pelvic pain: Level II-2.

Vaginal Cuff Revision

Patients with persistent or de novo pain at the vaginal cuff following hysterectomy may benefit from laparoscopic vaginal apex excision, although evidence for this procedure is limited to relatively small clinical trials with short follow-up. A case series of nine patients undergoing surgical excision of the vaginal apex for post-hysterectomy dyspareunia showed a decrease in mean coital VAS pain score from 9.22 presurgery to 3.11 postsurgery ($p < 0.001$), and an increase in coital frequency from 5.22 episodes per month to 11.11 episodes per month postsurgery ($p = 0.02$) [56]. A retrospective survey of 27 patients with vaginal apex pain and dyspareunia having undergone vaginal apex excision reported significant reduction in pain among 82%, with complete resolution of symptoms among 67% of patients for a median of 20 months, but only 26% of patients remained pain free at the end of the follow-up period [44]. A retrospective survey of 16 patients having undergone vaginal vault excision for post-hysterectomy dyspareunia and chronic pelvic pain reported improvement in dyspareunia among 81.25% of women at a mean postoperative interval of 1.8 months [57]. Evidence for vaginal apex excision: Level II–III.

Fertility-Sparing Pelvic Denervation Procedures

Surgical interruption of cervical sensory pain nerve fibers has been developed as a fertility-sparing treatment option for dysmenorrhea. Two techniques have been developed: laparoscopic uterine nerve ablation (LUNA), which involves the transection of the uterosacral ligaments at their attachment to the cervix,

and presacral neurectomy (PSN), which involves total resection of a segment of presacral nerves lying within the interiliac triangle. A Cochrane review from 2005 sought to determine the effectiveness of these two surgical interventions for management of dysmenorrhea: the meta-analysis suggested that LUNA is superior to the control arm for management of primary dysmenorrhea at 12 months, but success rates decline rapidly thereafter; long term, presacral neurectomy was significantly more effective at reducing pain from primary dysmenorrhea when compared to LUNA (OR 0.10) [58]. Presacral neurectomy is associated with greater adverse effects than LUNA, including constipation, urinary urgency, and painless labor. For patients with secondary dysmenorrhea from endometriosis, LUNA was equivalent to a control arm at up to 3 years postsurgery; evidence for presacral neurectomy for secondary dysmenorrhea was mixed, with significant improvement evident for patients with midline abdominal pain. The largest trial of presacral neurectomy for secondary dysmenorrhea compared laparoscopic treatment of endometriosis to laparoscopic treatment of endometriosis plus presacral neurectomy; cure rate was higher within the PSN group ($p < 0.05$) at 6 months (87.3% vs. 60.3%), at 12 months (65.7% vs. 57.1%), and at 24 months (83.3 vs. 53.3%) [59]. Evidence for presacral neurectomy: Level I.

Pelvic Vein Ligation

For women with pelvic congestion syndrome, chronic pelvic pain results from ovarian vein dilation; occlusive therapy of the dilated pelvic veins by ligation or embolic occlusion has emerged as a targeted therapy for this condition, with bilateral treatment showing superior results [60]. Several published case series of transcatheter embolotherapy of the ovarian veins have shown success rates ranging from 50% to 80% [61], with a more recent randomized controlled trial showing 40.2–61.5% pain decrease at 12-month follow-up among 52 patients stratified into groups on the basis of preoperative stress scores [52]. Laparoscopic bilateral transperitoneal vein ligation has shown promise within a pilot study of 23 women, with complete remission of pain reported in 74% of women at 12 months postsurgery [62]. Within our practice, transfundal venography immediately prior to surgery and using fluorescein with da Vinci Firefly™ fluorescence imaging is performed at the time of robotic-assisted laparoscopic ovarian vein ligation to assist in identification and dissection of dilated ovarian veins. Evidence for bilateral ovarian vein ligation: Level II-3. Evidence for bilateral ovarian vein percutaneous embolization: Level I.

Myomectomy

Pain is reported by 74% of women with symptomatic uterine fibroids, with up to 24% of women rating their pain as "severe" or "very severe" [63]. Among women desiring future fertility, myomectomy is considered the gold standard for surgical management of symptomatic fibroids. A systematic review of clinical and cost-effectiveness of uterine-preserving interventions for management of symptomatic uterine fibroids concluded that myomectomy was superior to uterine artery embolization for management of bulk symptoms, which may include pelvic pain, and for improving pregnancy outcomes; however, uterine artery embolization is superior for treatment of abnormal uterine bleeding [64]. Myomectomy has been demonstrated to improve quality of life and sexual function, regardless of surgical approach [65]. Evidence for myomectomy for management of pelvic pain: Level II.

Bladder Overdistension

Filling of the bladder to maximum capacity at a fixed pressure for a set period of time, known as cystodistension, hydrodistension, or bladder overdistension, is a common surgical technique for treatment of interstitial cystitis/bladder pain syndrome. A meta-analysis seeking to evaluate the evidence for use of this procedure included 17 heterogeneous trials and concluded that there was inadequate evidence to support the use of cystodistension for treatment of bladder pain syndrome [66]. The largest trial included within the meta-analysis was a prospective cohort study of 191 patients undergoing hydrodistension with and without electrical fulguration of Hunner's lesions if present, and showed mean time to therapeutic failure of 25.5 months in those without Hunner's lesions versus 28.5 months in those with Hunner's lesions; therapeutic failure was defined as "a necessity to repeat hydrodistension or initiating bladder instillation therapy and/or narcotic use for pain control [67]. In our practice, we perform bladder overdistension for 6 or for 30 minutes, often with spinal analgesia in addition to general anesthesia. Many of our patients undergo repeat bladder distension every 3–12 months due to recurrence of symptoms but find significant benefit

from the duration of symptom relief. Evidence for cystodistension: Level II–III.

Botox Injection of Pelvic Floor Muscles

Injection of botulinum toxin type A into pelvic floor muscles for management of chronic pelvic pain and dyspareunia is the most common procedure performed within our clinical practice. Reviews of the use of botulinum toxin for chronic pelvic pain have concluded that initial studies are promising, but that further clinical trials with robust methodology are needed to provide evidence for this procedure and to clarify the optimal dosing and administration technique for this application of botulinum toxin [68, 69]. The only RCT of botulinum toxic for pelvic pain included 30 women; among those receiving 80 units of onabotulinumtoxin A, significant improvement in nonmenstrual pain was demonstrated (VAS score 51 vs. 22, $p = 0.009$), with no significant difference for those receiving saline placebo; however, dyspareunia scores decreased significantly from baseline in both Botox and placebo groups, suggesting nonsuperiority of Botox [70]. Efficacy of onabotulinumtoxin A for chronic pelvic pain associated with pelvic floor tension myalgia was presented by our practice as a poster at the International Pelvic Pain Society: use of 200 units was associated with more than a 20-point VAS score improvement in 67% of patients, with 21% of patients electing to receive multiple injections, at an average of 162 days between serial injections [71]. A prospective study of 37 women undergoing injection of 100 units of botulinum toxin into the puborectalis and pubococcygeus muscles showed significant difference in dysmenorrhea or dyschezia from baseline scores in 26 women receiving their first injection as well as in 11 women receiving a second injection at an average of 33.4 weeks after the first, suggesting that repeat injections for symptom recurrence can be expected to have similar efficacy [72]. Evidence for botulinum toxin injection of pelvic floor muscles: Level I–II.

Mesh Removal

As a chronic pelvic pain referral center, we frequently see patients with chronic pelvic pain related to prior surgical placement of pelvic mesh, which causes pelvic floor muscular dysfunction and/or pudendal neuralgia. Candidates for removal of synthetic mesh grafts include patients with pain not relieved with conservative management, and in whom the risks of mesh removal are outweighed by the potential benefits of mesh excision [73]. Many patients present to our practice with pelvic pain that persists despite partial removal of mesh followed by treatment of spastic pelvic floor syndrome and/or pudendal neuralgia. Our practice regarding removal of pelvic mesh has evolved over time, and experience has increasingly led us to recommend total mesh removal for many patients, meaning removal of vaginal mesh as well as groin dissection performed for removal of transobturator mesh or laparoscopic transperitoneal dissection performed for removal of retropubic mesh. Conversely, the authors of a review on mesh removal report their experience with "trigger points" of pain localizing to areas of mesh arms or points of insertion, and report successful resolution of pain with partial removal of mesh from these areas [74]. There are no RCTs comparing partial and total mesh removal, but several retrospective surgical cohort studies show improvement in pain symptoms with both partial and complete removal of mesh. Many of these studies use the terminology "total" or "complete" mesh removal to refer to removal of all vaginally accessible mesh, not including mesh removal from the retropubic or groin and obturator spaces.

A series of 123 patients undergoing removal of the vaginal component of transobturator, retropubic, or vaginal prolapse mesh showed significant improvement in postoperative VAS scores for all groups, and reported a postoperative pain-free status in 81% of mid-urethral sling patients at an average of 35 months follow-up, and in 67% of prolapse mesh patients at an average of 22 months follow-up [75]. A series of 32 patients reported 17 cases of transperitoneal laparoscopic removal of retropubic mesh and 15 cases of vaginal removal of transobturator mesh, with 8 of these patients also undergoing groin dissection for mesh removal from the adductor muscle. At least 50% improvement in VAS score was reported among 68% of patients, with transobturator mesh patients who underwent groin dissection demonstrating a nonsignificant superior reduction in VAS score relative to patients undergoing only vaginal mesh removal (62% vs. 50%, $p = 0.5826$, $n = 15$) [76]. A retrospective study of 90 patients undergoing removal of pelvic mesh for a variety of indications included 58 patients with pain as the only indication for surgery; among these patients, 51% had persistent pain and of the 43 patients with preoperative dyspareunia, 30% reported persistent symptoms postoperatively [77]. A retrospective case series of 83 patients undergoing vaginal removal of a variety of mesh grafts, most commonly for vaginal pain (62%), dyspareunia (55%), and pelvic pain (50%), reported vaginal pain in 13% at 4–6 weeks postsurgery, and reoperation among 35% of patients, with 44% of these procedures being performed for additional mesh removal [78]. Evidence for removal of pelvic mesh: Level II. Evidence for removal of groin mesh: Level II–III.

Pudendal Neurolysis

Roger Robert and colleagues first described a transgluteal surgery for decompressing anatomic impingement of the pudendal nerve in patients with pudendal nerve entrapment syndrome. They report 150 cases with more than 10 years follow-up from which 45% of patients considered themselves cured, 22% who reported improved pain, and 33% of patients who derived no benefit from surgery [79]. A retrospective cohort of 55 heterogenous patients undergoing pudendal neurolysis via both a traditional posterior transgluteal approach and an anterior inferior ramus approach, including both neuroma transection and decompression methods, reported 86% of patients achieving an excellent result and 14% achieving a good result at an average of 14.3 months postsurgery [80]. A robotic-assisted laparoscopic approach to pudendal neurolysis has also been described, but the success rate of this procedure has been reported only for a single case as 50% reduction in pain at 2 and 10 weeks post-op [81]. Evidence for transgluteal pudendal neurolysis: Level II-3.

Vestibulectomy

A review of interventions for vulvodynia concluded that there is fair evidence for the efficacy of vestibulectomy surgery for treatment of vestibulodynia, with complete relief of symptoms reported as an outcome by 12 studies, with a median effect size of 67%; a median of 79% of patients reported improvement in symptoms, but this effect size ranged from 31% to 100% among the case series and randomized trials included in the meta-analysis [82]. Vestibulectomy is recommended for patients with provoked vestibulodynia, or possibly patients with mixed vulvodynia, but has not been shown to be effective for generalized vulvodynia [83]. Evidence for vestibulectomy for provoked vulvodynia: Level II.

Five Things You Need to Know

- Hysterectomy is an effective treatment for a variety of chronic pelvic pain conditions. There is strong evidence for hysterectomy in management of pelvic congestion syndrome. There is moderate evidence for hysterectomy in management of endometriosis or chronic pelvic pain of unknown etiology.

- There is strong evidence for the efficacy of excision or ablation of mild to moderate endometriosis, ovarian cyst wall excision for management of endometrioma, presacral neurectomy for management of midline dysmenorrhea, bilateral ovarian vein percutaneous ligation for pelvic congestion, and Botox injection of pelvic floor muscles for pelvic floor tension myalgia.

- There is moderate evidence for the efficacy of laparoscopy for evaluation of chronic pelvic pain, resection of DIE including urinary tract resection and discoid bowel resection, myomectomy for pelvic pain, appendectomy for chronic right lower quadrant pain, adhesiolysis for chronic pelvic pain, cystodistension for interstitial cystitis/bladder pain syndrome, removal of pelvic mesh, transgluteal pudendal neurolysis for pudendal nerve entrapment, and vestibulectomy for provoked vulvodynia.

- There is limited literature supporting the use of vaginal apex excision, bilateral ovarian vein ligation, and removal of groin mesh. Evidence does not support the efficacy of laparoscopic uterine nerve ablation (LUNA) for management of dysmenorrhea.

- For women under age 40 undergoing hysterectomy for treatment of endometriosis, bilateral oophorectomy does not reduce the risk of reoperation for recurrent pelvic pain. For women age 40 or older, there is moderate evidence for bilateral oophorectomy.

References

1. Stratton P. Evaluation of acute pelvic pain in nonpregnant adult women. UpToDate2016.

2. Kruszka PS, Kruszka SJ. Evaluation of acute pelvic pain in women. *Am Fam Physician.* 2010;**82**(2):141–7.

3. ACOG Committee on Practice Bulletins – Gynecology. Practice Bulletin 174: Evaluation and management of adnexal masses. *Obstet Gynecol.* 2016;**128**(5):e210–26.

4. Rivera Dominguez A, Mora Jurado A, Garcia de la Oliva A, de Araujo Martins-Romeo D, Cueto Alvarez L. Gynecological pelvic pain as emergency pathology. *Radiologia.* 2017;**59**(2):115–27.

5. Gaitán Hernando G, Reveiz L, Farquhar C, Elias Vanessa M. Laparoscopy for the management of acute lower abdominal pain in women of childbearing age. *Cochrane Database Syst. Rev.* 2014;(**5**).

6. Decadt B, Sussman L, Lewis MPN, Secker A, Cohen L, Rogers C, et al. Randomized clinical trial of early laparoscopy in the management of acute non-specific abdominal pain. *Br J Surg.* 1999;**86**(11):1383–6.

7. Tu F, As-Sanie S, Evaluation of chronic pelvic pain in women. UpToDate 2018.

8. Lamvu G, Williams R, Zolnoun D, Wechter ME, Shortliffe A, Fulton G, Steege JF. Long-term outcomes after surgical and nonsurgical management of chronic pelvic pain: one year after evaluation in a pelvic pain specialty clinic. *Am J Obstet Gynecol.* 2006;**195**(2):591–8.

9. Lamvu G, Robinson B, Zolnoun D, Steege JF. Vaginal apex resection: a treatment option for vaginal apex pain. *Obstet Gynecol.* 2004;**104**(6):1340–6.

10. Swanton A, Iyer L, Reginald PW. Diagnosis, treatment and follow up of women undergoing conscious pain mapping for chronic pelvic pain: a prospective cohort study. *BJOG.* 2006;**113**(7):792–6.

11. Holloran-Schwartz MB. Surgical evaluation and treatment of the patient with chronic pelvic pain. *Obstet Gynecol Clin North Am.* 2014;**41**(3):357–69.

12. Howard FM. The role of laparoscopy in chronic pelvic pain: promises and pitfalls. *Obstet Gynaecol Surv.*1993;**48**(6):357–87.

13. Howard FM. Laparoscopic evaluation and treatment of women with chronic pelvic pain. *J Am Assoc Gynecol Laparosc.* 1994;**1**(4 Pt 1):325–31.

14. Howard FM. The role of laparoscopy in the chronic pelvic pain patient. *Clin Obstet Gynecol.* 2003;**46**(4):749–66.

15. Kontoravdis A, Chryssikopoulos A, Hassiakos D, Liapis A, Zourlas PA. The diagnostic value of laparoscopy in 2365 patients with acute and chronic pelvic pain. *Int J Obstet Gynecol.* 1996;**52**(3):243–8.

16. de Almeida Filho DP, de Oliveira LJ, do Amaral VF. Accuracy of laparoscopy for assessing patients with endometriosis. *São Paulo Med J.* 2008;**126**(6):305–8.

17. Walter AJ, Hentz JG, Magtibay PM, Cornella JL, Magrina JF. Endometriosis: correlation between histologic and visual findings at laparoscopy. *Am J Obstet Gynecol.* 2001;**184**(7):1407–13.

18. Wykes CB, Clark TJ, Khan KS. Accuracy of laparoscopy in the diagnosis of endometriosis: a systematic quantitative review. *BJOG*. 2004;**111**(11):1204–12.

19. ElcombeL S, Gath D, Day A. The psychological effects of laparoscopy on women with chronic pelvic pain. *Psychol Med*. 1997;**27**(5):1041–50.

20. Duffy J, Arambage K, Correa F, Olive D, Farquhar C, Garry R, Barlow D. Laparoscopic surgery for endometriosis (Review). Summary Findings for the Main Comparison. *Cochrane Database Syst Rev*. 2014;(4).

21. Shakiba K, Bena JF, McGill KM, Minger J, Falcone T. Surgical treatment of endometriosis: a 7-year follow-up on the requirement for further study. *Obstet Gynecol*. 2008;**111**(6):1285–92.

22. Yeung PP, Shwayder J, Pasic RP. Laparoscopic management of endometriosis: comprehensive review of best evidence. *J Minim Invasive Gynecol*. 2009;**16**(3):269–81.

23. Healey M, Ang WC, Cheng C. Surgical treatment of endometriosis: a prospective randomized double-blinded trial comparing excision and ablation. *Fertil Steril*. 2010;**94**(7):2536–40.

24. Wright J, Lotfallah H, Jones K, Lovell D. A randomized trial of excision versus ablation for mild endometriosis. *Fertil Steril*. 2005;**83**(6):1830–6.

25. Chapron C, Chopin N, Borghese B, Malartic C, Decuypere F, Foulot H. Surgical management of deeply infiltrating endometriosis: an update. *Ann NY Acad Sci*. 2004;**1034**, 326–37.

26. Cao Q, Lu F, Feng WW, Ding JX, Hua KQ. Comparison of complete and incomplete excision of deep infiltrating endometriosis. *Int J Clin Exp Med*. 2015;**8**(11):21497–506.

27. Chopin N, Vieira M, Borghese B, Foulot H, Dousset B, Coste J, et al. Operative management of deeply infiltrating endometriosis: results on pelvic pain symptoms according to a surgical classification. *J Minim Invasive Gynecol*. 2005;**12**(2):106–12.

28. Ianieri MM, Mautone D, Ceccaroni M. Recurrence in deep infiltrating endometriosis: a systematic review of the literature. *J Minim Invasive Gynecol*. 2018.

29. Laganà AS, Vitale SG, Trovato MA, Palmara VI, Rapisarda AMC, Granese R, et al. Full-thickness excision versus shaving by laparoscopy for intestinal deep infiltrating endometriosis: rationale and potential treatment options. *BioMed Res Int*. 2016.

30. Darwish B, Stochino-Loi E, Pasquier G, Dugardin F, Defortescu G, Abo C, Roman H. Surgical outcomes of urinary tract deep infiltrating endometriosis. *J Minim Invasive Gynecol*. 2017;**24**(6):998–1006.

31. Roman H, Milles M, Vassilieff M, Resch B, Tuech JJ, Huet E, et al. Long-term functional outcomes following colorectal resection versus shaving for rectal endometriosis. *Am J Obstet Gynecol*. 2016;**215**(6),762.e1–e9.

32. Darwish B, Ron H. Surgical treatment of deep infiltrating rectal endometriosis: in favor of less aggressive surgery. *Am J Obstet Gynecol*. 2016;**215**(2):195–200.

33. American Urogynecologic Society and American College of Obstetricians and Gynecologists. Elective coincidental appendectomy. ACOG Committee Opinion No. 323. *Obstet Gynecol*. 2005;**106**:1141–2.

34. Fayez JA, Toy NJ, Flanagan TM. The appendix as the cause of chronic lower abdominal pain. *Am J Obstet Gynecol*. 1995;**172**(1), 122–3.

35. Lal AK, Weaver AL, Hopkins MR, Famuyide AO. Laparoscopic appendectomy in women without identifiable pathology undergoing laparoscopy for chronic pelvic pain. *JSLS*. 2013;**17**(1):82–7.

36. Moulder J, Siedhoff M, Melvin K, Jarvis E, Hobbs K, Garrett J. Risk of appendiceal endometriosis among women with deep-infiltrating endometriosis. *Int J Gynecol Obstet*. 2017;**139**:149–54.

37. Howard FM, El-Minawi AM, Sanchez RA. Conscious pain mapping by laparoscopy in women with chronic pelvic pain. *Obstet Gynecol*. 2000;**96**(6):934–9.

38. Gerner-Rasmussen J, Burcharth J, Gögenur I. The efficacy of adhesiolysis on chronic abdominal pain: a systematic review. *Langenbecks Arch Surg*. 2015;**400**(5):567–76.

39. Molegraaf MJ, Torensma B, Lange CP, Lange JF, Jeekel J, Swank DJ. Twelve-year outcomes of laparoscopic adhesiolysis in patients with chronic abdominal pain: a randomized clinical trial. *Surgery (US)*. 2017;**161**(2):415–21.

40. Cheong YC, Reading I, Bailey S, Sadek K, Ledger W, Li TC. Should women with chronic pelvic pain have adhesiolysis? *BMC Womens Health*. 2014;**14**(1):1–7.

41. Hart R, Hickey M, Maouris P, Buckett W, Garry, R. Excisional surgery versus ablative surgery for ovarian endometriomata: a Cochrane Review. *Cochrane Database Syst Rev*. 2008;(**2**).

42. Sinha A, Ewies AAA. Ovarian mature cystic teratoma: challenges of surgical management. *Obstet Gynecol Int*. 2016.

43. Parker WH, Broder MS, Liu Z, Shoupe D, Farquhar C, Berek JS. Ovarian conservation at the time of hysterectomy for benign disease. *Clin Obstet Gynecol*. 2007;**50**(2):354–61.

44. Kjerulff KH, Langenberg PW, Rhodes JC, Harvey LA, Guzinski GM, Stolley PD. Effectiveness of hysterectomy. *Obstet Gynecol*. 2000;**95**(3):319–26.

45. Casiano E, Trabuco E, Bharucha A, Weaver A, Schleck C, Melton LJ, Gebhart J. Risk of oophorectomy after hysterectomy. *Obstet Gynecol.* 2013;**121**(5):1069–74.

46. Namnoum AB, Hickman TN, Goodman SB, Gehlbach DL, Rock JA. Incidence of symptom recurrence after hysterectomy for endometriosis. *Fertil Steril.* 1995;**64**(5):898–902.

47. Wu J, Wechter M, Geller E, Nguyen T, Visco A. Hysterectomy rates in the United States, 2003. *Obstet Gynecol.* 2007;**110**, 1091–5.

48. Hillis SD, Marchbanks PA, Peterson HB. The effectiveness of hysterectomy for chronic pelvic pain. *Obstet Gynecol.* 1995;**86**(6):941–5.

49. Martin DC. Hysterectomy for treatment of pain associated with endometriosis. *J Minim Invasive Gynecol.* 2006;**13**(6):566–72.

50. Rizk B, Fischer AS, Lotfy HA, Turki R, Zahed HA, Malik R, et al. Recurrence of endometriosis after hysterectomy. *Facts Views Vision ObGyn.* 2014;**6**(4):219–27.

51. Beard RW, Kennedy RG, Gangar KF, Stones RW, Rogers V, Reginald PW, Anderson M. Bilateral oophorectomy and hysterectomy in the treatment of intractable pelvic pain associated with pelvic congestion. *BJOG.* 1991;**98**(10):988–92.

52. Chung M-H, Huh C-Y. Comparison of treatments for pelvic congestion syndrome. *Tohoku J Exp Med.* 2003.

53. Stovall TG, Ling FW, Crawford DA. Hysterectomy for chronic pelvic pain of presumed uterine etiology. *Obstet Gynecol.* 1990.

54. Lamvu G. Role of hysterectomy in the treatment of chronic pelvic pain. *Obstet Gynecol.* 2011;**117**(5):1175–8.

55. Hartmann KE, Ma C, Lamvu GM, Langenberg PW, Steege JF, Kjerulff KH. Quality of life and sexual function after hysterectomy in women with preoperative pain and depression. *Obstet Gynecol.* 2004;**104**(4):701–9.

56. Sharp HT, Dodson MK, Langer KM, Doucette RC, Norton PA. The role of vaginal apex excision in the management of persistent posthysterectomy dyspareunia. *Am J Obstet Gynecol.* 2000;**183**(6), 1385–9.

57. Trehan AK, Sanaullah F. Laparoscopic posthysterectomy vaginal vault excision for chronic pelvic pain and deep dyspareunia. *J Minim Invasive Gynecol.* 2009;**16**(3):326–32.

58. Proctor M, Latthe P, Farquhar C, Khan K, Johnson N. Surgical interruption of pelvic nerve pathways for primary and secondary dysmenorrhoea. *Cochrane Database Syst Rev.* 2005;(**4**).

59. Zullo F, Palomba S, Zupi E, Russo T, Morelli M, Sena T, et al. Long-term effectiveness of presacral neurectomy for the treatment of severe dysmenorrhea due to endometriosis. *Journal Am Assoc Gynecol Laparosc.* 2004;**11**(1):23–8.

60. Liddle A, Davies A. Pelvic congestion syndrome: chronic pelvic pain caused by ovarian and internal iliac varices. *Phlebology.* 2007;**22**(3):100–4.

61. Venbrux A, Lambert D. Embolization of the ovarian veins as a treatment for patients with chronic pelvic pain caused by pelvic venous incompetence (pelvic congestion syndrome). *Curr Opin Obstet Gynecol.* 1999;**11**(4):395–9.

62. Gargiulo T, Mais V, Brokaj L, Cossu E, Melis GB. Bilateral laparoscopic transperitoneal ligation of ovarian veins for treatment of pelvic congestion syndrome. *J Am Assoc Gynecol Laparosc.* 2003;**10**(4):501–4.

63. Borah BJ, Nicholson WK, Bradley L, Stewart EA. The impact of uterine leiomyomas: A national survey of affected women. *Am J Obstet Gynecol.* 2013;**209**(4):319.e1–e20.

64. Chen S, Pitre E, Kaunels D, Singh S. Uterine-preserving interventions for the management of symptomatic uterine fibroids: A systematic review of clinical and cost-effectiveness. Ottawa: CADTH Rapid Response Report, January 2016, 1–140.

65. Fortin C, Flyckt R, Falcone T. Alternatives to hysterectomy: the burden of fibroids and the quality of life. *Best Pract Res Clin Obstet Gynaecol.* 2018;**46**:31–42.

66. Olson LE, Dyer JE, Haq A, Ockrim J, Greenwell TJ. A systematic review of the literature on cystodistension in bladder pain syndrome. *Int Urogynecol J.* 2017;1–7.

67. Niimi A, Nomiya A, Yamada Y, Suzuki M, Fujimura T, Fukuhara H, et al. Hydrodistension with or without fulguration of Hunner lesions for interstitial cystitis: long-term outcomes and prognostic predictors. *Neurourol Urodyn.* 2016;**35**(8):965–9.

68. Bhide AA, Puccini F, Khullar V, Elneil S, Alessandro Digesu G. Botulinum neurotoxin type A injection of the pelvic floor muscle in pain due to spasticity: a review of the current literature. *Int Urogynecol J.* 2013;**24**(9):1429–34.

69. Purwar B, Khullar V. Use of botulinum toxin for chronic pelvic pain. *Womens Health* 2016;**12**(3):293–6.

70. Abbott JA, Jarvis SK, Lyons SD, Thomson A, Vancaille TG. Botulinum toxin type A for chronic pain and pelvic floor spasm in women: a

Nita Desai and Anna Reinert

randomized controlled trial. *Obstet Gynecol.* 2006;**108**(4):915–23.

71. Hibner M, et al. Poster presentation at International Pelvic Pain Society Annual Meeting; 2010.

72. Nesbitt-Hawes EM, Won H, Jarvis SK, Lyons SD, Vancaillie TG, Abbott JA. Improvement in pelvic pain with botulinum toxin type A – single vs. repeat injections. *Toxicon.* 2013;**63**(1):83–7.

73. Rogo-Gupta L, Castellanos M. When and how to excise vaginal mesh. *Curr Opin Obstet Gynecol.* 2016;**28**(4):311–15.

74. Wolff GF, Winters JC, Krlin RM. Mesh excision: is total mesh excision necessary? *Curr Urol Rep.* 2016;**17**(4):1–7.

75. Hou JC, Alhalabi F, Lemack GE, Zimmern PE. Outcome of transvaginal mesh and tape removed for pain only. *J Urol.* 2014;**192**(3):856–60.

76. Rigaud, J, Pothin, P, Labat, J J, Riant, T, Guerineau, M, Le Normand L, et al. Functional results after tape removal for chronic pelvic pain following tension-free vaginal tape or transobturator tape. *J Urol.* 2010;**184**(2):610–15.

77. Crosby EC, Abernethy M, Berger MB, DeLancey JO, Fenner DE, Morgan DM. Symptom resolution after operative management of complications from transvaginal mesh. *Obstet Gynecol.* 2014;**123**(1):134–9.

78. Cardenas-Trowers O, Malekzadeh P, Nix D, Hatch K. Vaginal mesh removal outcomes: eight years of experience at an academic hospital. *Female Pelvic Med Reconst* 2017;**23**(6):382–6.

79. Robert R, Prat-Pradal D, Labat JJ, Bensignor M, Raoul S, Rebai R, Leborgne J. Anatomic basis of chronic perineal pain: role of the pudendal nerve. *Surg Radiol Anat: SRA.* 1998;**20**(2):93–8.

80. Dellon AL, Coady D, Harris D. Pelvic pain of pudendal nerve origin: surgical outcomes and learning curve lessons. *J Reconstruct Microsurg.* 2015;**31**(4):283–90.

81. Moscatiello P, Carracedo CD, Yupanqui GL, Rivera Martinez ME, Mendiola de la Hoza A, Sanchez Encinas M. Robot-assisted pudendal neurolysis in the treatment of pudendal nerve entrapment syndrome. *Actas Urol Esp.* 2018;**42**(5):344–9.

82. Andrews JC. Vulvodynia interventions-systematic review and evidence grading. *Obstet Gynecol Surv.* 2011;**66**(5):299–315.

83. Stenson AL. Vulvodynia: diagnosis and management. *Obstet Gynecol Clin North Am.* 2017;**44**(3), 493–508.

Pelvic Pain Arising from Endometriosis

Mark Dassel and Alyssa Herrmann

Editor's Introduction

Endometriosis is the most common gynecological condition leading to pelvic pain and often it is the only one recognized by gynecologists. In many cases it coexists with pelvic floor muscle spasm, interstitial cystitis/bladder pain syndrome and irritable bowel syndrome and often all four are grouped as "evil quadruplets." Endometriosis can be diagnosed only surgically; and pathology confirmed tissue biopsy is by far the most accurate way of diagnosis. Unfortunately, all medical treatments of endometriosis are quite inadequate because they all rely on causing a hypoestrogenic state that only provides temporary relief of pain, and soon after medication is discontinued, symptoms return. Development of drugs addressing the cause of the disease is currently not possible because the cause of the disease is unknown. Multiple existing theories fail to unify an explanation of all cases, leading to the possibility that different etiologies may lead to a presence of endometrial glands and stroma in the peritoneal cavity and outside. Surgical resection of endometriosis in skilled hands is effective but patients need to be informed that disease will most likely return within a few years of initial surgery. Deep infiltrating endometriosis requires a very knowledgeable surgeon and often a specialized center for treatment. Additional procedures such as presacral neurectomy, although controversial and potentially risky, may alleviate dysmenorrhea symptoms in some patients. Meticulous removal of ovarian endometriomas is a must in all infertility patients and most pelvic pain patients as simple drainage will result in almost immediate return of endometrioma. Pre and postsurgical treatment with hormonal suppression is still debatable, and there is research to support it and research showing it ineffective. In my practice I do not use pre- and postsurgical hormonal suppression.

Introduction

Endometriosis is a common cause of pelvic pain, affecting an estimated 10% to 15% of women of reproductive age [1]. The disease has been associated with 70% of women who present to chronic pelvic pain clinics [2] and about 50% of all infertility patients [3]. *Despite its high prevalence, treatment methodologies for endometriosis remain controversial, even as the cannon of endometriosis literature continues to grow.* Traditionally, surgical evaluation and treatment of endometriosis were the mainstays of treatment; however, pain symptomatology associated with endometriosis is increasingly recognized as a syndrome of painful conditions rather than a single pain etiology to be corrected surgically. This greater recognition of comorbid disease states as (secondary pain generators) is providing a much better understanding of the etiology of pain associated with endometriosis and guiding less invasive and more effective treatment options.

In this chapter we will address the link between endometriosis and pain symptomatology including the ways that different types of endometriosis lead to pain symptoms. Furthermore, we will evaluate surgical and nonsurgical techniques that have been shown useful in the treatment of endometriosis-related pain.

Endometriosis is broadly defined as the presence of endometrioid glands and stroma ectopic to the uterus. This definition, though histologically accurate, does not fully describe the link between endometriosis and associated painful symptoms. Furthermore, endometriosis does not present as a singular phenotype; rather it presents in varied tissue architectures. There are superficial peritoneal blebs (superficial endometriosis), cystic lesions (endometriomas), and large fibrous nodules (deep infiltrating endometriotic nodules). The architecture of each endometriosis subtype dictates its own unique pain signature. Endometriosis subtypes can present in isolation or in combination with one another. As such, each patient's endometriosis disease must be evaluated and treated as a unique constellation of lesion subtypes. Further complicating pain resolution is the myriad of associated, downstream pain sequelae. These secondary pain generators are further described in this book and are commonly a reaction to the pain in the pelvis created by endometriosis. Frequently encountered secondary pain generators are pelvic floor tension myalgia, abdominal myofascial pain, vulvodynia, and centralized pain syndromes (irritable bowel syndrome, interstitial cystitis/bladder pain syndrome). Downstream sequelae of unchecked painful symptomatology can further lead to depression, anxiety, catastrophizing, and chronic widespread pain syndromes.

Recognizing the link between endometriosis subtypes and their accompanying pain syndromes is of vital importance in developing a plan to adequately address the complex milieu that defines pelvic pain arising from endometriosis. It is no longer acceptable to measure endometriosis cure rates solely by the absence of lesions in the pelvis at the time of surgery. True successful treatment of endometriosis should be measured by control of the disease itself as well as correction of its downstream sequelae.

Subtypes of Endometriosis

Superficial Endometriosis

Superficial endometriosis is the most common subtype of endometriosis and is most commonly found in the pelvis (Figure 8.1). It can present as dark purple-blue blebs, deep red splinter hemorrhages, gunpowder marks, and blister-like pustules. Though the varied appearance of each of these lesions is not completely understood in terms of etiology and clinical significance, the difference of appearance is likely due to the age and activity of the individual lesions [4]. Technically speaking, a lesion is considered to be superficial endometriosis when it histologically contains endometrioid glands and stroma and does not invade >5 mm into the surface on which it is attached. It is not possible to know for sure the depth of an endometriosis lesion by mere appearance, as studies have shown that up to 15% of lesions thought to be superficial invade >5 mm, making them technically deep infiltrating endometriotic lesions [5].

The etiology of superficial endometriosis is not beyond debate. Sampson's theory on endometriosis is the most widely accepted and appears to best describe superficial endometriosis. It states that reflux menstruation causes products of the menstrual cycle to spill into the peritoneal cavity. This ectopic tissue, aided by the natural counterclockwise flow of peritoneal fluid, travels and attaches to peritoneal surfaces within the abdomen and pelvis. Evidence of this reflux menstruation has been described in women with and without endometriosis, indicating reflux menstruation is a common occurrence. The reason some women develop endometriosis and others do not is believed to be related to a complex interplay of the intraperitoneal immune system, hormonal milieu, and the endometrial cells themselves.

Cystic Endometriosis

Cystic endometriosis, commonly known as endometrioma, is most commonly associated with the ovarian cortex. It occurs in 17%–44% of women who carry the diagnosis of endometriosis [6]. These cysts can range from subcentimeter intraovarian cystic structures to large cysts that completely encompass the ovary. They are typically filled with a thick brown semiviscous fluid that resembles liquid milk chocolate, hence the nickname "chocolate cysts." The cysts themselves are frequently thin walled and are easily ruptured surgically, though they rarely grossly rupture spontaneously. Quite often, endometriomas are associated with pelvic adhesive disease, scarring to the pelvic sidewall, loops of bowel, or posterior cul-de-sac. Because of their tendency to form as bilateral ovarian cystic structures (28%)[7], they commonly scar together in the midline, posterior to the uterus, forming "kissing ovaries." These adjoined ovaries are

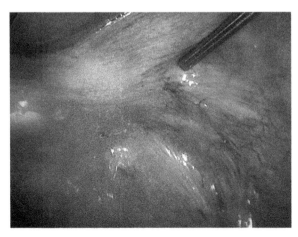

Figure 8.1 Superficial endometriosis.

frequently imbedded deep in the pelvis, scarred to the uterus, bilateral fallopian tubes, or the colon or rectum or both. Their presence can portend deep infiltrating nodules along the uterosacral ligaments, posterior cul-de-sac, or rectovaginal septum.

Endometriomas are thought to have a pathogenesis similar to that of superficial endometriosis. Consistent with Sampson's theory, Hughesdon suggested that endometrial cells are refluxed into the peritoneal cavity. These cells travel to the surface of an ovary that has just undergone ovulation. The endometrial cells implant and as the ovarian cortex heals over, thus trapping the endometriotic tissue within a superficial cystic structure on the surface of the ovary. These cells are bathed in the ovarian hormonal milieu and begin to cycle as typical endometrium. As this tissue is trapped, endometrial debris and blood products are contained within a cystic structure that continues to expand into an endometrioma [8].

Deep Infiltrating Endometriosis

Deep infiltrating endometriosis (DIE) is the most complex form of endometriosis in the way it interacts with tissues and pelvic organs. While numbers may be underreported given the difficulty of diagnosis, as many as 20% of patient with endometriosis have been reported to have DIE [9]. DIE typically presents as a thick fibrous nodule that contains smooth muscle tissues, fibroblasts, a fibrous matrix, and characteristic endometrial gland and stroma [10]. Because of the ability of endometriosis to secrete neural and epithelial growth factors, the lesions are rich in blood supply and neural tissue. The technical definition of deep infiltrating endometriosis is a lesion of endometrioid glands and stroma that invades >5 mm into its place of attachment; however, this definition is somewhat antiquated, as the histologic makeup of DIE more closely resembles adenomyosis than just a deeper invading form of superficial endometriosis lesion [11]. Interestingly, when DIE was primarily described by Karl von Rokitansky in 1860, it was termed "adenomyosis externa" because it contained endometrial tissue associated with extensive fibromuscular and loose connective tissue elements [12], resembling our current understanding of adenomyosis. This indicates that our increased understanding of endometriosis today may be leading back to the origins of its diagnosis.

The most common place to find deep infiltrating endometriosis is at the junction of the uterus and

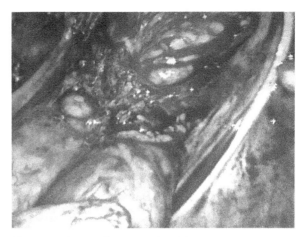
Figure 8.2 Deep infiltrating rectal nodule.

uterosacral ligament [13]. Because of its proximity to the gastrointestinal tract, this type often invades the colorectum (Figure 8.2). Other abdomino-pelvic sites of endometriosis include sites along the ureter, urinary bladder, appendix, and diaphragm. Endometriosis has also been discovered in remote locations including the lungs, heart, brain, and even the ear lobe. Theories suggest that these may be from stem cell rests that formed during embryonic development. Still other theories suggest a hematogenous or lymphatic spread of endometriosis is possible. The basic science of endometriosis is evolving at a rapid rate, and further discoveries continue to elucidate the etiology of the complex pathogenesis of this disease and its many subtypes.

Diagnosis of Endometriosis

In the setting of chronic pelvic pain, establishing a diagnosis of endometriosis may be important; however, establishing a definitive diagnosis often requires surgical intervention, which confers certain risks to the patient. Given a physician's duty to "first do no harm," it is important that one weighs the risks and benefits of performing a diagnostic procedure, especially if diagnosis will not alter management. There are certain situations in which surgical intervention will be superior to nonsurgical interventions and thus may justify an initial surgical approach. These situations will be highlighted later in the chapter. Surgery should not be the primary therapeutic approach when a patient has a high pretest probability of disease and conservative therapies are likely to be of therapeutic success. It is, however, important to recognize histology from directed biopsy is the gold standard in the diagnosis of endometriosis. Other diagnostics tests including imaging and serum blood tests have proven disappointing in the definitive diagnosis of endometriosis; however, some subtypes of endometriosis are more easily discernible with certain methods than others.

Superficial Endometriosis

Currently, neither serum blood testing nor imaging can successfully diagnose superficial endometriosis. Ultrasound, CT, and MRI do not have the fidelity to identify small, subcentimeter peritoneal lesions of superficial endometriosis. These modalities can occasionally identify coexisting intraabdominal adhesive disease that can suggest the diagnosis, but since extensive scarring seems to occur with less frequency among isolated superficial endometriosis, these noninvasive imaging techniques are nonspecific. Blood tests to date have been shown to be ineffective in the diagnosis of superficial endometriosis, though CA-125 a nonspecific marker of intraperitoneal inflammation, will often be elevated when endometriosis is present.

Apart from a surgical diagnosis, the most effective tool for diagnosis of endometriosis comes from the history and physical exam. The most common symptoms in women with endometriosis are dysmenorrhea and dyspareunia. Dysmenorrhea is typically present from the first few menstrual periods in a woman's reproductive lifecycle or sometime later in the teenage years. Differentiating pathologically painful periods from the typical period cramping can be difficult. It is important to ask patients about painful menses, as many women think the pain they experience is normal and may not report concerns without prompting. A typical differentiating factor is whether periods are painful enough to cause a patient to stay home from work or school. Additionally, young women with endometriosis may have more abnormal bleeding cycles than age-matched controls [14]. Dyspareunia is a common complaint in women with superficial endometriosis as well. This is sometimes linked to endometriosis at the junction of the uterus and the cervix, resulting in an area of tenderness that may be struck on deep insertion during intercourse. This pain is termed deep thrust dyspareunia and should be differentiated from entry dyspareunia. Alternatively, entry and deep thrust dyspareunia can develop as part of the sequelae of endometriosis-related pain, for example, in cases of vulvodynia or pelvic floor tension myalgia.

Table 8.1 Important anatomy to evaluate during diagnostic laparoscopy for endometriosis

Anterior cul de sac
Posterior cul de sac
Left ovarian fossa
Right ovarian fossa
Bilateral fallopian tubes and ovaries
Uterus
Uterosacral ligaments
Appendix
Colon and rectum
Diaphragm (both left and right sides)

From a physical exam standpoint, superficial endometriosis in isolation can be difficult to diagnose. There are no palpable lesions to confirm diagnosis; however, one can infer the presence of superficial endometriosis when retrocervical tenderness is present on bimanual exam. Similarly, DIE can also lead to this finding.

As previously mentioned, the gold standard in diagnosis of endometriosis is histological, which means a sample needs to be surgically collected. For diagnosis, it is important that endometriosis lesions be both directly visualized and biopsied, as visual identification of lesions alone can lead to a false-positive diagnosis [4]. Furthermore, it is important that a full survey of the abdomen and pelvis be completed and fully documented in the operative report. This level of detail ensures that future practitioners will have the confidence that a full evaluation of the abdomen and pelvis was completed to rule out endometriosis. The areas of the pelvis that should be separately visualized and commented on are in Table 8.1.

Endometrioma

The diagnosis of endometrioma is typically less enigmatic than superficial endometriosis because it typically presents as a cystic structure with characteristics findings on various imaging modalities. Pelvic ultrasound and MRI can both be employed to discern the etiology of an endometriotic cyst to a limited degree of efficacy. While an endometrioma has specific features on each of these modalities, it can appear similar to the hemorrhagic corpus luteal cyst, a common, nonpathological, self-limited finding. Persistence of a mass and clinical correlation to tenderness on bimanual exam are important adjunct findings to aid in the diagnosis of endometriomas. Malignancy must also be considered when a complex cystic structure is present and should be included in the differential diagnosis.

Symptomatology

Women with endometriomas tend to develop more noncyclic pelvic pain than those with superficial endometriosis alone. Frequently pain develops semiacutely and persists as the tender cyst grows and leads to increased mass effect. This pattern of slowly increasing pelvic pain not directly associated with menses may be easily confused with the development of pelvic floor tension myalgia, which also tends to lead to increased noncyclic point tenderness on contact such as is present with intercourse. Fortunately, these etiologies can be differentiated with physical exam and imaging. A pelvic exam that demonstrates a painful mass or adnexal tenderness that reproduces painful symptoms suggests the presence of endometrioma, which is not seen in hemorrhagic corpus luteal cysts. It is also important to examine the pelvic floor musculature in these cases. Isolated tenderness of the pelvic floor (especially that reproduces the patient's pain) may indicate that the pain is due solely to pelvic floor tension myalgia or dysfunction. When this test is equivocal ultrasound or MRI diagnosis can be helpful. We find that the information obtained from an exam for adnexal tenderness is most helpful when trying to decide whether to repeat imaging to establish persistence of a mass or whether to move to surgery more expeditiously.

Ultrasound and MRI

MRI sensitivity and specificity are just slightly better than ultrasound in the diagnosis of endometrioma [15]. Given the ability to further characterize cysts, MRI should be considered when transvaginal ultrasound (TVUS) is inconclusive or with concern for malignant transformation. MRI imaging with contrast enhancement should be utilized if question regarding potential neoplasm remains.

Deep Infiltrating Endometriosis

Diagnosis of DIE is more complex than the diagnosis of superficial endometriosis or endometrioma. No one methodology can definitively establish a diagnosis of DIE, though specificity can be high with certain findings on physical exam, ultrasound, and MRI. As with other subtypes of endometriosis, sensitivity of detection techniques is lacking in many cases. Colonoscopy has long been suggested to be an effective tool in the diagnosis of deep endometriosis, but studies have shown it to be of very little utility in detecting DIE of the bowel.

Because of the high cost of advanced imaging in endometriosis, the history and physical exam are very important in aiding diagnosis. A thorough history and physical examination can modify the pretest probability of finding DIE on imaging, allowing the practitioner to be judicious with testing. Patients with DIE frequently display organ-specific dysfunction. DIE that involves the bowel can cause increased pain with defecation, increasingly intense dysmenorrhea, and deep thrust dyspareunia [16] as well as constipation and rarely narrow-caliber stools. Similarly, DIE of the bladder often presents with higher rates of urinary urgency, frequency, and hematuria. Patients with DIE often complain of point tenderness at the sites of endometriotic nodules. For example, uterosacral ligament endometriosis commonly presents as deep thrust dyspareunia, specific to certain positioning during intercourse. Pain is frequently reproducible on physical exam with palpation of the nodule [17].

Physical exam findings with DIE can be quite impressive; often thick rubbery tissue is palpated on physical exam. Retrocervical nodules can be discovered along the uterosacral ligaments or along the bowel and are often described as uterosacral ligament nodularity. More rarely, an examiner may find tender nodularity in the inguinal fold or along the abdominal wall [17].

Ultrasound and MRI

Proper characterization of DIE is important, especially preoperatively. It is important to be able to properly counsel patients about steps that may need to be taken to partially or completely remove endometriotic lesions found intraoperatively. Abrao et al. demonstrated a sensitivity and specificity of 98% and 100% in TVUS for deep infiltrating endometriosis [13]. Given this accuracy, low cost, and ease of test, TVUS is the recommended initial test for those patients with suspected endometriosis, however, with the important caveat that the ultrasonographer is well versed in the identification of endometriosis.

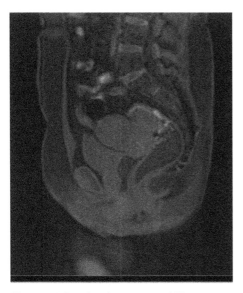

Figure 8.3 Bowel endometriosis on MRI.

Unfortunately, this level of expertise currently exists in only a few centers around the world. Additional methods, such as tender-point guided ultrasound, where attention is focused on areas previously found to be tender on physical exam, can increase diagnosis of endometriosis with TVUS [18].

MRI is also well studied as an imaging modality for the diagnosis of endometriosis (Figure 8.3). It has been shown that the sensitivity and specificity of MRI is 83% and 98% respectively for those patients with DIE[13]. MRI should be considered as a follow-up form of imaging in cases in which TVUS is equivocal. This is also true in patients who are symptomatic with negative ultrasound findings. MRI has also been found to improve diagnosis of endometriosis in areas difficult to visualize with TVUS including the rectovaginal septum.

Treatment Options for Endometriosis Subtypes

The variety of treatments of endometriosis are as broadly differing as the subtypes and presentations of the disease itself. All subtypes of endometriosis (including superficial, cystic, deep infiltrating; and more rare subtypes such as abdominal wall and catamenial endometriosis) require lesion-specific treatment planning. Importantly, the obliteration of the disease itself must not be the only treatment goal, as the guiding principle to the treatment of endometriosis should be the

obliteration of its sequelae including pain, subfertility, and organ dysfunction as they relate to overall quality of life.

Focused treatment strategies of endometriotic lesions fall into two general categories: medical treatment with the use of chemical compounds to suppress and diminish endometriosis and surgical management with the goal of destruction or resection of endometriotic lesions. Medical strategies include the induction of amenorrhea and suppression of disease through altering the hormonal milieu involved in menstrual cycle regulation. Destruction and diminution of lesions can be accomplished by halting the release and creation of hormones essential to endometriosis growth and menstrual cycle regulation. Surgical management focuses directly on destruction of lesions through fulguration and resection with a secondary goal of restoring normal anatomy by resolving and removing endometriosis-associated scar tissue.

Specific Treatments for Superficial Endometriosis

Superficial endometriosis is generally responsive to both medical and surgical management, each with distinct advantages and disadvantages. Medical management of endometriosis has the benefit of being noninvasive; however, many of the agents used may cause significant side effects, and their efficacy does not last long after cessation of use. Surgical treatment exposes the patient to increased risk; however, it may offer a longer interval of symptomatic relief. The side effects of surgery are predictable in terms of postoperative pain and recovery time; however, the recurrence of disease and coexisting pain is quite common. Focusing on treatment of downstream sequelae of endometriosis postsurgically is advantageous in slowing the recurrence of painful symptomatology. Postoperative menstrual suppressive therapy may be indicated. Furthermore, in choosing between medical and surgical management, a patient's goals must be considered with regard to restoration of organ function and the restoration (or maintenance) of fertility.

There are many medical therapeutic options used to suppress or neutralize endometriosis. Broadly, there are medications that provide gonadotropin hormone stabilization or suppression of gonadotropin production and release. In both cases the mainstay of treatment is menstrual suppression preventing cyclic inflammatory changes wrought by active endometriotic lesions. The efficacy of cycle control can be measured by the development of induced amenorrhea. Effective menstrual suppressive agents are injectable medroxyprogesterone acetate, and the levonorgestrel IUD, both of which have been studied and shown to improve outcomes in pain related to endometriosis. Further options include combined oral contraceptives, intravaginal contraceptive rings, and progestin-only treatments such as pills and implantable progestins.

Combined estrogen and progestin contraceptive methods, including the combined oral contraceptive pill and the combined vaginal ring, have been shown to reduce endometriosis-associated dysmenorrhea, dyspareunia, and noncyclic pain. As such, these formulations can be used in both a traditional (21-day active dose, with 7 days of placebo) and a continuous way. This formulation may be especially useful in women younger than 40 years of age who are not breastfeeding who desire oral therapy plus effective contraception. Theoretical concerns exist over the inclusion of estrogen in the treatment of endometriosis because estrogen is a known trophic factor for endometriosis lesions in vitro; however, in combination with progestins, studies have supported their use [19]. Their efficacy is likely due to overall control of the menstrual cycle, as opposed to the regulation of specific sex steroid hormones.

Progestin-only formulations have also shown efficacy in the treatment of endometriosis-related pain. There is research supporting the use of etonogestrel implants, levonorgestrel IUD, progestogen oral formulations, and injectable medroxyprogesterone. These formulations induce amenorrhea and may work directly to suppress the growth of endometriosis. However, no research to date supports the superiority of progestin-only therapies over combined hormonal contraceptives in the treatment of endometriosis-related pain.

Aromatase inhibitors are a unique formulation that may provide benefit in the treatment of endometriosis as well. This therapy, in conjunction with menstrual suppressive therapies, inhibits the peripheral conversion of androgens to estradiol. This suppresses menstrual cycles and thereby decreases the amount of estrogen available for growth of endometriotic implants. Menopause-like side effects of estrogen deprivation lead to intolerance of this medication in some women.

Complete suppression of the hypothalamic–pituitary–adrenal axis is also an effective method of inducing amenorrhea and suppressing the growth of endometriosis. For this reason, medications such as leuprolide acetate and gestrinone (gonadotropin-releasing hormone [GnRH] agonists and antagonists, respectively) are effective in women with superficial endometriosis. These medications are extremely effective at suppressing menstrual cycles and, therefore, suppressing dysmenorrhea. However, side effects can preclude their use in some women. Common side effects include hot flashes, mood changes, vaginal dryness, and other symptoms characteristic of estrogen deprivation. Side effects of GnRH agonists and antagonists can be partially attenuated with the use of progestin or estrogen add-back therapy. The loss of bone mineral density precludes these agents from being used as long-term therapeutic options in most women. New oral formulations of these medications have shown some recent promise and may have an increased role in the medical treatment of endometriosis.

Surgical intervention has been well established as an effective intervention for endometriosis pain related to isolated superficial endometriosis. A Cochrane review of the matter stated laparoscopic surgery was associated with decreased pain at both 6 months (odds ratio [OR] 6.58) and 12 months (OR 10.0) compared to those who underwent diagnostic laparoscopy alone [20]. Furthermore, studies have shown that fulguration and resection of endometriosis has proven superior to diagnostic laparoscopy alone in the resolution of pain. Disagreement still exists on whether resection is superior to fulguration; however, some studies [5] have indicated that resection is more effective. Others have advocated the use of plasma energy given the ability to control its depth of penetration [16], allowing full fulguration of lesions without damage to underlying structures. Despite disagreement in methodology, there seems to be strong evidence that destruction of endometriotic lesions decreases pain symptomatology, especially with regard to dysmenorrhea and dyspareunia. Furthermore, surgical intervention has the added benefit of establishing a histologic diagnosis of endometriosis.

Endometrioma

Medical treatment has not been proven as effective in treatment of cystic endometriosis as it has for isolated superficial endometriosis. The reason for this, while not well understood, is likely multifactorial. Endometriomas tend to be focally tender, so certain movements such as bending or vaginal penetration such as in sexual intercourse or pelvic exam can lead to increased noncyclic pain. Furthermore, mitotic activity has been found to be increased in endometriomas, which may limit regulation of its active glandular tissues by traditional medical therapies. Despite barriers to medical treatments, there is some evidence of decreasing endometrioma size with medical management; however, medication alone has not been shown to resolve endometriomas reliably and completely.

Surgical intervention is the mainstay in the treatment of endometrioma. Drainage, ovarian cystectomy, and oophorectomy have been shown to be effective in the relief of endometrioma with regard to dyspareunia, noncyclic pelvic pain, and dysmenorrhea. Deciding which surgical intervention to employ depends on patient desire for fertility balanced with risk of endometrioma recurrence. The recurrence of endometrioma is understandably lowest in oophorectomy. However, most women with endometrioma are of childbearing age, and maintaining the option for fertility and the overall health benefits of hormonal production is important. To this end, ovarian cystectomy has a substantially lower rate of recurrence than cyst drainage, 15%–40% versus 80%–90%. If suppressive therapy is initiated the postoperatively, the recurrence rate drops to 8% over a 2-year period [21, 22].

Despite higher recurrence rates associated with drainage, it may be preferred in relation to some fertility outcomes. Endometrioma drainage preserves ovarian cortex, making it an attractive option for women planning to undergo artificial reproductive technologies (ARTs) such as in vitro fertilization (IVF). It has been shown that ovarian cystectomy increases fertility rates compared to nonintervention; however, cystectomy may damage native ova. The risk of ovarian cystectomy in the reproductive population has been illustrated through studies that show decreased anti-Müllerian hormone (AMH) levels postcystectomy, a marker for ovarian reserve. However, with follow-up AMH levels have been shown to rebound to near pre-cystectomy levels. The optimal treatment for endometrioma is still debated. Many centers support ovarian cystectomy with careful preservation of maximum ovarian tissue, while others move to ART prior to surgical intervention.

Still endometrioma remains one of the major indications for surgical intervention in women with endometriosis because of its success with regard to pain relief and preservation of future fertility.

From the resolution of pain, the European Society of Human Reproduction and Embryology (ESHRE) recommends surgical resection of endometrioma if >3 cm in size, with ovarian cystectomy being superior to drainage. When an endometrioma is small, it may lack suitable planes with the ovarian cortex and removal may damage the ovary, altering the risk–benefit analysis of proceeding with ovarian cystectomy [22].

Hormonally mediated suppression of endometrioma recurrence has strong evidence for efficacy compared with other endometriosis subtypes. From a pathophysiologic standpoint, this is likely due to the invagination theory of endometrioma formation, which is contingent on ovulation occurring. From a practical standpoint, evidence of endometrioma suppression is more easily proven because recurrence can be seen with noninvasive imaging techniques. Conversely, detection of superficial or deep infiltrating endometriosis is difficult to detect and may require surgical evaluation.

Deep Infiltrating Endometriosis

The treatment of deep infiltrating endometriosis remains quite complex. Interventions differ significantly based on lesion location and are determined through risk–benefit analysis on an individual basis. A major point of decision is the degree to which surgical excision should be pursued, balancing outcomes between full excision, partial excision, and suppressive therapies. Risks and benefits of excisional surgery vary based on a patient's pain symptomatology, degree of organ dysfunction, and the potential of complications that may develop. A generally applicable maxim is that suppressive therapies halt progression of the size of DIE lesions but do not destroy it. Resection is the only definitive treatment for removal of these thick, fibrous, deeply invasive nodules.

When resection of DIE proves undesirable, either by patient preference or clinical risk–benefit analysis, medical interventions can be applied. Though hormonal agents inducing amenorrhea such as combined hormonal contraceptives or progestins may suppress the growth of DIE, efficacy of these medication remains difficult to establish. Medications that downregulate the hypothalamic–pituitary–adrenal axis, however, such as GnRH agonists and GnRH antagonists have been shown to decrease lesion size. This has been associated with a decrease in pain symptomatology that may recur after cessation of treatment.

As a result of incomplete resolution of deep infiltrating lesions with medical management, surgical intervention is largely considered the mainstay of therapeutic intervention. Sites most commonly affected by DIE are the uterosacral ligaments, the bowel, urinary bladder, ureters, and diaphragm. However, growth in distant sites has also been reported such as pulmonary and neurological sites. Furthermore, the iatrogenic spread of endometriosis can cause cystic and deep infiltrating lesions invading hysterotomy scars (from caesarean delivery) and abdominal wall incisions (following both laparotomy and laparoscopy). The diverse and unique characteristics of these lesions require individualized planning regarding risks and benefits of medical versus surgical intervention, involving the expertise of the physician and the desires of the patient.

Uterosacral Ligament Endometriosis

The uterosacral ligament is the most common anatomical site for the growth of DIE. Its involvement is recognized clinically as retrocervical tenderness or nodularity. Patients will often report deep thrust dyspareunia well localized to lesion location. This pain is commonly reproducible on pelvic examination and is typically exquisitely tender to palpation. Imaging studies report that they represent 83% of DIE lesions [13]. These lesions are the most common to occur in isolation and are frequently adhered to the colorectum but may concomitantly infiltrate into the bowel, complicating removal. Resection of the isolated uterosacral ligament nodule involves separating the bowel from the lesion, isolating the uterine artery and ureter, and then excising the full nodule. When lesions are bilateral, close attention should be paid to resecting only the nodular component, avoiding collateral damage to parasympathetic nerves from the inferior gluteal plexus. These nerve fibers run toward the bladder in this location, and damage to these nerves can result in temporary or permanent difficulty in emptying the bladder.

Bowel Endometriosis

Treatment of bowel endometriosis elicits contentious arguments among endometriosis experts. This is due to the high frequency with which it occurs and the high impact and frequency of complications that surround surgery on the intestinal structures. Endometriosis affecting the small intestine is relatively rare and will not be discussed in great detail.

Some experts suggest that treatment of colorectal endometriosis can be managed conservatively with medical management. Largely, treatment with GnRH analogs has proven to shrink deep infiltrating lesions of the bowel, decrease organ dysfunction, and decrease pain, but perhaps not as fully and reliably as resection of the deep lesions. Furthermore, side effects associated with long-term use of these medications limit their functionality as a long-term solution. They are frequently used to decrease nodule size in resective treatments in an attempt to limit the surgical morbidity.

Deep infiltrating colorectal endometriosis is generally treated surgically. The bulk of the argument among expert endometriosis surgeons centers on the technique for removal of these lesions. Some authors have suggested that shaving of endometriosis lesions from the surface of the bowel should be pursued when possible, only moving toward discoid resections and segmental bowel resections upon deep lesion invasion. Other authors have recommended more liberal use of segmental resection to ensure complete removal of endometriosis that may not be seen except microscopically. Still others have recommended the use of plasma technology either in conjunction with or in lieu of these methods. The decision regarding which technique of colorectal endometriosis excision to choose is based on the completeness of resection, restoration of proper bowel function, resolution of pain (mainly dyschezia, dyspareunia, and dysmenorrhea), and incidence of major complications (including bowel perforation, anastomotic leak, and development of obstruction).

Support for shaving of rectal endometriosis is demonstrated by a review of 500 cases published by Donnez et al. It was reported that the resection of a majority of DIE can significantly reduce pain symptoms, even without complete resection. Only 8% of women reported recurrence and 84% of women were able to conceive following the shaving procedure. Compared to rectal resection complications including laparoconversion, repeat surgery, sepsis, and rectovaginal fistulas were all found to be lower [11]. Given the increasing number of studies supporting improvement in quality of life with fewer complications, consideration of less aggressive shaving techniques should be considered when appropriate.

Appendiceal Endometriosis

Appendiceal endometriosis is a relatively common finding when other forms of DIE are present. The disease most frequently involves the terminal extent of the organ and its removal is very effective in reducing right lower quadrant pain. Because of the relatively high association between appendiceal involvement and stage 3 and 4 endometriosis some authors recommend removal of the appendix in these circumstances even when the appendix appears grossly normal [23].

Urinary Bladder Endometriosis

Making up 4%–20% of DIE, lesions affecting the urinary bladder are difficult to detect on imaging (Figure 8.4). Urinary bladder DIE often presents as urinary frequency, urgency, dysuria, and hematuria [24]. These symptoms can be confused with interstitial cystitis/bladder pain syndrome, recurrent urinary tract infections, or other bladder conditions, delaying diagnosis for many years. Cystoscopy can be helpful in diagnosis even when imaging techniques miss these lesions. Medical treatments have been largely ineffective in treatment of this pathology; however, surgical intervention involving full resection of the lesion has been quite successful. Complication rates are low, and long-term pain relief and improvement of urinary function are often excellent [24]. Part of the success of treatment can be attributed to the frequency at which DIE solely affects the dome of the bladder. DIE lesions that interfere with the insertion of the ureter and the urinary trigone have the potential to lead to long-term urinary frequency and urgency symptoms postsurgically.

Endometriosis near the ureter is relatively common. Surgeons commonly separate disease from this structure; however, true infiltration of the ureter is rare, in less than 1% of all DIE [25]. Pain symptomatology is often noncyclic and may result in obstructive sequelae including costovertebral angle tenderness, hydronephrosis, and even kidney failure. Like bladder and colorectal endometriosis, medical management of ureteral DIE tends to be beneficial in the short term but surgery is often required for definitive treatment. Resection of endometriosis, abutting the ureter can often resolve obstruction, but the surgeon should be prepared to fully resect a portion of the ureter when hydronephrosis is present. Ureteroscopic biopsy can be useful in diagnosis of DIE invading into the ureteral parenchyma when imaging is not definitive. Ureteral stents may be placed for treatment or presurgically to aid in surgical ureteral identification.

Diaphragmatic Endometriosis

Determining the best treatment strategy for diaphragmatic endometriosis can be challenging because it is not always obvious when a lesion is superficial or deeply infiltrating. This uncertainty results in greater risk because the distance from the abdominal peritoneum through the thin muscular diaphragm and into the pleura of the thoracic cavity is small. Incidental infiltration into this space can expose the patient to pulmonary complications including pneumothorax lung collapse and infection. As a result, many surgeons employ conservative fulguration techniques, but these interventions can be insufficient to resolve lesions. Resective treatments should be performed with a practitioner confident in managing pleurotomy. Anesthesia should be prepared to ventilate the patient

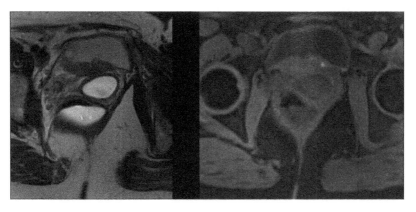

Figure 8.4 Bladder endometriosis on MRI.

using a single lung, and preemptive antibiotic dosing should be considered. If endometriosis is suspected in the pleural cavity, especially if the patient has increased pulmonary symptomatology such as menstrual pattern cough hemoptysis associated with menstruation, or suggestive imaging findings, a video-assisted thoracoscopy (VATS) should be considered.

Iatrogenic Endometriosis

Iatrogenically produced lesions of endometriosis tend to involve incisions of the uterine scar following caesarean delivery or the abdominal wall. (Though abdominal wall endometriosis is almost always from iatrogenic causes, one notable exception is endometriosis of the umbilicus that can be naturally occurring called a Villar's nodule.) The predominant treatment of these lesions is surgical, though shrinkage of the lesions may be accomplished with GnRH analogs. Excision need occur only in the symptomatic patient.

Common associated symptomatology with abdominal wall endometriosis is noncyclic abdominal pain that occurs with movement and tenderness of the abdominal wall (Figure 8.5). The pain typically worsens with menses and a nodule is often palpable in the subcutaneous tissue. Imaging commonly shows thick scarring and characteristic appearance of DIE on MRI or CT. However, lesions can also appear cystic and contain blood products. Resection of these lesions in conjunction with physical therapy can help to resolve the painful sequelae from these lesions. Surgical planning must be careful and preoperative imaging should ascertain the

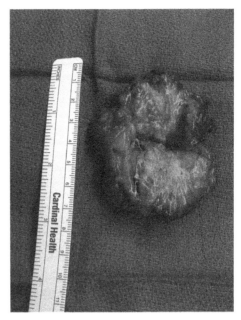

Figure 8.6 Resected Cesarean section deep infiltrating endometriosis.

extent of affected structures, so that the correct expertise is present in case of a larger fascial defect.

Cesarean scar endometriosis makes up about 0.3%–0.4% of endometriosis cases. It can have a long incubation period with mean time from surgery to symptoms ranging from 30 months to 30 years. Lesions may be cutaneous, raised, and discolored or deep in the pelvic scar and palpable with deep pressure. Drainage of dark "chocolate brown" fluid from the scar site has been reported (Figure 8.6). Diagnosis is often made on history and physical exam; however, ultrasound and MRI can be useful. Fine-needle aspiration (FNA) can be considered if there is significant concern for malignancy. Medical treatment with GnRH analogs or danazol does not provide absolute symptom relief. Gold standard treatment remains wide excision, as any cells left behind will increase the risk of recurrence [26].

Conclusion

When treating the patient suffering from endometriosis, a practitioner must have a sound understanding of the variable nature of the disease. Each subtype and affected organ system will have a unique set of symptoms that will vary with each patient. Taking into consideration the medical and surgical options, a patient-specific treatment plan should be developed, keeping in mind that the ultimate goal should be

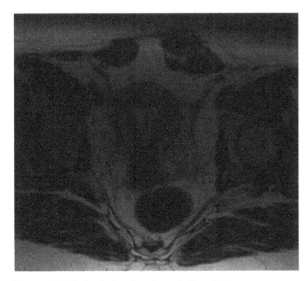

Figure 8.5 Abdominal wall endometriosis on MRI.

symptom management rather than reduction of disease burden alone.

> **Five Things You Need to Know**
> - Approximately 20% of women with endometriosis will have deep infiltrating endometriosis.
> - Gold standard histological endometriosis via biopsy confirms a diagnosis of endometriosis; however, many patients can find relief with empiric menstrual cycle suppression.
> - Colonoscopy is low utility in detecting endometriosis involving the bowel, though it has been used historically.
> - Both medical and surgical options have demonstrated efficacy for pain related to all endometriosis subtypes: superficial, cystic, and deep infiltrating lesions.
> - In the case of endometrioma, ovarian cystectomy followed by menstrual suppression substantially decreases recurrence rates.

References

1. Giudice LC, Kao LC. Endometriosis. *Lancet.* 2004;**364**(9447):1789–99.

2. Carter JE. Laparoscopic treatment for chronic pelvic pain: results from three-year follow-up. *J Am Assoc Gynecol Laparosc.* 1994;**1**(4, Part 2):S6–7.

3. Eskenazi B, Warner ML. Epidemiology of endometriosis. *Obstet Gynecol Clin North Am.* 1997;**24**(2):235–58.

4. Walter AJ, Hentz JG, Magtibay PM, Cornella JL, Magrina JF. Endometriosis: correlation between histologic and visual findings at laparoscopy. *Am J Obstet Gynecol.* 2001;**184**(7):1407–11; discussion 1411–13.

5. Healey M, Cheng C, Kaur H. To excise or ablate endometriosis? A prospective randomized double-blinded trial after 5-year follow-up. *J Minim Invasive Gynecol.* 2014;**21**(6):999–1004.

6. Jenkins S, Olive DL, Haney AF. Endometriosis: pathogenetic implications of the anatomic distribution. *Obstet Gynecol.* 1986; **67**(3):335–8.

7. Vercellini P, Aimi G, De Giorgi O, Maddalena S, Carinelli S, Crosignani PG. Is cystic ovarian endometriosis an asymmetric disease? *Br J Obstet Gynaecol.* 1998;**105**(9),1018–21.

8. Hughesdon PE. The structure of endometrial cysts of the ovary. *J Obstet Gynaecol Br Emp.* 1957;**64**(4):481–7.

9. Kavallaris A, Köhler C, Kühne-Heid R, Schneider A. Histopathological extent of rectal invasion by rectovaginal endometriosis. *Hum Reprod.* 2003;**18**(6):1323–7.

10. van Kaam KJ, Schouten JP, Nap AW, Dunselman GA, Groothuis PG. Fibromuscular differentiation in deeply infiltrating endometriosis is a reaction of resident fibroblasts to the presence of ectopic endometrium. *Hum Reprod.* 2008;**23**(12):2692–700.

11. Donnez J, Squifflet J. Complications, pregnancy and recurrence in a prospective series of 500 patients operated on by the shaving technique for deep rectovaginal endometriotic nodules. *Hum Reprod.* 2010; **25**(8):1949–58.

12. Cornillie FJ, Oosterlynck D, Lauweryns JM, Koninckx PR. Deeply infiltrating pelvic endometriosis: histology and clinical significance. *Fertil Steril.* 1990 ;**53**(6):978–83.

13. Abrao MS1, Gonçalves MO, Dias JA Jr, Podgaec S, Chamie LP, Blasbalg R. Comparison between clinical examination, transvaginal sonography and magnetic resonance imaging for the diagnosis of deep endometriosis. *Hum Reprod.* 2007;**22**(12):3092–7. Epub 2007 Oct 18.

14. Laufer MR, Goitein L, Bush M, Cramer DW, Emans SJ. Prevalence of endometriosis in adolescent women with chronic pelvic pain not responding to conventional therapy. *J Pediatr Adolesc Gynecol.* 1997;**10**:199–202.

15. Hottat N, Larrousse C, Anaf V, et al. Endometriosis: contribution of 3.0-T pelvic MR imaging in preoperative assessment-initial results. *Radiology.* 2009;**253**:126–34.

16. Nezhat C, Kho KA, Morozov V. Use of neutral argon plasma in the laparoscopic treatment of endometriosis. *JSLS.* 2009;**13**(4):479–83.

17. Carneiro MM, Filogônio ID, Costa LM, de Ávila I, Ferreira MC. Clinical prediction of deeply infiltrating endometriosis before surgery: Is it feasible? A review of the literature. *Biomed Res Int.* 2013;**2013**:564153.

18. Turocy J, Benacerraf B. Transvaginal sonography in the diagnosis of deep infiltrating endometriosis: a review. *J Clin Ultrasound.* 2017; **45**(6):313–18.

19. Baranov V, Malysheva O, Yarmolinskaya M. Pathogenomics of endometriosis development. *Int J Mol Sci.* 2018;**19**(7).

20. Duffy J, Arambage K, Correa F, et al. Laparoscopic surgery for endometriosis. *Cochrane Database Syst Rev.* 2014;(4).

21. Seracchioli R, Mabrouk M, Frascà C, Manuzzi L, Montanari G, Keramyda A, Venturoli S. Long-term cyclic and continuous oral contraceptive therapy and endometrioma recurrence: a randomized controlled trial. *Fertil Steril.* 2010;**93**(1):52–6.

22. Dunselman GA, Vermeulen N, Becker C, Calhaz-Jorge C, D'Hooghe T, De Bie B, ; European Society of Human Reproduction and Embryology. ESHRE guideline: management of women with endometriosis. *Hum Reprod.* 2014;**29**(3):400–12.

23. Moulder JK, Siedhoff MT, Melvin KL, Jarvis EG, Hobbs KA, Garrett J.I. Risk of appendiceal endometriosis among women with deep-infiltrating endometriosis. *nt J Gynaecol Obstet.* 2017;**139**(2):149–54.

24. Knabben L, Imboden S, Fellmann B, Nirgianakis K, Kuhn A, Mueller MD. Urinary tract endometriosis in patients with deep infiltrating endometriosis: prevalence, symptoms, management, and proposal for a new clinical classification. *Fertil Steril.* 2015;**103**(1):147–52.

25. Maccagnano C, Pellucchi F, Rocchini L, et al. Ureteral endometriosis: proposal for a diagnostic and therapeutic algorithm with a review of the literature. *Urol Int.* 2013;**91**:1–9.

26. Yildirim D, Tatar C, Doğan O, et al. Post cesarean scar endometriosis. *Turk J Obstet Gynecol.* 2018;**15**:33–8.

Bladder Pain Syndrome

Katherine de Souza and Charles Butrick

Editor's Introduction

Interstitial cystitis/bladder pain syndrome (IC/BPS) is one of the evil quadruplets – diseases coexisting with endometriosis. Etiology and even the way to obtain proper diagnosis is very debatable among providers. One of the mainstays of IC/BPS is pain with full bladder, and patients with this condition urinate often because they want to avoid pain and not because they have urgency. Diagnosis of IC/BPS may be done based on the symptoms but some practitioners would use potassium sensitivity test or cystoscopy with bladder hydrodistension if necessary. Treatment consists of avoiding foods that irritate the bladder and increase the pain. Oral medications such as pentosan polysulfate sodium do not seem to be as effective. Patients with IC/BPS also very often have pelvic floor muscle spasm that may be primary to the onset of bladder pain, and treatment of this spasm may be the most effective way to treat IC/BPS. Pelvic floor physical therapy and botulinum toxin A injections to pelvic floor muscles (not bladder) may be very helpful.

What Is Bladder Pain Syndrome?

Definition

First described in the 1800s, bladder pain syndrome is a chronic disorder characterized by pelvic pain and voiding symptoms. This condition is known by several epithets and corresponding acronyms including interstitial cystitis (IC), painful bladder syndrome (PBS), bladder pain syndrome (BPS), and hypersensitive bladder syndrome (HBS). For simplification in this book chapter, we will refer to this syndrome as bladder pain syndrome or BPS. In 1987, the National Institute of Arthritis, Diabetes, Digestive and Kidney Diseases proposed diagnostic criteria for clinical trials;

however, that definition is meant to be used in the research setting and does not translate well to clinical practice. In 2009, the Society for Urodynamics and Female Urology defined BPS with the following criteria:

- An unpleasant sensation (pain, pressure, discomfort) perceived to be related to the urinary bladder
- Associated with lower urinary tract symptoms of more than 6 weeks duration
- In the absence of infection or other identifiable cause [1]

Ultimately, BPS is a clinical diagnosis based on symptoms that cannot be explained by more traditional problems such as bladder infection, bladder cancer, or other pelvic/bladder pathology. This definition does present BPS as a diagnosis of exclusion in part because the etiology of the disorder is still being explored.

Pathophysiology

Much progress has been made toward better understanding of the pathophysiology of BPS in the past two decades. While there are many theories as to the etiology of BPS, it is generally thought to be a pain disorder that likely has many potential triggers that initiate the symptoms. Even with the heterogeneity of this pain disorder there are certain characteristics that tend to be present in the majority of patients who have BPS. As in all patients with chronic pain there is generally a centralized pain component that results in allodynia, and urinary frequency is the hallmark of this central sensitization. Most patients also demonstrate evidence of urothelial dysfunction as well as peripheral sensitization with biopsy evidence of increased neural density and mast cell activation.

The urothelial dysfunction results in a deficiency of the glycosaminoglycan (GAG) layer of the bladder surface. Normal bladder epithelium is impermeable to irritants and urinary solutes, so the GAG layer deficiency in patients with BPS allows irritating solutes to penetrate into the bladder tissue, which is thought to result in localized inflammatory changes and localized upregulation (inflammatory cytokines, nerve growth factors, etc.). Several studies have suggested that there is an immune component in which upregulation of mast cell activation causes activation of capsaicin-sensitive nerve fibers that leads to inflammation which in turn damages the GAG layer of the bladder epithelium. This also leads to neurogenic upregulation [2].

Central sensitization plays a role in the development of BPS, as the prolonged exposure to noxious stimuli (i.e., bladder irritants) leads to activation of N-methyl-D-aspartate (NMDA) receptions in the dorsal horn of the spinal cord. NMDA receptor activation decreases the inhibition of dorsal horn neurons, which lowers the threshold for a stimulus to be perceived as painful. The process of central sensitization is key to many chronic pain disorders that are often associated with patients who have IC/BPS. Classic examples include fibromyalgia, vulvodynia, and endometriosis (see Chapter 2). These sensory processing abnormalities are self-perpetuating as nonpainful stimuli in sensitized patients are increasingly perceived as painful (e.g., 2 ounces of urine in the bladder feels like 20 ounces) leading to further C-fiber upregulation in the periphery as well as glial cell activation centrally. Some authors feel the persistence of neurogenic inflammation results in damage of bladder muscle fibers and bladder fibrosis [2, 3] that results in the contracted small capacity bladder that is seen in patients with long-standing untreated BPS.

There is no unified theory for the inciting event that leads to the development of BPS. There are many potential triggers with "insults" that can occur in the periphery or centrally that can result in the cascade of events that ultimately results in the symptoms of BPS. Theories include bacterial infections, autoimmune disorder, and environmental factors including stress and diet, as well as association with other pain disorders such as fibromyalgia, irritable bowel syndrome, and panic disorders. There appear to be significant genetic factors that contribute to the development of BPS as well as other chronic pain disorders [4]. Regardless of the original trigger, the end result is typically the same constellation of symptoms. One exception to this is ulcerative BPS, which is likely a unique entity requiring specific therapy [5].

Ulcerative Bladder Pain Syndrome

Also known as classic interstitial cystitis, Hunner-type IC, ulcerative IC, and BPS European Society for Study of Interstitial Cystitis (ESSIC) type 3C, ulcerative BPS has emerged as a discrete condition within the disease spectrum of BPS. This condition is defined by the presence of Hunner's lesions on cystoscopy and occurs rarely in approximately 4% of cases [6]. This disease presentation tends to respond more reliably to specific therapies versus BPS in general [7]. There has been the proposal to treat BPS ESSIC type 3C as a discrete inflammatory disease process within the syndrome of BPS [5]. Patients with BPS ESSIC type 3C tend to have more severe pain and lower bladder capacity when they have a larger number of lesions. Despite increased symptom severity with increased lesions, this is not predictive of long-term response to interventions [8]. There are a number of interventions that benefit patients with Hunner's lesions such as fulguration of lesions, steroid injection into lesions, and cyclosporine A [7]. (See the section "How Is Bladder Pain Syndrome Treated?)

How Common Is Bladder Pain Syndrome?

The prevalence of BPS differs widely depending on the manner in which epidemiological studies are conducted. Billing data, self-reported diagnosis, patient questionnaires, and medical record extractions have all been used in order to quantify the number of people affected by BPS. There is a significant difference in the prevalence of the syndrome in women versus men; the ratio of female to male individuals affected by BPS is five to one. For this reason, many studies have focused on the prevalence of BPS in women [7].

One of the most referenced studies on BPS prevalence is the RAND Interstitial Cystitis Epidemiology (RICE) Study. This population-based study showed that 2.70%–6.53% of adult women in the United States meet the criteria for BPS. Approximately 87% of women had sought medical care of their symptoms, and many had been evaluated by multiple providers, with a mean number of 3.5 physicians consulted among study participants. However, fewer than 50% had been given any diagnosis associated with their bladder symptoms and only 9.7% of the women who met the criteria for BPS based on the study definition had been assigned a diagnosis of BPS. This study highlights the fact that BPS is more prevalent than many clinicians recognize [9].

What Is the Typical Course and Impact of Bladder Pain Syndrome?

Based on available data, it is typical for BPS to be diagnosed in the fourth decade of life; however, there may be confounding factors of delayed diagnosis as detailed earlier. Many patients present with culture-positive urinary tract infections, but their symptoms fail to resolve with adequate treatment of infections. Patients may present with one symptom and then eventually develop all of the typical symptoms in BPS. It is common for patients to have "flares" of their symptoms that may last hours to weeks at a time [7].

The negative impact of BPS on quality of life is significant. Patients have high rates of poor sleep, depression, social functioning difficulties, and sexual dysfunction. The rate of moderate to severe sexual dysfunction is much higher in these patients and serves as a strong predictor of poor quality of life. The psychosocial impact of BPS is worse than in women with endometriosis, overactive bladder, and vulvodynia. Effective treatment of BPS is associated with improved sleep and sexual function and in turn associated with improved quality of life.

The economic impact of BPS is difficult to ascertain because of its unknown prevalence. The direct cost of doctor visits, hospitalizations, and therapies is greater than the mean annual per-person cost of disease such as diabetes and hypertension [10]. The more abstract costs such as lost economic contribution and productivity are also significant considering that most patients are diagnosed while they are working age and the condition is chronic. The cost to individuals should be considered as well. Patients with BPS typically have two to four times higher annual medical costs than age-matched controls [10]. Those individuals also suffer the economic burden of lost wages [7].

How Is Bladder Pain Syndrome Diagnosed?

History

Obtaining a detailed patient history is the first step in diagnosing bladder pain syndrome. Patients may

initially present with only one complaint such as urinary frequency or dysuria and eventually develop additional features of BPS with urinary symptoms as well as pain. One defining feature of BPS is increased pain with increasing fluid volume in bladder. In addition to pain pattern, clinicians should evaluate for urinary frequency, urinary urgency, nocturia, and sexual dysfunction. Voiding patterns should be defined. A hallmark of BPS is frequent voiding for the purpose of pain relief. This must be differentiated from frequent voiding due to urge or avoidance of incontinence. Additionally, voiding volume is pertinent because patients with BPS have pain with bladder filling and void at lower bladder volumes (less than 120 mL) in order to relieve pain. Patients with PBS may describe "flares" of pain that may be associated with a number of stressors including diet, seasonal allergies, or sexual activity. Therefore, timing of symptoms can also be helpful in both initial diagnosis and choice of intervention [7].

Bladder diaries can be helpful in diagnosis of BPS and also serve as useful documentation when deciding whether or not an intervention for BPS is effective. Bladder diaries should include number of voids in a 24-hour period as well as details regarding urine volume, presence of pain, incidence of nocturia, presence of urgency, and episodes of incontinence. A bladder diary for one 24-hour period is adequate [11].

When reviewing past medical history, several conditions occur more frequently in patients with bladder pain syndrome than in the general population. Irritable bowel syndrome, fibromyalgia, vulvodynia, endometriosis, depression, anxiety, and systemic lupus erythematosus are all more common. Patients with BPS have a high rate of previous pelvic surgery although it is unclear whether this is a contributing factor or an intervention for an incorrect diagnosis in the past. A history of sexual abuse is more common in patients with pelvic pain compared to the general population. These conditions should be identified and treated as appropriate [7].

BPS has symptoms that overlap with those of other urologic conditions and pelvic pain syndromes, and a thorough history can distinguish it from those conditions. While patients with overactive bladder (OAB) will have symptoms of urinary frequency, patients will typically report that this symptom is associated with the fear of leakage of urine. Patients with BPS have frequency because of discomfort that is typically relieved by voiding. There is an overlap between these two disorders; it is thought that approximately 20% of patients with BPS will be found to have detrusor instability. Therefore, these mixed symptoms sometimes require therapy directed toward both etiologies. Patients with BPS will occasionally report leakage of urine yet the leakage that is reported is small in amount and often occurs without the patient experiencing severe urgency or undergoing stress maneuvers. This atypical loss of urine will often resolve with correction of the inflammatory changes within the bladder and treatment of the pelvic floor hypertonic dysfunction. BPS can present either as the patient's chief complaint and source of pelvic pain or it can be a component of a complex pain disorder that might include other pain generators such as endometriosis (patients with endometriosis are four times more likely than controls to have BPS) or vulvodynia (50% of patients with BPS have vulvodynia). Patients with low voiding frequency and high-volume voids likely have another etiology for pain [2].

Supplemental Questionnaires

Like voiding diaries, questionnaires can be very helpful in both diagnosis and assessment for effectiveness in treatments. When initially diagnosing BPS, questionnaires improve efficiency and accuracy of diagnosis. The Pelvic Pain and Urgency/ Frequency Patient Symptom Scale (PUF)[12] and O'Leary-Sant Symptom Screener (OLS)[13] both elicit information about urinary symptoms essential to diagnosis of BPS. (See Appendix.)

Examination

Pelvic examination of a patient with symptoms suggestive of BPS involves a careful assessment of each pain generator and the determination of its involvement in the patient's symptomatology. Patients with bladder pain syndrome typically will be found to have tenderness at the bladder base as well as hypertonic pelvic floor muscles that also are tender and reproduce the feeling of pressure or the need to urinate. The clinician can use this information to determine the potential source of the primary pain generator. Many patients have both a pelvic floor muscle contribution as well as bladder tenderness. Many patients will also report urethral burning yet with pain mapping the "urethral" burning is often elicited by light touch above the urethral meatus – this is a classic finding of BPS. Pain mapping is an essential component of the physical exam. Patients should be evaluated for

vaginitis, tenderness, and other potential source of pain or infection. Absence of bladder pain with palpation should decrease suspicion for BPS. Examination also identifies other factors that may be causing a patient's symptoms such as fibroids, vulvar disease, urethral diverticuli, or pelvic organ prolapse. All of these conditions may potentially lead to high-frequency, low-volume voiding. A post-void residual should be determined at the time of exam to rule out urinary retention as a cause of symptoms [7].

Diagnostic Testing

Diagnostic evaluation beyond a thorough history and physical exam is not required, with the exception of urinalysis and urine culture. However, if there are any questions regarding the diagnosis, additional testing can be helpful.

Urinalysis/Urine Culture/Urine Cytology Bladder pain and urgency are characteristic of acute cystitis and therefore urinalysis and culture are warranted in patients whose symptoms are suggestive of BPS. Patients with evidence of urinary tract infection (UTI) should be treated and reevaluated for symptoms when the infection has resolved because UTIs are relatively common among patients with BPS. Additionally, urinalysis showing microhematuria may prompt further evaluation with urine cytology, especially in patients at risk for bladder malignancies (e.g., tobacco users)[7]. When patients present with new bladder pain symptoms that started after a new sexual partner, evaluation of the vaginal canal for the presence of *Mycoplasma* or *Ureaplasma* should be considered. Some suggest all patients need to be tested, yet that is not universally accepted [14].

Cystoscopy Although cystoscopic evaluation is a requirement for the restrictive definition of BPS intended for research, it is not necessary for clinical diagnosis. Performing cystoscopy has not been found to provide additional diagnostic information beyond that elucidated via history and physical exam. Multiple authors have demonstrated both false negatives and false positives when presence of glomerulations is used to rule in or rule out BPS. While cystoscopy alone can be misleading, it is essential in identifying those patients with ulcerative disease. Cystoscopy also allows the clinician to rule out other etiologies for the persistent bladder symptoms [6].

Urodynamics Like for cystoscopy, the utility of urodynamics in BPS is ruling out other etiologies such as bladder outlet obstruction and detrusor overactivity. Therefore, if there is a question regarding the presence of these other conditions, urodynamic testing should be performed. Although patients with BPS have been found to have common findings such as early first sensation to void and decreased bladder capacity, these characteristics are not necessary for diagnosis [15]. Evaluation of urethral pressures during urodynamics will often demonstrate urethral pressures that are elevated (greater than 130 cm H_2O) in patients who have pelvic floor hypertonicity. Voiding dysfunction due to the inability to completely relax the pelvic floor muscles is common in patients with hypertonicity and BPS [16].

Bladder Anesthetic Challenge Test When the clinician suspects the bladder to be a source of pain, a relatively simple anesthetic challenge will often demonstrate for both the patient and the clinician that at least temporary relief of pain can be achieved. The placement of 20 mL of 2% lidocaine combined with 20,000 units of heparin can result in at least 2 hours of marked improvement in pain when pain is originating from the bladder. This diagnostic test has replaced the use of potassium chloride in many practices as a test of bladder hypersensitivity and pain [17].

How Is Bladder Pain Syndrome Treated?

The management of BPS should be guided by the following principles:

- The initial treatment level should be tailored to the individual patient based on severity of symptoms, patient preference, and clinician judgment.
- The clinician should target each pain generator and thus therapy will be individualized. Most patients will have both bladder and pelvic floor pain. Therapy should address both.
- If in the best interest of the patient, multiple treatments may be started simultaneously.
- Ineffective treatments should be stopped.
- Pain management should be a central consideration throughout treatment, as the ultimate goal of intervention is to minimize pain and therapy side effects while maximizing patient function.
- Treatment should be implemented from most to least conservative. Surgical intervention should be reserved for patients who are not responsive to conservative therapy with an exception for patients who are discovered to have Hunner's lesions.
- If there is no improvement of symptoms in a clinically meaningful timeframe, diagnosis should be reevaluated.

Recommendations for treatment of BPS are based on the American Urologic Association (AUA) guidelines for the diagnosis and treatment of BPS. The hierarchy of the treatment recommendations is based on potential benefit, risk–benefit profile, and severity and reversibility of adverse effects. Treatment is challenging because there is no one treatment that is reliably effective for the majority of patients. Therefore, a trial of multiple treatment approaches including multimodal therapy may be required before an effective regimen is identified for an individual patient.

First-Line Interventions

All patients should be offered these interventions when diagnosed with BPS [7].

Patient Education (Clinical Principle)

This element of treatment is important in setting patient expectations for their disease course and options for therapy. Patients should be counseled on normal bladder function and BPS including the fact that there is much still unknown about this condition. Patients should be educated about the various triggers to their symptoms and why treatment is typically multimodal. The concept of multiple pain generators and the need to treat each one is stressed so that the patient understands the reasoning behind each of the treatment modalities and gets her involved in her treatment decisions. Additionally, it is important for patients to understand that BPS is a chronic condition that may have periodic flares interspersed with asymptomatic periods.

General Relaxation/Stress Management (Clinical Principle)

It is well established that stress is associated with heightened pain sensitivity. Therefore, development of relaxation exercises and coping mechanisms can provide relief from symptoms of BPS. As this type of intervention is beyond the scope of practice for most gynecologists, a multidisciplinary approach is recommended with coordination of care with counselors.

Self-Care/Behavior Modification (Clinical Principle)

Behavior modification typically includes appropriate fluid management (48–64 ounces per day). Dietary manipulation is beneficial in approximately two thirds of patients. Patient education concerning avoidance of bladder irritants such as acidic foods, alcoholic beverages, and caffeine should be reviewed. The use of over-the-counter supplements is poorly studied but calcium glyceryl phosphate seems to benefit many patients with BPS. This appears to work by neutralizing the acid in certain foods and beverages.

Second-Line Interventions

Appropriate Manual Physical Therapy Techniques (Grade A Evidence)

More than 80% of patients with PBS have a component of hypertonic pelvic floor muscle dysfunction [7]. This hypertonicity results both in voiding dysfunction as well as myofascial pain. The constant pressure caused by the muscles results in the constant feeling of needing to urinate, which then makes the patient "hold urine" and therefore tends to perpetuate the hypertonicity and pain. This hypertonic dysfunction is easily identified on pelvic examination as well as during the performance of urodynamics. If pelvic floor hypertonicity and pain are thought to be components then referral to physical therapy for further evaluation and management of this symptomatology is required. It is important to note that strengthening (e.g., through Kegel exercises) is not the goal of pelvic floor physical therapy. These patients need to learn to relax their pelvic floor muscles and the exercise techniques are sometimes referred to as "reverse Kegels." Multiple studies have shown the benefit in symptom resolution through the use of manual therapy, sometimes referred to as myofascial release. Identification of a qualified pelvic floor physical therapist is important, as these providers are not available in every community. The availability of this type of physical therapy in your community can be determined by a visiting www.womenshealthapta.org or www.pelvicpain.org.

Oral Medications

Amitriptyline (Grade B Evidence) Amitriptyline is a tricyclic antidepressant that has been shown to improve symptoms of BPS in more than 60% of patients in multiple studies [7]. Medication side effects such as sedation and nausea have been observed in up to 79% of patients. These adverse effects were a major reason for discontinuation of the medication, so starting patients at a low dose such as 10 mg daily and up-titrating to 75–100 mg daily over time is recommended.

Cimetidine (Grade B Evidence) Cimetidine is a histamine H2 antagonist. Several studies including a randomized controlled trial (RCT) have shown that this medication can improve BPS symptoms, although no long-term follow-up data are available [7]. However, there were no adverse effects reported in trials investigating cimetidine as a potential treatment for BPS, so it has the potential to be a low-riskintervention. Dosing of this medication varies in studies from 200 mg three times daily to 300–400 mg twice daily.

Hydroxyzine (Grade C Evidence) Hydroxyzine is a histamine H1 antagonist that has been shown to improve symptoms in some patients [7]. However, the only study that demonstrated statistically significant symptom relief included only patients with systemic allergies. The existence of systemic allergies may be considered when selecting patients for this medication. A large number of patients reported side effects including short-term drowsiness and weakness. These adverse effects were considered serious by patients and were similar to side effects described by patients receiving placebo medications. In studies, patients were started on a lower dose and titrated up with regimens such as 10 mg daily increased to 50 mg over weeks and 25 mg daily increased to 75 mg daily over weeks.

Pentosanpolysulfate (PPS; Grade B Evidence) PPS is a urinary analgesic that has been widely studied for the treatment of BPS including multiple RCTs [7]. Results of these studies are conflicting, but aggregations of data from all RCTs evaluating efficacy of PPS does show that the medication significantly improves symptoms of BPS. Of note, there is some evidence to support that PPS is less useful in patients with ulcerative BPS. Dosing of this medication is 100 mg three times daily.

Intravesical

Dimethyl Sulfoxide (DMSO; Grade C Evidence) DMSO is a urinary tract analgesic that has resulted in improvement in BPS symptoms in multiple studies

[7]. The medication is instilled in the patient's bladder and retained for 15–20 minutes. Longer intravesical retention of the medication is not recommended because it is associated with severe pain due to the medication's rapid absorption into bladder tissue. There are several regimens for these bladder instillations, although the principle is for treatments every 2 weeks for 4–8 weeks with assessment for response to therapy. Additional instillations can be performed as needed with the idea that there will be progressively longer intervals of pain relief. There are no known significant adverse effects for this treatment.

Heparin (Grade C Evidence) Heparin is an anticoagulant that has been shown to improve symptoms of BPS both when used alone and when combined with other agents. There are several regimens that have been shown to improve symptoms including 10,000 IU heparin in 10 mL of sterile water three times a week for 3 months with retention of 1 hour and 25,000 IU in 5 mL of distilled water twice a week for 3 months. There are no known serious adverse effects; however, the risk–benefit profile of this intervention has not been fully evaluated, as there are no placebo-controlled trials available.

Lidocaine (Evidence Grade B) Lidocaine is a topical anesthetic that has been most extensively investigated in combination with other agents for relief of BPS symptoms. Lidocaine can be administered with or without alkalinization. In theory, alkalinization should improve efficacy of treatment because it improves the penetration of lidocaine into the urothelium; however, this is controversial. One of the advantages to anesthetic-based intravesical therapy is the use of this approach not only as a "rescue" intervention but also as one that can be used by the patient for maintenance therapy in more severe cases or when a patient cannot easily reach the clinician involved in the management of her BPS.

Most clinicians use intravesical therapy that involves a combination of ingredients that potentially provide more benefit than intravesical installations that involve only one ingredient [18]. The efficacy of combination intravesical therapy (often referred to as "bladder cocktails") has been reported by many authors. (See Appendix: Rescue / therapeutic cocktails for bladder pain syndrome flare.)

Pain Management

As evidenced by the recommendations for treatment in this section, there is a large range of both pharmacological and surgical interventions for BPS [7]. Because of the severe impact of pain on patients' quality of life, improvement in pain is a central aim when treating this disorder. While providers should use treatment algorithms and work with patients to find appropriate therapy, additional pain control with systemic analgesics may be considered in order to improve functionality. Again, a multidisciplinary approach may be advantageous. Referral to anesthesia or pain specialists for management of analgesics such as narcotic pain medication can be very helpful for providers who do not have experience with these medications in chronic pain patients. Regardless of whether the primary provider for PBS decides to provide systemic analgesics or refer to another provider, pain management should adhere to the following principles:

- Oral analgesics should be used in conjunction with other medications that address BPS with the aim of minimizing the reliance on narcotics for pain control. In addition to medication, psychological therapy should be integrated to reduce the requirement for narcotic pain medications.
- Narcotics and other medications with high potential abuse should only be prescribed by one provider/clinic. Pain management agreements between patients and providers should set guidelines for use of these medications and how they are prescribed including responsibilities that patients must fulfill in order to continue medications.
- If narcotics are being used, long-acting agents are preferred over short-acting narcotics except for breakthrough pain.

Medications should be trialed in a systematic manner with addition and titration of one medication at a time so that efficacy of individual treatments for patients can be correctly identified. Medications should be initiated at the lowest possible dose and increased in a stepwise manner as is appropriate based on symptoms, pain scores and patient tolerance of medication adverse effects. This requires clinicians to be in close contact with patients.

Although pain relief is an important component of BPS management, it is important for underlying bladder dysfunction to be addressed concurrently in order to improve function and decrease the need for pain medication. Patients should be counseled that adequate pain relief is the goal of pain management as complete pain relief is not always possible.

Third-Line Interventions

Cystoscopy with Hydrodistention (Evidence Grade C)

If more conservative therapies have failed, cystoscopy with hydrodistention under anesthesia can be considered if one has not been done in the recent past [7]. This procedure allows for visual inspection of the bladder epithelium for any abnormalities including Hunner's lesions and to rule out the possibility of other pathology that might explain the persistent symptoms. Management of Hunner's lesions is discussed in the text that follows. The bladder capacity determined at the time of cystoscopy with hydrodistention is also thought to be a prognostic indication of patients who are at risk for poor response to traditional therapies. Volume under anesthesia of less than 300 mL is a sign of severe disease.

Hydrodistension can be a helpful diagnostic tool as well as a therapeutic intervention. Its use solely as a diagnostic tool for cannot be recommended [7]. Ideal hydrodistension has yet to be determined but most authors advocate low-pressure, from 60 to 80 cm H_2O with a duration of less than 10 minutes, although longer duration low-pressure hydrodistension has been used by some providers. The duration of symptom relief is variable across multiple studies. The major adverse effects experienced by patients in these studies were temporary flare of symptoms and rare episodes of bladder rupture. Providers and patients must determine if the benefit of hydrodistension is worth the risk of a short-term increase in symptoms.

Treatment of Hunner's Lesions (Grade C Evidence)

If identified, Hunner's lesions can managed at the time of cystoscopy via either fulgration or steroid injection [7]. Fulguration can be achieved via laser or electrocautery and this intervention has shown significant improvement in pain, including complete resolution of pain, in more than 75% of patients. Patients also experienced relief from urinary frequency. The duration of effectiveness for fulguration of Hunner's lesions is not clearly defined. Adverse effects from this intervention are rare but do include the rare risk of bladder perforation and need for subsequent repair. Similarly, studies on laser fulguration of lesions have shown high response rates, with 80%–100% of patients experiencing improvement in both pain and bladder function. The treatment effect lasted for up to 23 months in these studies. One serious adverse effect unique to laser fulguration is possible delayed bowel perforation due to scatter of laser to the bowel. Regardless of method of fulguration, patients should be counseled that they may require repeat treatment, approximately 46% in laser studies.

Treatment of Hunner's lesions with intralesional steroid injections is advocated by some clinicians. Submucosal injection of triamcinolone using either 10 mg/mL concentration or 40 mg/mL concentration with a maximum total injection of 60 mg triamcinolone is recommended. Larger doses of triamcinolone have been studied but are not recommended because of a lack of high-quality safety information. This intervention has yielded symptom relief from 7 to 12 months in studies.

Fourth-Line Interventions

Neuromodulation (Grade C Evidence)

Use of permanent sacral or pudendal neurostimulation devices is not FDA-approved for BPS; however, sacral neurostimulator devices are approved for management of urinary frequency [7]. Regarding sacral versus pudendal nerve stimulation, a single randomized crossover trial did show patient preference toward pudendal nerve stimulation. Overall, there is a relatively high response rate to implants, from 66% to 94%. Patients with BPS appeared to have a higher incidence of implant site pain requiring revision of pulse generator site or even removal. In recent studies, removal of devices occurred in up to 28% of patients due to low efficacy of treatment or intolerable side effects. There are multiple cohort studies in the literature, while not typically randomized and often with follow-up of 1 year, showing symptom improvement including urinary frequency, pelvic pain, and voiding dysfunction [19].

Fifth-Line Interventions

Intradetrusor Botulinum Toxin A (Grade C Evidence)

Botulinum toxin A (BTX-A) can be used either alone or in conjunction with hydrodistension [7]. There is not strong evidence to support recommendation for or against contaminant treatment with bladder hydro-distension. Studies have shown up to 86% efficacy for BTX-A; however, almost all patient experienced return to baseline pain and function after a certain time interval, commonly 3 months. There is a range of intervals between repeat treatments as well as a range of locations for injection including the trigone alone, the bladder walls alone, and a combination of both. No definitive recommendation for site of bladder injection of BTX-A exists. The recommended dose is 100 U BTX-A, as there are significant potential adverse effects that increase with higher doses. Adverse effects include dysuria as well as urinary retention. Retention can range from mild, requiring abdominal straining in order to void, to severe with the need intermittent self-catheterization. These effects generally resolved in 1 to 3 months, but in some cases, they persisted. Patients should be thoroughly counseled and accept the risk of severe urinary retention requiring self-catherization prior to use of BTX-A. Additionally, patients with known urinary retention may not be good candidates for this therapy given the adverse effect profile.

Cyclosporin A (Grade C Evidence)

Cyclosporine A (CyA) is an immunosuppressive agent that has been shown to be particularly effective for patients with ulcerative BPS [7]. The recommended dose is 2–3 mg/kg/day in two divided doses with a maximum dose of 300 mg daily. If symptom control is established yet side effects such as an increase in blood pressure or creatinine occur, some patients will require a reduction in dose. A dose reduction to as little as 1 mg/kg/day should be considered. Clinicians should carefully follow the concerning side effects, which include hypertension and deterioration of renal function. In a trial comparing CyA to pentosanpolysulfate, 75% of patients experienced improvement of symptoms in 6 months with CyA. Other studies have shown that this medication is effective in as little as 6 weeks, with 87% of patients reporting markedly improved urinary function and resolution of pain. While adverse effects are quite common, present in 94% of patients in one study, most are minor. Serious adverse effects include hypertension, renal impairment, and cutaneous lymphoma. Therefore, the use of this medication should be done with carefully performed informed consent as well as a program of close follow-up especially as it relates to blood pressure and renal function changes.

Sixth-Line Interventions

Major Surgery (Evidence Grade C)

Surgical management of BPS should be reserved for patients with severe disease that has been unresponsive to other treatments [7]. Surgical interventions are irreversible and lead to significant changes in lifestyle that patients may not wish to undertake considering that they may not experience symptoms relief following surgery even if the bladder is completely removed. The likelihood of favorable outcomes can be increased by carefully selecting the patients to whom these procedures are offered. Patients who have small bladder capacity under anesthesia and failed to improve with more conservative measures are most likely to benefit from surgery. Additionally, patients with little or no neuropathic pain are more likely to experience symptom relief from surgery.

Diversion with or without Cystectomy This procedure involves diversion of urine to an alternative to the bladder such as an ileal conduit. Because of the possibility of persistent pain following removal of the bladder, cystectomy may or not be performed at the time of diversion. Creation of a diversion has the potential to effectively improve urinary frequency, so patients for whom this is a major complaint may be good candidates if they have failed conservative measures.

Substitution Cystoplasty : This procedure involves excising a portion of the bladder thought to be contributing to BPS. In some cases, the trigone is excised while in other cases it is preserved. The benefit of trigone excision is that the area is thought to be a source of pain and is a common location for Hunner's lesions; however, trigone excision increases the risk of urinary retention, requiring chronic self-catheterization. Patients with Hunner's lesions and small bladder capacity under anesthesia are more likely to benefit from substitution cystoplasty. Patients who identify the urethra as their main site of discomfort are less likely to benefit.

Treatments That Should Not Be Offered

Although there is no reliable intervention that will improve the BPS for every patient, several therapies have shown no benefit and should not be offered to patients because the risk of the intervention outweighs potential benefits.

- **Long-Term Antibiotics (Grade B Evidence)** Antibiotics should be reserved for patients with positive urine cultures. There has not been any benefit to antibiotic therapy for bladder pain of noninfectious etiology. Given the serious potential adverse outcome of antibiotic resistance, this therapy should not be offered [7].
- **Intravesical Bacillus Calmette-Guérin (BCG; Grade B Evidence)** There have been several studies that demonstrated no significant difference between BCG instillation and placebo. Because there is no evidence of benefit and there have been serious adverse effects such as sepsis and death associated with BCG, this therapy should not be offered [7].
- **High-Pressure Long-Duration Hydrodistension (Grade C Evidence)** There has been no reliable benefit to performing hydrodistension at pressures greater than 80 to 100 mm H_2 O. Similarly, longer durations of hours or repeated 30-minute intervals have shown no reliable benefit. However, these interventions place patients at greater risk for complications such as sepsis and bladder rupture. Therefore, this technique of hydrodistension is recommended against [7].
- **Long-Term Systemic Glucocorticoid Administration (Grade C Evidence)** Although studies have shown that this intervention can provide symptoms relief, long-term steroid use is associated with diabetes, hypertension, and immunocompromise. For this reason, this treatment is not recommended [7].

Experimental/Future

Many current studies are focusing on whether it is beneficial to "phenotype" individuals with BPS in order to more effectively guide treatment regimens. There are several investigatory treatments that are targeting immune modulation that contribute to bladder inflammation. Nerve growth factor (NGF) is more common in animal models, and anti-NGF with monoclonal antibodies is one of the treatments currently under investigation. Although studies in humans have not shown significant improvement, larger population studies may reveal this to be an effective treatment. Likewise, antitumor necrosis factor-α (TNF-α) is under investigation using adalimumab to block the cytokine's proinflammatory effect. Treatment revealed significant improvement in symptoms although there was significant placebo effect as well. Activation of SH2-containing inositol-5'-phosphatase 1, P2X3 receptor antagonists, and α1 adrenoceptor antagonists is also under investigation and has shown success in improving symptoms of BPS. These potential treatments may have a systemic effect addressing neurogenic inflammation. There are also trials of bladder treatments such as intravesical liposomes and toll-like receptor antagonists. These two areas of study would affect only the symptoms of BPS that arise from the bladder itself and not address symptoms due to central sensitization [5].

Summary

Bladder pain syndrome affects approximately 5% of all women. As our understanding of this pain disorder advances we now realize that patients can present with many clinical phenotypes. Some will present with isolated bladder symptoms but some will present with a history of various types of chronic pain disorders with multiple pain generators. Given our understanding of centralized pain, the management of this visceral pain syndrome requires that the clinician identify each pain generator, and using a multimodal approach, attempt to downregulate each component of the pain using the therapeutic options that we have discussed. Most patients will benefit from this approach, especially if identification of BPS and initiation of therapy are undertaken in a timely fashion. As with any pain disorder, the longer the delay in the diagnosis and initiation of therapy the more difficult it will be to manage.

Five Things You Need to Know

- Hallmarks of bladder pain syndrome (BPS) are bladder pain and urgency in the setting of frequent small-volume voids for the purpose of pain relief.
- This condition causes severely diminished quality of life but is frequently underdiagnosed by clinicians despite simple clinical criteria for diagnosis.
- Although all patients should be offered education, stress management, and behavioral modification as first-line treatment, no single reliable pharmaceutical or surgical intervention will work for all patients. Treatments should be individualized based on assessment of active pain generators. Most patients with BPS have both bladder and pelvic floor myofascial components to their pain.

- The goal of therapy is to identify triggers to their pain disorder and to treat each pain generator. Most patients will have marked improvement in symptomatology but intermittent flares are common even after appropriate therapy.
- While ulcerative IC is relatively rare, approximately 4%, it represents a unique form and typically is associated with persistent symptoms despite appropriate therapy. Cystoscopy is required to identify and treat active Hunner's lesions.

References

1. Hanno P, Dmochowski R. Status of International Consensus on Interstitial Cystitis/Bladder Pain Syndrome/Painful Bladder Syndrome: 2008 snapshot. *Neurourol Urodyn.* 2009;**28**(5):274–86. DOI: 10.1002/nau

2. Bharucha AE, Lee TH. Anorectal and pelvic pain. *Mayo Clin Proc.* 2016;**91**(10):1471–85. DOI: 10.1037/a0038432.Latino

3. Butrick CW. Interstitial cystitis/bladder pain syndrome. Management of the pain disorder: a urogynecology perspective. *Urol Clin North Am.* 2012;**39**(3):377–87. DOI: 10.1016/j.ucl.2012.06.007

4. Jhang J, Kuo H. Pathomechanism of interstitial cystitis/bladder pain syndrome and mapping the heterogeneity of disease. *Int Neurourol J.* 2016;**20**(Suppl 2):S95–S104.

5. Andersson KE, Birder L. Current pharmacologic approaches in painful bladder research: an update. *Int Neurourol J.* 2017;**21**(4):235–42. DOI: 10.5213/inj.1735022.511

6. Ottem DP, Teichman JMH. What is the value of cystoscopy with hydrodistension for interstitial cystitis? *Urology.* 2005;**66**(3):494–9. DOI: 10.1016/j.urology.2005.04.011

7. Hanno PM, Burks DA, Clemens JQ, et al. American Urological Association (AUA) guideline: diagnosis and treatment of interstitial cystitis/bladder pain syndrome. *J Urol.* 2011;**185**(6):2162–70.

8. Akiyama Y, Niimi A, Nomiya A, et al. Extent of Hunner lesions: the relationships with symptom severity and clinical parameters in Hunner type interstitial cystitis patients. *Neurourol Urodyn.* 2018;(August):1–7. DOI: 10.1002/nau.23467

9. Berry SH, Elliott MN, Suttorp M, et al. Prevalence of symptoms of bladder pain syndrome/interstitial cystitis among adult females in the United States. *J Urol.* 2011;**186**(2):540–4. DOI: 10.1016/j.juro.2011.03.132

10. Clemens JQ, Meenan RT, Keeffe MCO, Kimes T, Calhoun EA. Costs of interstitial cystitis in a managed care population. *Urology.* 2008;**71**(5):776–81. DOI: 10.1016/j.urology.2007.11.154.COSTS

11. Mazurick CA, Landis JR. Evaluation of repeat daily voiding measures in the national interstitial cystitis data base study. *J Urol.* 2000;**163**(4):1208–11. DOI: 10.1016/S0022-5347(05)67725-7

12. Powell CR, Kreder KJ. Long-term outcomes of urgency-frequency syndrome due to painful bladder syndrome treated with sacral neuromodulation and analysis of failures. *J Urol.* 2010;**183**(1):173–6. DOI: 10.1016/j.juro.2009.08.142

13. O'Leary MP, Sant GR, Fowler FJ, Whitmore KE, Spolarich-Kroll J. The interstitial cystitis symptom index and problem index. *Urology.* 1997;**49**(5 Suppl.):58–63. DOI: 10.1016/S0090-4295(99)80333-1

14. Combaz-Söhnchen N, Kuhn A. A systematic review of Mycoplasma and Ureaplasma in urogynaecology. *Geburtshilfe Frauenheilkd.* 2017;**77**(12):1299–1303.

15. Kuo Y-C, Kuo H-C. The urodynamic characteristics and prognostic factors of patients with interstitial cystitis/bladder pain syndrome. *Int J Clin Pract.* 2013;**67**(9):863–9. DOI: 10.1111/ijcp.12116

16. Butrick C, Sanford D, Hou Q, Mahnken J. Chronic pelvic pain syndromes: clinical, urodynamic, and urothelial observations. *Int Urogynecol J Pelvic Floor Dysfunct.* 2009;**20**(9):1047–53.

17. Evans RJ, Sant GR. Current diagnosis of interstitial cystitis: an evolving paradigm. *Urology.* 2007;**69**(Suppl. 4A):64–72. DOI: 10.1016/j.urology.2006.05.048

18. Cvach K, Rosamilia A. Review of intravesical therapies for bladder pain syndrome/interstitial cystitis. *Transl Androl Urol.* 2015;**4**(6):629–37. DOI: 10.3978/j.issn.2223-4683.2015.10.07

19. Laviana A, Jellison F, Kim JH. Sacral neuromodulation for refractory overactive bladder, interstitial cystitis, and painful bladder syndrome. *Neurosurg Clin North Am.* 2014;**25**(1):33–46. DOI: 10.1016/j.nec.2013.08.001

Appendix

To help your physician determine if you have interstitial cystitis, please put a check mark to the most appropriate response to each of the questions below. then add up the numbers to the left of the check marks and write the total below.

Symptom index

During the past month:

Q1. How often have you felt the strong need to urinate with little or no warning?

0. ❑ Not at all.
1. ❑ Less than 1 time in 5.
2. ❑ Less than half the time.
3. ❑ About half the time.
4. ❑ More than half the time.
5. ❑ Almost always.

Q2. Have you had to urinate less than two hours after you finished urinating?

0. ❑ Not at all.
1. ❑ Less than 1 time in 5.
2. ❑ Less than half the time.
3. ❑ About half the time.
4. ❑ More than half the time.
5. ❑ Almost always.

Q3. How often did you most typically get up at night to urinate?

0. ❑ None.
1. ❑ Once.
2. ❑ Two times.
3. ❑ Three times.
4. ❑ Four times.
5. ❑ Five or more times.

Q4. Have you experienced pain or burning in your bladder?

0. ❑ Not at all.
1. ❑ A few times.
2. ❑ Almost always.
3. ❑ Fairly often.
4. ❑ Usually.

Add the numeric values of the checked entries: total score: _____

Problem index

During the past month, how much has each following been a problem for you?

Q1. Frequent urination during the day?

0. ❑ No problem.
1. ❑ Very small problem.
2. ❑ Small problem.
3. ❑ Medium problem.
4. ❑ Big problem.

Q2. Getting up at night to urinate?

0. ❑ No problem.
1. ❑ Very small problem.
2. ❑ Small problem.
3. ❑ Medium problem.
4. ❑ Big problem.

Q3. Need to urinate with little warning?

0. ❑ No problem.
1. ❑ Very small problem.
2. ❑ Small problem.
3. ❑ Medium problem.
4. ❑ Big problem.

Q4. Burning, pain, discomfort, or pressure in your bladder?

0. ❑ No problem.
1. ❑ Very small problem.
2. ❑ Small problem.
3. ❑ Medium problem.
4. ❑ Big problem.

Add the numeric values of the checked entries: total score: _____

Figure 9.1 O'Leary-Sant symptom screener.

Katherine de Souza and Charles Butrick

PELVIC PAIN and URGENCY/FREQUENCY
PATIENT SYMPTOM SCALE

Patient's Name: ———————————— Today's Date: ——————

Please circle the answer that best describes how you feel for each question,

		0	1	2	3	4	SYMPTOM SCORE	BOTHER SCORE
1	How many times do you void during the waking hours?	3-6	7-10	11-14	15-19	20+		
2	a. How many times do you void at night?	0	15-19 / 1	2	3	4+		
	b. How many times do you void so what extent does it usually bother you?	None	Mild	Moderate	Severe			
3	Are you currently sexually active. YES ____ NO ____							
4	a. IF YOU ARE SEXUALLY ACTIVE, do you now or have you ever had pain or symptoms during or after sexual intercourse?	Never	Occasionally	Usually	Always			
	b. Has pain or urgency ever made you avoid sexual intercourse?	Never	Occasionally	Usually	Always			
5	Do you have pain associated with your bladder or in your pelvis (vagina, lower abdomen, urethra, perineum)?	Never	Occasionally	Usually	Always			
6	Do you still urgency shortly after urinating?	Never	Occasionally	Usually	Always			
7	a. If you have pain, is it usually		Mild	Moderate	Severe			
	b. How often does your pain bother you?	Never	Occasionally	Usually	Always			
8	a. If you have urgency, is it usually		Mild	Moderate	Severe			
	b. How often does your urgency bother you?	Never	Occasionally	Usually	Always			

SYMPTOM SCORE (1, 2a, 4a, 5, 6, 7a, 8a)		
BOTHER SCORE (2b, 4b, 7b, 8b)		
TOTAL SCORE (Symptom Score + Bother Score) =		

Figure 9.2 Pelvic pain and urgency/frequency patient symptom scale.

Therapeutic Cocktail for Bladder Pain Syndrome Flare

Supplies:

- Lidocaine 2% – 20mL
- 1mL Triamcinolone 40mg/1mL
- 1mL Heparin Sodium 20,000 units/mL
- 30mL syringe

- 3mL syringe
- 18 gauge needle
- #8 French Pediatric feeding tube
- 10mL Lidocaine Hydrochloride Jelly USP, 2%
- Catheter Tray

Procedure:

- Draw up 20mL of Lidocaine in 30 mL syringe
- Draw up 120mL of Triamcinolone in 3 mL syringe followed by 1mL of Heparin
- Inject into 30mL syringe
- Explain procedure to patient
- Have patient void before procedure

    If _symptoms_ of bladder infection present, dipstick urine to rule out infection

    If positive do not proceed, if negative proceed

    While patient is in Lithotomy position, open catheter tray and supplies

    Cleanse labia and urethra for catheterization

    Insert small amount of Lidocaine Jelly to use as lubricant, can use regular lubricant

    Insert Pediatric catheter – check for post void residual

- Then inject Appell Cocktail slowly
- Pull catheter out
- Instruct to try not to void for 2 hours

May reschedule weekly or up to three times week if needed. Average is 6 weeks of treatment and then as needed

Figure 9.3 Rescue/therapeutic cocktails for bladder pain syndrome flare. When patients have a flare in their bladder symptoms the clinician should always consider the possibility that they have a bladder infection. Also in the differential is a flare of myofascial pain that often accompanies BPS. After evaluation, if a component of a flare is thought to be due to bladder pain, a rescue cocktail should be administered. The patient's response to this will also clarify for the patient and the clinician if the bladder is a significant pain generator at this time. This can also be used during the initial evaluation of the patient's symptoms of pelvic pain, to determine if the bladder is involved.

Chapter 10

Pelvic Pain Arising from Pelvic Congestion Syndrome

Nita Desai and Mark Dassel

Editor's Introduction

Pelvic congestion syndrome is another condition causing pelvic pain for which there is no consensus on diagnosis or treatment; moreover, some physicians don't even believe it causes pelvic pain. Pain from pelvic congestion is multifactorial and may be caused by hypoxia and mechanical stretching of pelvic veins. It usually occurs after pregnancy (may be full term, ectopic, or miscarriage) and presents as a sensation of heaviness in the lower abdomen with upright body position. On the background of this sensation there is intermittent sharp lower pelvic pain. In our practice we diagnose pelvic pain based on symptoms but confirm it with transfundal venography preformed in the operating room immediately prior to surgery. We treat pelvic congestion syndrome either by referring the patient to interventional radiology for embolization of the pelvic veins or by surgical selective pelvic vein ligation. In this procedure we separate ovarian veins from arteries and ligate them and any significantly enlarged veins in the broad ligament. Outcomes from this treatment are effective; however, pain and congestion may return with time, especially if the patient becomes pregnant again.

Introduction

Pelvic congestion syndrome (PCS), also known as pelvic venous insufficiency, is a chronic condition causing pelvic pain. PCS occurs when varicose veins develop around the ovaries in the setting of chronic pelvic pain (CPP). Similar to varicose veins in the legs, pelvic varicosities are thought to result from a combination of dysfunctional venous valves, retrograde blood flow, and venous engorgement [1].

Prevalence

PCS, or pelvic venous insufficiency, initially described around the 1850s, and correlated with pelvic pain in the 1940s–50s, is now a well-characterized etiology of PCS [2]. PCS typically affects women of reproductive age. Worldwide, rates of CPP, for women of childbearing age, range from 14% to 43% [2, 3]. CPP rates in the United States are approximately 15% for women of childbearing age [4]. Congested pelvic veins can be quite painful and can account for a range of 10%–40% of cases of CPP [1,2,5]. No cases have been reported in postmenopausal women [5].

Anatomical Considerations

The complex arena of venous circulation of the female pelvis must be considered when evaluating patients for PCS, as these plexuses are uniquely interconnected: the left renal and ovarian veins, the iliac veins (common, external, and internal), and the lower extremity veins. In addition to communications between these systems, there is also frequent crossover, from side to side. In the female pelvis, the ovarian veins drain blood flow from the parametrium, cervix, mesosalpinx, and pampiniform plexuses, which may also drain through the internal iliac as a collateral pathway [6]. These plexuses form the ovarian vein, which may have two to three trunks before becoming a single trunk at the level of L4–L6. The ovarian vein has a mean diameter of approximately 3 mm, which increases with pregnancy, and usually has two or three valves, which are incompetent in about 50% of women [6]. Although variations may occur, the right ovarian vein usually drains directly into the inferior vena cava (IVC), whereas the left drains into the left renal vein. The ovarian veins collateralize extensively with the ascending lumbar and peritoneal veins [5]. The internal iliac veins receive inflow from the utero-ovarian, vesicular, hemorrhoidal, and sacral venous plexuses [5]. The two systems, the ovarian, and internal iliac veins, run together in the broad ligament with extensive communication [5].

Pathophysiology

Insufficiency of the pelvic veins arises when there is abnormal dilation or distention of the venous territories between the iliac and ovarian veins. While the precise etiology of PCS remains uncertain, it is likely multifactorial. Valvular insufficiency, venous obstruction, and hormones all may play a role in the development of congestion of the pelvic veins [5]. The cause of pain due to the pelvic congestion remains unclear, but the most likely possibility is that increased dilatation, concomitant with stasis, leads to the release of local pain-producing substances [5]. Insufficiency can be delineated further into primary/intrinsic causes and secondary/extrinsic causes.

Primary venous insufficiency occurs due to either the absence of venous valves or the incompetence of such valves. Congenital absence of ovarian vein valves has been shown in 13%–15% of patients on the left side and in 6% on the right side [5]. Venous valves are incompetent in 41%–43% of women on the left side, and in 35%–46% on the right side [5]. There is higher prevalence of PCS in multiparous women, which may be related to the 50% increase in pelvic vein capacity during pregnancy [5]. This phenomenon can result in valvular incompetence as well as retrograde blood flow. These changes may persist for up to 6 months following pregnancy [5].

Secondary pelvic vein incompetence is related to venous outflow obstruction by extrinsic compression. Possible causes are nutcracker syndrome, wherein the left renal vein is compressed due to entrapment between the abdominal aorta and the superior mesenteric artery, or May–Thurner syndrome, in which the left common iliac vein is compressed by the right internal iliac artery [5]. Rarely, PCS may develop from regional venous overload from congenital venous and arteriovenous malformations due to cirrhosis, retroaortic left renal vein, tumor thrombosis of the inferior vena cava, portal vein thrombosis, and renal cell carcinoma with left renal vein thrombosis [5].

Diagnosis

A thorough history and physical examination are paramount to achieve proper diagnosis in the case of PCS, especially given that patients with incompetent pelvic veins can be asymptomatic. Other causes of pelvic pain, both chronic and acute, should be ruled in or out based on the clinical history, such as, but not limited to, ovarian torsion, endometriosis, painful

bladder syndrome, spastic pelvic floor syndrome, and others. Typical features are shown in Table 10.1 [5].

In a patient with characteristic symptoms, the diagnosis is supported by bimanual examination exhibiting cervical motion tenderness, uterine tenderness, and/or ovarian tenderness. However, patients can also have no pain on exam. A study by Beard reported the combination of tenderness on abdominal palpation over the adnexa compounded by a history of postcoital ache was 94% sensitive and 77% specific for discriminating pelvic congestion from other causes of pelvic pain [5, 7]. Unfortunately, no clear diagnostic algorithm exists for PCS, and therefore a multidisciplinary approach for pelvic pain, utilizing gynecological, urological, vascular, or interventional radiological input may be helpful. Imaging should be performed to support but not define diagnosis, especially given that incompetent and dilated ovarian veins are common, nonspecific findings. Further, although dilatation of the ovarian vein is necessary but not sufficient for diagnosis, there is no consensus on the optimum cut-off for ovarian vein diameter in PCS and no validated measures for venous congestion and tortuosity. Furthermore, the reported cut-off values for ovarian vein diameter differ between the imaging techniques [5].

Predisposing risk factors for the development of PCS are those of most women alive today: being of reproductive age. Pregnancy and its changes on total blood volume, and the distribution of said volume, are an obvious predisposing factor. However, there are cases of PCS in patients without prior pregnancy. This

Table 10.1 Common symptoms of pelvic congestion syndrome

Noncyclical pain for at least 3–6 months

Pain presenting during or after pregnancy, with worsening pain with subsequent pregnancies

Unilateral dullness, achiness, and/or heaviness sensations; can be present bilaterally or alternate sides

Pain aggravated before or during menstrual bleeding because of any factor leading to increased intraabdominal pressure such as standing for long periods of time, walking, lifting, and postural changes

Pain worse during or after intercourse

Pain least severe at start of day, worse at end of day

Symptom improvement by lying in supine position

Pain takes several hours to subside

Possible presence of vulvovaginal, gluteal, perineal, or lower limb varicosities may be due to intrinsic issues with the veins, or lifestyle choices in which intraabdominal pressure is routinely increased, such as patients who must stand for prolonged periods of time, routinely lift heavy objects, or engage in extreme sports, such as skydiving or bungee-jumping. In all these cases, increased intraabdominal pressure is common denominator. However, we must note here the effect of estrogen, which can act as a vasodilator, causing smooth muscle relaxation and loss of vascular responsiveness [5]. This effect may explain why these symptoms improve with time and the parallel decline of estrogen, as there is complete regression of symptoms after menopause [5].

Imaging

Ovarian venography is, and has been, the gold standard for diagnosis [6]. Initially published by Beard et al. in 1984, these criteria included ovarian diameter of 6 mm or greater, contrast retention in the pelvic venous plexus of more than 20 seconds, congestion of the pelvic venous plexus and/or opacification of the ipsilateral (or contralateral) internal iliac vein, and/or filling of vulvovaginal and thigh varicosities.

Each variable was assigned a value of 1 to 3, depending on the degree of abnormality, with a score greater than 5 indicating PCS [7]. A benefit of contrast venography is that the tool is both diagnostic and therapeutic, after which sclerotherapy or embolization may be performed. These treatments will be discussed later in the chapter. However, numerous less invasive imaging options are available.

Ultrasound

Ultrasound imaging is the least invasive imaging testing available to date. It is helpful in that it can thoroughly evaluate pelvic anatomy, as well as include or exclude other etiologies of pain. PCS can be suspected in patients with dilation of ovarian vein greater than 4 mm, reversed or retrograde blood flow, slow blood flow (<3 cm/second), presence of tortuous and or dilated veins, dilated arcuate veins crossing the uterine myometrium, or variable duplex waveform in the varicoceles during Valsalva maneuver [5]. However, the ability to obtain such detail is operator dependent, so further workup may be warranted.

Both CT and MRI offer detailed cross-sectional imaging of both anatomy and pelvic vasculature. Both modalities are sensitive for pelvic varices, ovarian vein dilation, and compression of iliac and renal veins [5]. Unfortunately, CT requires radiation, and neither modality provides hemodynamic information, a clear benefit of duplex ultrasonography. Duplex ultrasound has become the diagnostic test of choice in most venous centers [6]. Additionally, as these two modalities typically require the patient to be positioned in the supine position, there is concern for less specificity of results.

Laparoscopy is often performed in patients with pelvic pain. The rate of any pathological findings at time of laparoscopy, in women with CPP, is 35%–83%, however, the rate of PCS seen at time of laparoscopy is 20% [5]. PCS is likely to be missed at the time of laparoscopy due to CO_2 insufflation and Trendelenburg position causing venous collapse [5]. Therefore, laparoscopy should not be considered a first-line diagnostic tool for PCS [5].

Table 10.2 summarizing these imaging modalities as described by Borghi et al details these issues.

Complications/Fertility

There is scant information in the literature regarding rate of pregnancy and associated outcomes after treatment for PCS, regardless of modality. The procedure appears to do no harm to ovarian function, as no significant differences in hormone levels were observed before and after therapy [8]. Additionally, reports about pregnancy and ovary hormone levels after embolization are also rare [8]. Further studies are warranted.

Treatment

PCS is as enigmatic to treat as it is to diagnose; however, many reported successful treatments have shown varying degrees of efficacy. Treatments range from hormonal to a variety of surgical and nonsurgical procedures. Moreover, as PCS is a vascular disorder found in the pelvis, traditionally separated specialties have each developed unique approaches to the condition, including treatment from gynecology, vascular surgery, and interventional radiology. It should be kept in mind that as PCS is often found concurrently with other pelvic pain related disorders (i.e., endometriosis, high-tone pelvic floor dysfunction, centralized pain syndromes, among others), treatment options will vary in regard to outcome. Therefore, a thorough pelvic pain workup should be completed so the correct disease will be

Table 10.2 Advantages and disadvantages of various radiological tests performed in patients with pelvic congestion syndrome

Technique	Pros	Cons
US	First-line screening tool Exclude other causes Noninvasive No radiation	False positives False negatives Operator dependent Technically difficult
CT	Detailed anatomical overview Exclude other causes	Radiation exposure Low specificity Expensive Intervention not possible
MRI	Detailed anatomical overview Exclude other causes No radiation	Low specificity Expensive Intervention not possible
Venography	Gold standard Intervention possible	Radiation exposure Invasive
Laparoscopy	Detailed anatomical overview Exclusion of other causes Intervention possible	Invasive Expensive Low specificity CO_2 insufflation and Trendelenberg may cause vein collapse

specifically treated. The generally complicated and multifaceted nature of chronic pelvic pain syndromes can make evaluating treatment efficacy of a single disease process difficult, as unintended treatment of concurrent syndromes can alter important outcome measures. Keeping this in mind, there is much published data regarding treatment for PCS, and many interventions have been shown to be effective in the treatment of this condition.

Medical Therapies

Progestins have shown benefit in the treatment of PCS with regard to decreased congestion of vessels on ultrasound and relief of pain, likely via partial suppression of ovarian function [9]. Though the exact mechanism of action is unknown, the treatment seems to be paradoxical because progestins are suspected to be responsible for dilation of blood vessels in bodily processes, particularly during pregnancy. Nevertheless, oral progestin-only contraceptives, as well as the etonogestrel implant, have both demonstrated efficacy in the treatment of pain in women with PCS [9–11]. Of note, in one study, both patient satisfaction and pelvic venography scores improved with etonogestrel implant at 1 year [10]. At 6 months, pain scores with the implant decreased from a visual analog score (VAS) of 7.7 to 4.6, and 83% of women were satisfied to very satisfied with the result [10]. Objective repeat per-uterine venography scores improved, decreasing 4.5 points from 8.6 in treatment

versus control groups. There was also a corresponding decrease in monthly quantified blood loss from 204 mL to 90 mL on a pictorial menstrual blood loss tool [10]. This could suggest that a decreasing duration of dysmenorrhea symptoms may have been the major contributor to pain improvement [10].

The efficacy of these hormonal medications may also be linked to interruption of the menstrual cycle, since there are known changes to both uterine and ovarian blood flow during the course of the menstrual cycle [12].

Similarly, goserelin acetate, a gonadotropin-releasing hormone (GnRH) agonist, has shown efficacy in the treatment of PCS. This medication also induces amenorrhea, but perhaps the blockage of the hypothalamic–pituitary–adrenal (HPA) axis and subsequent decrease in overall female hormone levels plays a role. This theory may be supported by evidence that PCS seems to resolve in postmenopausal women [10] with the decrease in estrogen, which has been proposed to be a venous dilator [11]. In a randomized controlled trial comparing goserelin acetate to medroxyprogesterone acetate, goserelin acetate was superior with respect to pelvic venography, sexual functioning, anxiety, and depressive states, as well as pelvic symptoms score (a scale including pelvic pain, dyspareunia, dysmenorrhea, and pelvic tenderness on exam) [11]. Other medical treatments that may show some efficacy for the treatment of PCS include danazol, phlebotonics, dihydroergotamine, and nonsteroidal anti-inflammatory drugs (NSAIDs), but there is a paucity of data on these treatments [13].

One consistent issue with medical treatment is the return of symptoms upon patient discontinuation of therapy. When patients are *peri*-menopausal or are willing and able to use these medications as long-term therapy, this treatment course can be highly successful. However, many of these medications have side effects. Progestins, namely medroxyproges-terone acetate, have been associated with mood changes, emotional lability, headaches, abnormal uterine bleeding, and a variety of other symptoms [14]. When a patient requires this medication for a short period of time, or there is an absence or limited side effects, it may make sense for her to continue this treatment course. Goserelin acetate also may develop issues of intolerability, producing side effects linked to a low estrogen state, for example, hot flashes, night sweats, emotional lability, vaginal dryness, with resulting dyspareunia [14]. Furthermore, goserelin acetate is not indicated for long-term use, as the low estrogen state it induces can lead to decreased bone mineral density. One should balance the quality of life considerations related to medication side effects versus those associated with pain relief, as well as patient desires for future fertility.

Procedural Interventions

When conservative medical therapy fails, there are a variety of effective procedures that can be considered. These have the advantage of not having the long-term side effects of medical management; however, they are not free of risk. Procedural interventions are either radiologically directed or surgical procedures performed under general anesthesia.

Physicians trained in interventional radiology can perform a variety of therapies with the aim of obliterating the dilated, dysfunctional pelvic veins associated with PCS, typically the ovarian and iliac veins, targeting the plexuses around the uterus itself. Treatment for PCS has historically involved placement of endothelial scler-osing or embolic agents by accessing pelvic venous structures through entry points in the femoral, jugular, or radial arteries [15]. Sclerosing agents produce occlusion by causing severe inflammation and thrombosis, some inducing immediate endothelial cell death. As a result, these agents act immediately and irreversibly, and include absolute alcohol, sodium tetradecyl, ethyl-ene vinyl alcohol (Onyx), and other agents [15]. Because

sclerosants are liquid and not radiopaque, to better control placement, many interventionalists treating PCS will use them in conjunction with embolic agents, which can be better visualized on imaging and deployed more specifically [15]. For this reason, embolization agents are typically used in larger vessels with the added advantage of radio-opacity to localize their place-ment more precisely. These agents include vascular coils, Amplatzer plugs (nitinol mesh), and microembolic particles, among others [15]. In the literature, transcath-eter embolization may be used to describe an interven-tional procedure that includes the use of both a sclerosing and embolic agent [16]. Selection of a specific agent is provider dependent and can depend on vessel size, desire for permanence of effect, and whether or not cell death is desired [15]. The Society for Vascular Surgery and the American Venous Forum "suggest treatment of pelvic congestion syndrome with coil embolization, plugs, transcatheter sclerotherapy can be used alone or together" [17].

The mainstay of interventional radiologic treatment of PCS is transcatheter embolotherapy (TCE). Introduced for the treatment of PCS in the early 1990s by Edwards et al. [18], the procedure has been modified from a unilateral approach to include bilateral embol-ization of ovarian veins using coils and sclerosant foam, either from a jugular or femoral approach [19]. With the left-sided unilateral approach, approximately one-third of patients reported no or only partial relief; however, the bilateral approach has excellent success rates [19]. The procedure is technically successful 98% of the time and efficacious in decreasing pain in 65%–85% of patients with recurrence rates of 8% [19]. A trial of long-term follow up showed that 83% of patients had clinical improvement 4 years post-procedurally [20]. TCE is generally low risk related to complications, ranging from 3% to 8%, and can include foam or coil migration; recurrence of varices; and thrombophlebitis, gonadal vein perforation, or cardiac arrhythmia [13]. A 2016 systematic review of 22 studies ($n = 1,308$ patients) reported significantly decreased pain scores on a visual analog scale (VAS) with a follow-up of at least 12 months [16].

Overall, the interventional radiologic approach using TCE is beneficial in that it is very effective, has a low risk profile, and can be performed concomi-tantly with the procedure that confirms the diagnosis of PCS. Furthermore, its long-term success rate and rapid return to full function for patients makes it an attractive therapy for the treatment of PCS.

Surgical Procedures

A variety of surgical therapies have been used to treat PCS with positive results. These procedures range from ovarian vein ligation to extirpative therapies such as hysterectomy, with or without bilateral salpingo-oophorectomy (BSO).

Studies have shown efficacy with regard to minimal impact laparoscopic procedures such as ovarian vein ligation procedures, efficacy shown both with ligation near the infundibulopelvic ligament, as well as a higher vein ligation [21]. Care must be taken with these procedures to recognize that there can be multiple main trunks (instead of the usual single trunk) providing venous drainage from the ovary, 40% on the time on the left and 25% on the right [13]. One small cohort study reported efficacy with this treatment, with approximately 80% of women reporting total elimination of pain [21]. At 1 year, all of the remaining study cohort (74% after dropout) reported resolution of pain [21]. Though attractive, the reported procedure requires an experienced laparoscopic surgeon with excellent knowledge of the anatomy, as accessing the ovarian venous vasculature is performed at various locations along its course, not restricted to the infundibulopelvic ligament where it is most easily accessible.

Extirpative procedures such as hysterectomy with and without removal of one or both ovaries have shown to be effective as well. Some patients with PCS have experienced marked pain relief with these therapies, with VAS scores decreasing from 10 to 0 over 1 year following hysterectomy with BSO [22, 23]. In the same cohort, however, one in three women reported residual pain [22] with a return of symptomatology for some, 30%, at 1 year [13]. The confirmation of PCS in these patients, however, was not well established, and in one trial 25% were shown to have adenomyosis on postsurgical histology [22]. All in all, though hysterectomy appears beneficial, it is difficult to recommend hysterectomy or hysterectomy with BSO over other treatment modalities given the current data.

There is an important caveat to this conclusion. Although surgical therapies have less evidence to support their efficacy and may put patients at higher risk when compared to interventional radiological techniques, surgical evaluation allows for the identification and treatment of concomitant pelvic pathologies such as endometriosis; and this is not trivial because 70% of patients with chronic pelvic pain have been shown to have endometriosis [24]. As a result, surgical intervention has relevance among the current treatment modalities. Additionally, some authors suggest surgical intervention may be further indicated when the etiology of PCS is obstructive, such as in May–Thurner syndrome, or nutcracker syndrome [25]. In these circumstances, treatments with embolotherapy or sclerotherapy may not be as effective because these treatments focus on the incompetent valves and not the anatomical obstructive etiology [25].

Discussion

After confirmed diagnosis, medical management is the most conservative effective therapy with the least amount of risk for patients with PCS. These therapies can include progestins, GnRH agonists, danazol, phlebotonics, dihydroergotamine, and NSAIDs. However, these therapies can be ineffective in some patients or side effects may prohibit and or limit their use. These patients should subsequently be offered surgical or nonsurgical procedural interventions. Transcatheter embolotherapy (TCE) is effective and low risk and should be considered next line therapy; however, in patients who have suspected concomitant pelvic pathology, surgical evaluation and treatment may be a more effective option.

From published series in the 1990s, success rates for reduction of chronic pelvic pain ranged from 50% to 80%; however, with advancements in technique, significant relief is now reported in 60%–100% of patients [1]. This improvement may stem from multiple factors such as advancements in diagnostic imaging modalities, as well as innovations in surgical and radiological techniques. While these results are encouraging, the overarching data outcomes are contradictory. For example, 6%–31.8% of patients do not get substantial relief following ovarian embolization [6]. We believe this discrepancy is due to a number of reasons. First, pathophysiology is poorly understood, and symptoms can overlap with other diseases, thereby leading to either incorrect and/or underestimated diagnosis. Next, confirmatory diagnostic testing itself is quite variable, depending on not only patient access to testing, but also variability in these imaging results, reliant on both the testing operator and subsequent radiological interpretation. Adding to diagnostic confusion is that ovarian dilation, though associated with and predictive of PCS, is not itself synonymous with venous incompetence or symptoms [2]. So how next should one proceed?

In all cases of pelvic pain, as noted throughout this publication, the quality of life of the patient must be taken into consideration when determining the treatment plan, and if intervention is warranted and/or desired. Most studies employ either a subjective degree of improvement or VAS to assess outcomes. It is clear, however, based on the inconsistency of outcomes, that further study is warranted, and a disease-specific evaluation tool, as it relates to both the physical and psychosocial aspects of the disease, is needed and will be paramount in effectively assessing future treatment outcomes.

In conclusion, PCS is a common condition, with significant impact on both the physical and psychological facets of patient quality of life. Overall, there is great promise in treatment options, especially in regard to pain improvement, although an optimum treatment modality is yet to be determined. In many cases, complete pain relief is noted. However, in the cases where it is not, care should be taken to ensure proper diagnosis was achieved as well as a comprehensive search for other sources of chronic pelvic pain.

Five Things You Need to Know

- Pelvic congestion syndrome (PCS) often starts after pregnancy.
- Congested vessels may be difficult to diagnose on laparoscopy because of abdominal/pelvic insufflation and Trendelenburg position.
- The medical treatment of pelvic congestion syndrome focuses on medications that alter the hypothalamic–pituitary–adrenal axis; however, these treatments have side effects and on discontinuation symptoms typically return.
- Transcatheter embolotherapy of pelvic venous vasculature is associated with a high cure rate and low risk.
- A variety of surgical treatments for PCS have been shown to be effective and are most indicated when another surgical intervention is performed concomitantly..

References

1. Phillips D, Deipolyi AR, Hesketh RL, Midia M, Oklu R. Pelvic congestion syndrome: etiology of pain, diagnosis, and clinical management. *J Vasc Interv Radiol.* 2014;**25**(5):725–3. DOI: 10.1016/j.jvir.2014.01.030.
2. Brown CL, Rizer M, Alexander R, Sharpe EE, Rochon PJ. Pelvic congestion syndrome: systematic review of treatment success. *Semin Interv Radiol.* 2018;**35**(1):35–40. DOI: 10.1055/s-0038-1636519.
3. Mathias SD, Kuppermann M, Liberman RF, Lipschutz RC, Steege JF. Chronic pelvic pain: prevalence, health-related quality of life, and economic correlates. *Obstet Gynecol.* 1996;**87**:321–7.
4. Andrews J, Yunker A, Reynolds WS, Likis FE, Sathe NA, Jerome RN. Noncyclic chronic pelvic pain therapies for women: comparative effectiveness. *Comp Effect Rev.* 2012;**41**. Rockville, MD: Agency for Healthcare Research and Quality (US). Report No. 11(12)-EHC088-EF.
5. Borghi C, Atti LD. Pelvic congestion syndrome: the current state of literature. *Arch Gynecol Obstet.* 2016;**293**(2):291–301. DOI: 10.1007/s00404-015-3895-7.
6. Meissner MH, Gloviczki P. Pelvic venous disorders. In *Atlas of Endovascular Venous Surgery*, 2nd ed. Philadelphia: Elsevier; 2019, 567–99.
7. Beard RW, Highman JH, Pearce S, Reginald PW. Diagnosis of pelvic varicosities in women with chronic pelvic pain. *Lancet.* 1984; **2**(8409):946–9.
8. Liu J, Han LH, Han X. The effect of a subsequent pregnancy after ovarian vein embolization in patients with infertility caused by pelvic congestion syndrome. *Acad Radiol.* 2019;**pii**: S1076-6332(19)30017-0. DOI: 10.1016/j.acra.2018.12.024.
9. Farquhar CM, Rogers V, Franks S, Pearce S, Wadsworth J, Beard RW. A randomized controlled trial of medroxyprogesterone acetate and psychotherapy for the treatment of pelvic congestion. *Br JObstet Gynaecol.* 1989;**10**:1153–62.
10. Shokeir T, Amr M, Abelshaheed M. The efficacy of Implanon for the treatment of chronic pelvic pain associated with pelvic congestion: 1-year randomized controlled pilot study. *Arch Gynecol Obstet.* 2009;**280**:437–43.
11. Soysal ME, Soysal S, Vicdan K, Ozer S. A randomized controlled trial of goserelin and medroxyprogesterone acetate in the treatment of pelvic congestion. *Hum Reprod.* 2001;**16**(5):931–9.
12. Tan SL, Zaidi J, Campbell S, Doyle P, Collins W. Blood flow changes in the ovarian and uterine arteries during the normal menstrual cycle. *Am J Obstet Gynecol.* 1996;**175**(3 Pt 1):625–31.
13. Ignacio EA, Dua R, Sarin S, Harper AS, Yim D, Mathur V, Venbrux AC. Pelvic congestion syndrome: diagnosis and treatment. *Semin Interv Radiol.* 2008;**25**(4):361–8.
14. PDR (Prescriber's Digital Reference). Drug Summary. ConnectiveRx. May 28, 2019. www.pdr.net/drug-summary/Provera-medroxyprogesterone-acetate-1015

15. Ray CE, Bauer JR. Embolization agents. In Mauro MA (ed.), *Image-Guided Interventions*. Philadelphia, PA: Saunders Elsevier; 2008,131–9.

16. Daniels JP, Champaneria R, Shah L, Gupta JK, Birch J, Moss JG. Effectiveness of embolization or sclerotherapy of pelvic veins for reducing chronic pelvic pain: a systematic review. *J Vasc Interv Radiol.* 2016;**27**(10):1478–86.

17. Gloviczki P, Comerote AJ, Dalsing MC, et al. The care of patients with varicose veins and associated chronic venous diseases: clinical practice guidelines of the Society for Vascular Surgery and the American Venous Forum. *J Vasc Surg.* 2011;**53**(5 Suppl):2S-48S. DOI: 10.1016/j.jvs.2011.01.079.

18. Edwards RD, Robertson IR, MacLean AB. Case report: pelvic pain syndrome: successful treatment of a case by ovarian vein embolization. *Clin Radiol.* 1993; **47**:429–31.

19. Freedman J, Ganeshan A, Crowe PM. Pelvic congestion syndrome: the role of interventional radiology in the treatment of chronic pelvic pain. *Postgrad Med J.* 2010;**86**(1022):704–10. DOI: 10.1136/ pgmj.2010.099473.

20. Kim HS, Malhotra AD, Rowe PC, et al. Embolotherapy for pelvic congestion syndrome: long-term results. *J Vasc Interv Radiol.* 2006;**17**:289.

21. Gargiulo T, Mais V, Brokaj L, Cossu E, Melis GB. Bilateral laparoscopic transperitoneal ligation of ovarian veins for treatment of pelvic congestion syndrome. *J Am Assoc Gynecol Laparosc.* 2003;**10** (4):501–4.

22. Beard RW, Kennedy RG, Gangar KF, et al. Bilateral oophorectomy and hysterectomy in the treatment of intractable pelvic pain associated with pelvic congestion. *Br J Obstet Gynaecol.* 1991;**98**:988.

23. Carter JE. Surgical treatment for chronic pelvic pain. *JSLS.* 1998;**2**(2):129–39.

24. Propst AM, Laufer MR. Endometriosis in adolescents: incidence, diagnosis, and treatment. *J Reprod Med.* 1999;**44**(9):751–8.

25. Bookwalter CA, VanBuren WM, Neisen MJ, Bjarnason H. Imaging appearance and nonsurgical management of pelvic venous congestion syndrome. *Radiographics.* 2019;**39**(2):596–608.

Irritable Bowel Syndrome

Maryam R. Kashi and Seetha Lakshmanan

Editor's Introduction

Irritable bowel syndrome (IBS) is another condition of the "evil quadruplets." It often coexists with endometriosis and adds to the pain of this condition. The mainstay is pain associated with change in bowel habit. It is also important to remember that IBS is diagnosed based on symptoms, and endoscopy is often performed in those patients is done to rule out any other bowel disease. This condition is best managed by a gastroenterologist but it is important to note that quite a large number of patients with this condition have spasm of pelvic floor muscles and treatment of that spasm may improve some of the IBS symptoms.

Introduction

Irritable bowel syndrome (IBS) is an important member of disorders of gut–brain interaction. It is a chronic disease with recurring periods of exacerbation. It is defined by the presence of abdominal pain in association with change in bowel habits in the absence of detectable organic disease. As the most commonly diagnosed gastrointestinal (GI) condition, it is often part of the differential diagnosis in the evaluation of chronic pelvic pain. Globally, the prevalence of IBS varies greatly, with South America having the highest prevalence (21%) and Southeast Asia the lowest (7%). The prevalence of IBS in North America is 12% [1]. It is most commonly found in women, and prevalence seems to decline with age, decreasing by 25% in patients older than age 50 [1, 2. In a survey of 1,924 patients with a history of GI symptoms, 56.9% met criteria for IBS; however, 43.1% of these had not been formally diagnosed. Still, the impact on quality of life is significant [3]. In some studies, up to 70% of patients with IBS symptoms do not consult a physician; nevertheless, the disease accounts for

$20 billion annually in total direct and indirect costs, including medications [41, 4].

Pathophysiology

The pathogenesis of IBS is heterogeneous, complex, and, likely, multifactorial. Traditionally, the focus has been on GI motility, visceral hypersensitivity, and psychosocial factors. More recently, studies have focused on alternate potential causes of IBS, including inflammation, alterations in microbiota, bacterial overgrowth, and food sensitivity. Studies evaluating the role of genetics are being pursued.

Gastrointestinal Dysmotility

Normally after meals, increase in colonic motility occurs by an irregular alternation of quiescence, sporadic non-propagating contractions, and progression of intestinal contents by propagating movements. In IBS, however, there is increased frequency and irregularity of luminal contractions. In constipation-dominant IBS, transit time is prolonged, whereas in diarrhea-dominant IBS, there is exaggerated motor response to cholecystokinin and meal ingestion, leading to decreased bowel transit time. Recent data show that pelvic floor dyssynergia can mimic non-diarrhea predominant IBS symptoms, suggesting anorectal function tests should be considered in these patients [5]. Serotonin (5-hydroxytryptamine [5-HT]) plays a central role in GI motility, secretion, and pain modulation. Patients with IBS-C have been shown to have decreased levels of 5-HT, while patients with IBS-D have been found to have increased levels. Serotonin activity is modulated through 5-HT3 and 5-HT4 receptors, which have been a focus for some therapeutic initiatives [6].

Visceral Hypersensitivity

Visceral hypersensitivity has been postulated to be linked with various issues, including psychosocial events, prior history of abuse, and small and large bowel permeability. The interaction may be through the brain–gut axis and/or mucosal immunity [1]. Increased intestinal sensitivity in IBS causes abdominal pain and GI motor disorder, which provokes alterations in defecation patterns; that is, diarrhea or constipation. Several studies suggest that this selective hypersensitization of visceral afferent nerves in the gut are triggered by bowel distention or bloating. Abnormal visceral perception is suggested by excessive sensitivity to balloon distention documented at the rectosigmoid and the anorectum [7].

Intestinal Inflammation (Including Postinfectious IBS)

Postinfectious IBS (IBS-PI) has been reported to occur in 3%–36% of patients with enteric infections. Up to 10% of IBS patients report that their symptoms began with an acute infectious process. Intestinal mucosa from IBS patients have demonstrated activation of the immune system. An increased number of activated immunocompetent cells, such as T-lymphocytes, neutrophils, and mast cells, were seen in immunohistological assessment of intestinal mucosa, suggesting persistent inflammation in mucosa and enteric nerves, possibly contributing to the pathogenesis of IBS. IBS-PI attributed to viral infections seem to have only short-term effects; however, those attributed to bacterial, protozoan, or helminth infections seem to have a prolonged course. Some studies report that half of IBS-PI patients develop spontaneous recovery within 6 to 8 years [1]. IBS-PI is often associated with female gender, younger age, prolonged duration of infection, use of antibiotics, smoking, anxiety, and depression. The bowel symptoms following this acute infectious enteritis could be due to malabsorption, increased colonic mucosal lymphocytes, and enteroendocrine cells secreting high levels of serotonin [61, 6].

Altered Microbiota and Bacterial Overgrowth

A range of host factors may account for the differences in fecal microbiota of IBS patients compared to controls. These factors may include diet, genetics, and recent antibiotic use. Luminal- and mucosa-associated microbiota can affect the host via immunomicrobial interactions contributing to IBS symptoms. Emerging data suggest that the fecal microbiota in individuals with IBS differ from those of healthy controls and vary with their predominant symptom. In some studies, small intestinal bacterial overgrowth (SIBO) is more prevalent in IBS patients and its eradication with antibiotics may alleviate some symptoms. SIBO is typically diagnosed by indirect methods with diagnostic limitations. Reports on the prevalence of SIBO in IBS patients vary quite largely, ranging from 10% to 84%. Due to significant inconsistencies among studies, the relationship between IBS and SIBO remain unclear [61, 6, 8, 9].

Food Sensitivity

Many patients identify certain food items as triggers for their IBS symptoms. As such, food is a central issue for some patients. As many as 70% of patients report that IBS symptoms are associated with or exacerbated by certain foods in their diet. Although true food allergies play a small part in IBS symptomatology, food intolerances are quite common. Multiple studies have shown that poorly absorbed carbohydrates can have osmotic effects and lead to fermentation and gas production, contributing to various symptoms [1, 10].

More recent studies have explored the role of several other mechanisms, including genetic predisposition, altered intestinal permeability, disordered bile salt metabolism, and abnormalities in 5-HT metabolism. A better understanding of the pathophysiology of IBS will pave the way for novel therapies.

Diagnosis

Diagnosis of IBS rests heavily on a symptom-based criteria. Ensuring the absence of GI alarm signs is an important step in distinguishing between a chronic IBS issue and an acute problem, which may require more urgent evaluation. Alarm signs include evidence of GI bleeding, anemia, and weight loss. Patients often have several GI symptoms simultaneously. It is important to validate their concerns by ensuring them that all of their symptoms will be evaluated; however, it is sometimes best to explore each separately.

Understanding when a patient's pain began is important in determining if the issue is acute or chronic. The location of the pain is helpful for similar reasons. A diffuse pain, or one with a migratory

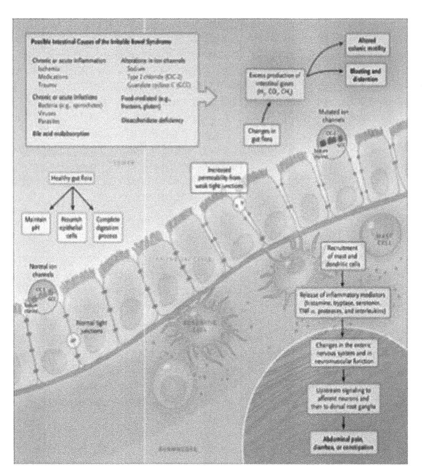

Figure 11.1 Theoretical model of the pathophysiology of IBS, representing the common intestinal causes of IBS. (www .nejm.org/doi/full/10.1056/NEJMr a1607547" www.nejm.org/doi/full/10.1056 /NEJMra1607547).

pattern, may be more consistent with IBS than a focal pain. Pain that is constant is likely not IBS, which is usually intermittent. Severity of pain can vary significantly in IBS and may range from mild to quite severe. Frequency of pain is a helpful indicator for the care provider, as it helps one understand how often this issue is disruptive to the patient. Treatment for a patient whose pain occurs only two or three times per year will vary quite significantly from that for a patient whose discomfort is daily. With this same concept in mind, the length of time that the pain lasts is quite important, as well. Pain that lasts only seconds will likely not benefit from medications as needed (prn) basis because it is likely gone by the time the patient finds his or her medication bottle. Determining if certain factors, such as food and bowel movement, exacerbate or alleviate the abdominal pain can be significant. Lastly, associated factors may be helpful, such as nausea and vomiting, fever and chills, diarrhea and constipation, and evidence of GI bleeding.

Rome IV criteria were developed in 2016 to assist in the diagnosis of IBS in clinical practice and to ensure consistency in patient selection for clinical trials. The Rome IV criteria define IBS as recurrent abdominal pain at least once per week in the prior 3 months with symptom onset at least 6 months before diagnosis. Abdominal pain must be associated with at least two of the following: defecation, change in stool frequency, and change in stool form.

Physical exam is helpful to elicit pain that is focal and to rule out rebound tenderness, which may indicate appendicitis. Patients with IBS range from benign, nontender abdomen to diffuse tenderness on exam. As IBS is a functional disorder, there are no laboratory or radiological findings to help with diagnosis. Laboratory evaluation may be used to help exclude conditions such as inflammatory bowel disease (IBD) and celiac disease, which may mimic IBS [11]. Radiological evaluation may be used to exclude

Table 11.1 Rome criteria for irritable bowel syndrome

Rome III criteria for diagnosing IBS[a]

Recurrent abdominal pain or discomfort[b] at least 3 days/month in the prior 3 months associated with two or more of the following:
- Improvement with defecation
- Onset associated with a change in frequency of stool
- Onset associated with a change in form (appearance) of stool

Rome IV criteria for diagnosing IBS[c]

Recurrent abdominal pain, on average, at least 1 day/week in the prior 3 months, associated with two or more of the following criteria:
- Related to defecation
- Associated with a change in frequency of stool
- Associated with a change in form (appearance) of stool.

[a] Criterion fulfilled for the prior 3 months with symptom onset at least 6 months before diagnosis.

[b] "Discomfort" means an uncomfortable sensation not described as pain.

[c] Criteria fulfilled for the prior 3 months with symptom onset at least 6 months before diagnosis.

Source: Lacy BE, et al. Bowel disorders. Rome III Diagnostic Criteria for Functional Gastrointestinal Disorders.*Gastroenterology*. 2016;150:1393–1407.

structural issues that may be in the provider's differential diagnosis. We often use an abdominal radiograph to evaluate retained stool burden, which may be contributing to patient symptoms. In the same manner, there are no specific endoscopic signs for IBS. Endoscopic evaluation may be used only to exclude processes, such as peptic ulcer disease, celiac disease, and IBD.

IBS is a heterogeneous disease with multiple subtypes that likely exist along a continuum. Patients may have predominance of constipation (IBS-C) or diarrhea (IBS-D). Still others may show a mixed pattern (IBS-M) with which they alternate between constipation, diarrhea, and "normal" bowel habits. There is great fluidity between these subtypes, where patients may have different patterns at different stages in life. Rome IV defines that IBS-C at having more than 25% hard or lumpy stools and less than 25% soft or loose stools. IBS-D is defined as less than 25% hard or lumpy stools and more than 25% soft or loose stools. IBS-Mixed is defined as more than 25% hard or lumpy stools and more than 25% soft or loose stools. Stool patterns that do not meet these diagnostic criteria are defined as IBS-Unclassified.

Treatment

Treatment of IBS is often based on control of dominant symptoms. As there may be variability in symptoms over time, the focus of treatment may need to change periodically. A wide range of dietary and

pharmacological treatments are available. As many patients associate consumption of certain foods with IBS symptoms, more emphasis is now placed on the diet than in previous years. Management of IBS should include a combination of both. In addition, a good doctor–patient relationship, reassurance, and continuity of care are critical to the management of IBS. The British Society of Gastroenterology highlighted the influence of placebo on the outcome of IBS.

Diet

Patients commonly report that dietary factors play an important role in their GI symptoms. Until relatively recently, few studies were available to demonstrate a relationship. As more data have become available, there has been greater support for dietary manipulation as a means of treatment of IBS symptoms. Our approach is often to start with the least restricting diets first. Lactose intolerance is a common disorder, where lactose is not properly digested and absorbed in the small bowel, leading to fermentation by colonic bacteria, which produce various gases, including hydrogen, carbon dioxide, and methane. Symptoms of lactose intolerance (abdominal pain, nausea, bloating, diarrhea) may overlap with symptoms with IBS; as such, it is important to rule out this condition early in the evaluation process [12]. Diagnosis of lactose intolerance may be made with the hydrogen breath test or simple trial of dairy avoidance for 2–4 weeks.

Bristol Stool Chart

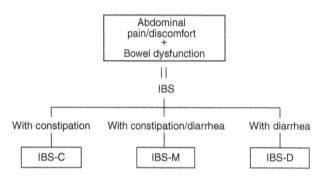

Type 1 Separate hard lumps, like nuts (hard to pass)

Type 2 Sausage-shaped, but lumpy

Type 3 Sausage-shaped, but with cracks on surface

Type 4 Sausage or snake like, smooth and soft

Type 5 Soft blobs with clear-cut edges (easy to pass)

Type 6 Fluffy pieces with ragged edges, mushy

Type 7 Watery, no solid pieces (entirely liquid)

Figure 11.2 (A) The Bristol Stool Form Scale (BSFS) is a useful tool to evaluate bowel habits. The BSFS has been shown to be a reliable surrogate marker for colonic transit. (B) IBS subtypes can be established according to stool consistency, using the BSFS. (*Source*: Lacy, BE et al. Bowel disorders. *Gastroenterology*. 2016;150(6), 1393–1407.e5)

Abdominal pain/discomfort + Bowel dysfunction

||

IBS

With constipation — IBS-C

With constipation/diarrhea — IBS-M

With diarrhea — IBS-D

Figure 11.3 Clinical relationship among abdominal pain and bowel movement abnormalities in functional bowel disorders. Current and classical model where the presence of abdominal pain is mandatory to make the diagnosis of irritable bowel syndrome (IBS) and subtyped according to the association of constipation or diarrhea. (*Source*: Mearin F, Lacy BE. Diagnostic criteria in IBS. *Neurogastroenterol Motil*. 2012;24:791–801)

FODMAPS (fermentable oligosaccharides, disaccharides, monosaccharides, and polyols) are a group of short-chained carbohydrates that are incompletely absorbed in the small bowel. As such, fermentation of these substrates, which include legumes, lactose, fructose, and sorbitol, leads to increased gas production and osmotic luminal water content. The result is increased luminal distention and possible symptoms of pain, bloating, and diarrhea. Practical use of a FODMAP diet includes avoidance of such foods for several weeks and then return of one food item per week with close observation of recurrent symptoms. This method helps patients avoid unnecessary over-restriction of foods and identification of those foods that truly do cause symptoms.

Fiber has traditionally been a staple among treatments for IBS; however, strong evidence is not only lacking but there has also been significant discrepancy among studies. Clinically, fiber does seem to be very helpful in some patients; however, not all patients are responsive to fiber.

Probiotics

There has been great interest in intestinal microbiota and their effect on IBS symptoms. Probiotics are microorganisms that have the potential to change gut microflora, leading to possible alterations in gut barrier function and potential for antiinflammatory effects. Studies on probiotics have been very difficult to compare owing to great heterogeneity among studies. Studies differ in type of strains used and whether treatment is monotherapy or uses multiple strains. Doses seem to vary significantly among them and duration of treatment is yet another variance. Nevertheless, most studies show a benefit in IBS patients. A meta-analysis of 21 randomized controlled trials (RCTs) found that probiotics were associated with greater improvement in overall symptom response when compared to placebo. In addition, quality of life scores were greater in the probiotics groups. In addition, single-strain probiotics resulted in greater

Table 11.2 Characteristics and source of common FODMAPs

F	Fermentable		By colonic bacteria	
O	Oligosaccharides	Fructans, galacto-oligosaccharides	No absorption (of small intestinal hydrolyzes)	Wheat, barley, rye, onion, leek, white part of spring onion, garlic, shallots, artichokes, beetroot, fennel peas, chicory, pistachio, cashews, legumes, lentils and chickpeas
D	Disaccharides	Lactose	↓Digestion, therefore ↓ absorption in 10%–95%	Milk, custard, ice cream, and yoghurt
M	Monosaccharides	"Free fructose"(fructose in excess of glucose)	Slow, active absorption; poor in 1 in 3	Apples, pears, mangoes, cherries, watermelon, asparagus, sugar snap peas, honey, high-fructose corn syrup
A	And			
P	Polyols	Sorbitol, mannitol, and xylitol	Slow passive absorption	Apples, pears, apricots, cherries, nectarines, peaches, plums, watermelon, mushrooms, cauliflower, artificially sweetened chewing gum and confectionery

Source: Shepherd SJ, Lomer MC, Gibson PR. Short-chain carbohydrates and functional gastrointestinal disorders. *Am J Gastroenterol.* 2013;108:707.

overall symptom response than combination probiotics [13].

Gluten

Not uncommonly, patients without celiac disease independently begin gluten-free diets and find significant improvement in their GI symptoms. This is referred to as nonceliac gluten sensitivity. A randomized, double-blind, placebo-controlled, rechallenge trial studied the effect of gluten in 34 IBS patients with gluten sensitivity. Gluten was noted to worsen pain, bloating, and stool consistency, as well as "tiredness" [14]. Although it is more challenging to rule out celiac disease in patients already on a gluten-free diet, it is important to at least check genetic markers for celiac disease, as patients with possible celiac disease may be at risk for other conditions, such as iron deficiency anemia, osteoporosis, and small bowel malignancy.

IBS-C

Decreased fluid secretion and motility result in infrequent and hard stools, characteristic of IBS-constipation (IBS-C). Pharmacological treatments of

IBS-C thus focus on prokinetics that decrease intestinal transit time and antispasmodics that alleviate cramping as a result of intestinal wall pressure. Osmotic laxatives such as polyethylene glycol are frequently recommended as first-line therapy. Other treatment options include docusate, bisacodyl, senna, psyllium, lactulose, lubiprostone, plecanatide, and linaclotide. Stool softeners, such as docusate, are helpful in patients with mild symptoms. Stimulant laxatives, such as bisacodyl and senna, are usually avoided for long-term use due to possible development of melanosis coli.

In two RCTs, a prostaglandin analog, lubiprostone, a locally acting chloride channel activator that enhances chloride-rich intestinal fluid secretion, showed a significant response rate of 17.9% to global symptoms compared to 10.1% in IBS-C placebo group [8].

In the small intestine uroguanylin, a naturally occurring peptide hormone, binds to GC-C receptors, propelling cGMP to activate CFTR channels to open. This cascade leads to increased fluid secretion and intestinal transit. In the large intestine, guanylin binds to the same receptors with a similar response. GC-C receptor agonists, such as linaclotide and plecanatide, lead to an increased number of spontaneous bowel movements. In addition to this primary effect, they decrease visceral hypersensitivity of the gut, as do their naturally occurring analogs, uroguanylin and guanylin. In two double-blind, randomized, placebo-controlled multicenter studies with more than 1,600 patients, linaclotide was able to meet the primary endpoint, decrease abdominal pain 30% from baseline, and increase the frequency of spontaneous bowel movements in 33.6% and 33.7% compared to 21.0% and 13.9% in placebo groups [16, 17].

In two randomized clinical trials of IBS-C, using similar primary endpoints, 30.2% and 21.5% were responders to plecanatide compared to 17.8% and 14.2% in the placebo groups, respectively [8].

IBS-D

Patients with diarrhea-dominant irritable bowel syndrome (IBS-D) are burdened with significant diarrhea and abdominal pain, which often impact their lives in a multitude of ways. Patients may be limited in their ability to leave home and/or may have limited restroom access at work. Their symptoms and fears of stool urgency often cause them to have multiple absences from work or school. Treatment options for IBS-D include over-the-counter medications such as bismuth subsalicylate and loperamide. Prescription medications for IBS-D include alosetron, rifaximin, diphenoxylate + atropine, and eluxadoline.

Antidiarrheal agents inhibit peristalsis, prolong transit time, and reduce fecal volume. Loperamide is an over-the-counter agent, frequently used by patients prior to seeking care; its use is limited by its significant constipating effect. Its mechanism of action is mediated primarily by peripheral mu receptors that reduce gut motility and secretions, allowing for greater fluid absorption and improved stool consistency. As a result, it should be avoided in patients with IBS-C and should be used in limited doses (prn) in patients with alternating bowel habits.

Although data for alosetron (5-hydroxytryptamine-3 receptor antagonist) showed improvement in abdominal pain and global IBS symptoms, post-marketing data suggested increased risk of ischemic colitis. Alosetron was voluntarily withdrawn from the market but returned with specific and limited prescribing requirements. RCTs showed improvement in global IBS symptoms with use of xifaxan for 14 days [18]. However, a need for repeat treatment is not uncommon.

Eluxadoline binds to opioid receptors (mu, kappa, and delta) in the gut. Although the exact mechanism of action is not clear, it is believed that eluxadoline slows GI motility and decreases visceral hypersensitivity. Two RCTs showed 29% and 33% of treatment patients improvement in abdominal pain and diarrhea on at least 50% of days in the trial compared to 19% and 20% in the placebo group. Eluxadoline should be avoided in patients with history of pancreatitis, sphincter of Oddi spasm, cholecystectomy, advanced liver disease, or significant alcohol consumption [19].

Antispasmodics provide short-term relief in symptoms of abdominal pain in patients with IBS, but their long-term efficacy has not been established. Antispasmodics may directly affect intestinal smooth muscle relaxation (e.g., mebeverine and pinaverine), or act via anticholinergic or antimuscarinic properties (e.g., dicyclomine and hyoscyamine). In clinical practice, antispasmodics are best used on an as-needed basis for acute pain.

Numerous small clinical trials suggest that enteric peppermint oil, an antispasmodic with calcium-channel blocking properties, has benefit in some IBS patients. Antidepressants are also used as a treatment for patients with moderate to severe IBS due to their effects on pain perception, mood, and motility. TCAs and SSRIs appear to be more effective than placebo in the overall reduction of symptoms associated with IBS. However, the degree of tolerability and safety vary [20].

Psychotherapeutic interventions (e.g. cognitive behavioral therapy, dynamic psychotherapy, hypnotherapy, biofeedback and relaxation therapy) are adjunctive therapeutic options in IBS. Effective interventions include hypnotherapy and stress management with concomitant treatment of underlying depression or anxiety.

Five Things You Need to Know
- IBS is defined by the presence of abdominal pain in association with change in bowel habit in the absence of detectable organic disease.
- The three most common factors associated with IBS include GI motility, visceral hypersensitivity, and psychosocial factors.
- Post-infectious IBS (IBS-PI) has been reported to occur in 3%–36% of patients with enteric infections who were previously asymptomatic.
- Many patients identify certain food items as triggers for their IBS symptoms.
- Treatment of IBS is often based on control of dominant symptoms.

Table 11.3 Summary of therapies for irritable bowel syndrome

Treatment	Quality of evidence	Treatment benefits	Most common adverse events
Over-the-counter			
fiber: psyllium	Moderate	Best suited for IBS-C	Bloating, gas
Laxatives: polyethylene glycol	Very low	Beneficial for constipation but not global symptoms or pain in IBS-C	Bloating, cramping, diarrhea
Antidiarrheals: loperamide	Very low	Beneficial for diarrhea but not global symptoms or pain in IBS-D	Constipation
Probiotics	Low	Possible benefits for global symptoms, bloating, and gas as a class but unable to recommend specific probiotics	Similar to placebo
Antispasmodics: peppermint oil	Moderate	Benefits for global symptoms and cramping	GERD, constipation
Prescription			
antidepressants: TCAs, SSRIs	High	TCAs and SSRIs improve global symptoms and pain; leverage adverse effects to choose TCAs for IBS-D patients and SSRIs for IBS-C patients	Dry eyes/mouth, sedation, constipation, or diarrhea
Antispasmodics	Low	Some drugs offer benefits for global symptoms and pain	Dry eyes/mouth, sedation, constipation
Prosecretory agents			
Linaclotide	High	Improves global, abdominal, and constipation symptoms in IBS-C	Diarrhea
Lubiprostone	Moderate	Improves global, abdominal, and constipation symptoms in IBS-C	Nausea, diarrhea
Antibiotics: rifaximin	Moderate	Improves global symptoms, pain, and bloating in nonconstipated IBS patients	Similar to placebo
5-HT receptor	Moderate	Improves global, abdominal, and diarrhea symptoms in	Constipation, rare
Antagonists: alosetron		women with severe IBS-D	ischemic colitis
Other therapies			
Psychological behavioral therapy	Very low	benefits for global IBS symptoms in all subgroups	Similar to placebo

5-HT, 5-hydroxytryptamine; IBS, irritable bowel syndrome; IBS-C, IBS-constipation; IBS-D, IBS-diarrhea; SSRIs, selective serotonin reuptake inhibitors; TCAs, tricyclic antidepressants.

Source: Ford AC, Moayyedi P, Lacy BE, et al. Task Force on the Management of Functional Bowel Disorders. American College of Gastroenterology monograph on the management of irritable bowel syndrome and chronic idiopathic constipation.

References

1. Chey WD, Kurlander J, Eswaran S. Irritable bowel syndrome: a clinical review. *JAMA*. 2015;**313** (9):949–58.

2. Lovell RM, Ford AC. Global prevalence of and risk factors for irritable bowel syndrome: a meta-analysis. *Clin Gastroenterol Hepatol*. 2012;**10**:712.

3. Sayuk GS, Wolf R, Chang L. Comparison of symptoms, healthcare utilization, and treatment in diagnosed and undiagnosed individuals with diarrhea-predominant irritable bowel syndrome. *Am J Gastroenterol*. 2017;**112**:892–9.

4. Olafsdottir LB, Gudjonsson H, Jonsdottir HH, Jonsson JS, et al. Irritable bowel syndrome: physicians' awareness and patients' experience. *World J Gastroenterol*. 2012;**18** (28):3715–20.

5. Suttor VP, Prott GM, Hansen RD, Kellow JE, Malcolm A. Evidence for pelvic floor dyssynergia in patients with irritable bowel syndrome. *Dis Colon Rectum*. 2010;**53**(2):156–60.

6. Saha L. Irritable bowel syndrome: pathogenesis, diagnosis, treatment, and evidence-based medicine. *World J Gastroenterol*. 2014;**20** (22):6759–73.

7.   Alaradi O, Barkin J. Irritable bowel syndrome: update on pathogenesis and management. *Med Princ Pract.* 2002;**11**(1):2–17.

8.   Camilleri M. Peripheral mechanisms in irritable bowel syndrome. *N Engl J Med.* 2012;**367** (17):1626–35. DOI: 10.1056/NEJMra1207068.

9.   Lee YJ, Park KS. Irritable bowel syndrome: emerging paradigm in pathophysiology. *World J Gastroenterol.* 2014;**10**(20):2456–69. DOI: 10.3748/wjg.v20. i10.2456.

10.   Altobelli E, Del Negro V, Angeletti PM, et al. Low-FODMAP diet improves irritable bowel syndrome symptoms: a meta-analysis. *Nutrients.* 2017;**9**:940; DOI: 10.3390/nu9090940.

11.   Lacy BE. Rome criteria and a diagnostic approach to irritable bowel syndrome. *J Clin Med.* 2017;**6**(11):99.

12.   Yang J, Deng Y, Chu H, et al. Prevalence and presentation of lactose intolerance and effects on dairy product intake in healthy subjects and patients with irritable bowel syndrome. *Clin Gastroenterol and Hepatol.* 2013;**11**:262–8.

13.   Zhang Y, Li L, Guo C, et al. Effects of probiotic type, dose and treatment duration on irritable bowel syndrome diagnosed by Rome III criteria: a meta-analysis. *BMC Gastroenterol.* 2016;**16**(1):62.

14.   Vazquez-Roque MI, Camelleri M, Smyrk T, et al. A controlled trial of gluten-free diet in patients with irritable bowel syndrome-diarrhea: effects on bowel frequency and intestinal function. *Gastroenterology.* 2013;**144**(5):903–11. e.3.

15.   Camilleri M, Ford AC. Pharmacotherapy for irritable bowel syndrome. *J Clin Med.* 2017;**6**:101. DOI: 10.3390/jcm6110101.

16.   Rao S, Lembo AJ, Shiff SJ, et al. A 12-week, randomized, controlled trial with a 4-week randomized withdrawal period to evaluate the efficacy and safety of linaclotide in irritable bowel syndrome with constipation. *Am J Gastroenterol.* 2012;**107**:1714–24. DOI: 10.1038/ajg.2012.255.

17.   Chey WD, Lembo AJ, Lavins BJ, et al. Linaclotide for irritable bowel syndrome with constipation: a 26-week, randomized, double-blind, placebo-controlled trial to evaluate efficacy and safety. *Am J Gastroenterol.* 2012; **107**:1702–12; DOI: 10.1038/ajg.2012.254.

18.   Weinberg DS, Smalley W, Heidelbaugh JJ, et al. American Gastroenterological Association Institute guideline on the pharmacological management of irritable bowel syndrome. *Gastroenterology.* 2014;**147**:1146–8.

19.   Lembo AJ, Lacy BE, Zuckerman M, et al. Eluxadoline for irritable bowel syndrome with diarrhea. *N Engl J Med.* 2016;**374**:242–53. DOI: 10.1056/ NEJMoa1505180.

20.   Soares RL. Irritable bowel syndrome: a clinical review. *World J Gastroenterol.*

Vulvodynia

Jorge Carrillo and Georgine Lamvu

Editor's Introduction

Vulvodynia is chronic vulvar pain caused by a variety of conditions outlined in this chapter. Vulvodynia is similar to other chronic pelvic pain conditions in that it requires biopsychosocial evaluation and is best addressed by multi-modal interventions.

Introduction

Vulvar pain is a symptom that was described in the literature as early as the first century AD, by Soranus of Ephesus when he wrote about "Satyriasis in females" [1]. Few publications referred to this type of pain until 1987, when Friedrich described vulvar vestibulitis syndrome as "severe pain on vestibular touch or vaginal entry" [2]. Subsequently, there was little advancement in the classification of chronic vulvar pain trough the 1990s. However, in 2003, the International Society for the Study of Vulvovaginal Diseases (ISSVD) recommended that vulvodynia be defined as chronic vulvar pain occurring for at least 3 months [3]. Additionally, the ISSVD indicated that vulvodynia can be further characterized by location (generalized or localized to the vaginal entrance or clitoris), by whether the pain is provoked by contact or unprovoked, by onset (primary from first genital contact or secondary if it occurred after a pain-free period), and by whether the pain is intermittent or persistent [4]. After recognizing that vulvodynia is a condition experienced by millions of women, the National Institutes of Health convened consensus meetings on the state of vulvodynia research in 2004 and 2011 [5, 6]. These consensus meetings, and subsequent research, suggested that vulvodynia is a heterogeneous disorder and the 2003 diagnostic criteria did not sufficiently describe the spectrum of disease. Therefore, in 2015 the ISSVD, the International Society for the Study of Women's Sexual Health (ISSWSH), and the International Pelvic Pain Society (IPPS) developed new consensus terminology for the classification of persistent vulvar pain [7].

Currently, vulvar pain can be classified as (1) pain caused by a specific disorder, that is, acute or chronic pain with an identifiable cause such as vaginal infections, neoplasms, or neurological disorders; and (2) vulvodynia, which is defined as chronic pain, lasting 3 months or longer without an identifiable cause [7]. Vulvodynia may may be further subtyped based on location, onset, timing, and provocation. Additionally, it is important to note that in this new classification, vulvodynia may also coexist with other disorders such as pelvic floor muscle dysfunction, specific skin disorders such as lichen sclerosus; other comorbid pain syndromes such as interstitial cystitis/bladder pain syndrome (IC/BPS) or irritable bowel syndrome (IBS); and emotional distress such as anxiety, depression, and poor coping [7]. In addition to psychiatric, musculoskeletal, neurological, and inflammatory factors, vulvodynia severity may also be impacted by hormonal, genetic, and environmental factors that are poorly understood [8].

Epidemiology and Burden of Disease

It is estimated that by age 40, 7%–8% of women experience vulvar pain consistent with vulvodynia, making the lifetime prevalence of vulvodynia among women 18–64 years of age approximately 16% [11]. Hispanics are 1.4 times more likely to develop vulvar pain symptoms compared to white women [12]. Research shows that most women who are able to access care self-identify as white (and are educated and employed). Hispanic women are underrepresented in clinical and research settings, suggesting that for nonwhites there may be a significant disparity in access to care and inclusion in research [13, 14].

Table 12.1 Diagnostic criteria for vulvodynia
2015 Consensus Terminology and Classification of Persistent
Vulvar Pain and Vulvodynia

A. Vulvar pain caused by a specific disorder[a]

1. Infectious (e.g., recurrent candidiasis, herpes)
2. Inflammatory (e.g., lichen sclerosus, lichen planus, immunobullous disorders)
3. Neoplastic (e.g., Paget disease, squamous cell carcinoma)
4. Neurological (e.g., postherpetic neuralgia, nerve compression or injury, neuroma)
5. Trauma (e.g., female genital cutting, obstetrical)
6. Iatrogenic (e.g., postoperative, chemotherapy, radiation)
7. Hormonal deficiencies (e.g., genitourinary syndrome of menopause [vulvovaginal atrophy], lactational amenorrhea)

B. Vulvodynia: vulvar pain of at least 3 months' duration, without clear identifiable cause, which may have potential associated factors

The following are the descriptors:

1. Localized (e.g., vestibulodynia, clitorodynia) or generalized or mixed (localized and generalized)
2. Provoked (e.g., insertional, contact) or spontaneous or mixed (provoked and spontaneous)
3. Onset (primary or secondary)
4. Temporal pattern (intermittent, persistent, constant, immediate, delayed)

[a] Women may have both a specific disorder (e.g., lichen sclerosus) and vulvodynia.

Table 12.2 Factors associated with vulvodynia

Potential factors associated with vulvodynia[a]

- Comorbidities and other pain syndromes (e.g., painful bladder syndrome, fibromyalgia, irritable bowel syndrome, temporomandibular disorder; level of evidence 2)
- Genetics (level of evidence 2)
- Hormonal factors (e.g., pharmacologically induced; level of evidence 2)
- Inflammation (level of evidence 2)
- Musculoskeletal (e.g., pelvic muscle overactivity, myofascial, biomechanical; level of evidence 2)
- Neurological mechanisms
- Central (spine, brain; level of evidence 2)
- Peripheral: neuroproliferation (level of evidence 2)
- Psychosocial factors (e.g., mood, interpersonal, coping, role, sexual function; level of evidence 2)
- Structural defects (e.g., perineal descent; level of evidence 3)

[a] Factors could co-occur in patients. The challenge of classifying vulvodynia, and differentiating it from other conditions that can cause (or be associated with) vulvar pain, is further complicated by the fact that some of these inflammatory, neuropathic, and environmental conditions are not easily identified, making vulvodynia difficult to diagnose and consequently difficult to treat [9, 10].

The burden of this disease on women, their partners, families, and communities has been extensively studied and research consistently shows that this disorder can have devastating effects. Women with vulvodynia suffer significant distress and poor quality of life. More than 50% of women experience pain with intercourse and more than 80% fear intercourse or report disabling sexual dysfunction [15]. Women with vulvodynia also tend to have higher somatic awareness, environmental stress, catastrophizing, and psychological distress when compared to pain-free controls [14]. Vulvodynia is four times more likely in women with a mood or anxiety disorder, and women with vulvodynia are seven times more likely to develop a new mood or anxiety disorder [16]. Thus far, it is not yet clear whether psychological symptoms promote the development of vulvodynia, or they develop mostly as a consequence of being in chronic pain.

Research also shows a significant overlap between vulvodynia and other chronic pain conditions such as IBS, IC/BPS, fibromyalgia, chronic fatigue syndrome, migraines, and temporomandibular joint disorders (TMD) [14]. Approximately 20% of vulvodynia patients report being additionally diagnosed with one or more of these disorders [14] and the odds of screening positive for vulvodynia are to three times higher in women who report having IC/BPS, IBS, fibromyalgia, or TMD [17, 18]. Although we do not know with certainty whether the presence of other chronic pain syndromes promotes the development of vulvodynia, the evidence suggests that vulvodynia patients with fewer comorbid pain conditions have a greater chance of responding successfully to treatment [19, 20].

The costs to the US healthcare system have also been studied. A 2012 study reported that a patients with vulvodynia has an average of 8.8 office visits/year [21]. Researchers calculated an annual cost of $17,724.80 per patient with vulvodynia, which converts to an estimated annual national expenditure that ranges from $31 billion to $72 billion (higher than the estimated cost for endometriosis, fibromyalgia, and IC/BPS combined) [21].

Despite the immense burden of disease and personal distress reported by patients, almost 50% of patient never seek care [12]. Of those who seek treatment, 41% see three or more doctors before receiving a diagnosis [12]. On average, women suffer with pain for 2–5 years and fewer than 50% receive a diagnosis. It is estimated that even after being diagnosed with a chronic pain syndrome, fewer than 1.5% of women receive an actual diagnosis of vulvodynia [12, 22]. Anecdotal patient reports and multiple studies confirm that women are not only impacted by the pain, which causes them suffering and distress, but they are also negatively affected by feelings of social isolation and dismissive or invalidating attitudes from their healthcare providers [23, 24].

Anatomy of Vulvar Pain

Anatomically the vulva is the region extending inferiorly from the pubic arch and the inguinal and femoral creases to the perineal body (Figure 12.1). Important anatomical structures within this area include the mons pubis, labia majora, labia minora, clitoris, and clitoral bulbs and the vestibule (Figure 12.1) [25]. Although vulvodynia can be described as pain in any of these areas, the terms vestibulitis, vulvar vestibulitis syndrome, focal vulvitis, vestibular adenitis, and provoked vestibulodynia (PVD) are used to describe a subtype of vulvodynia in which the pain is localized only to the vulvar vestibule and provoked by contact [8]. By contrast, the terms generalized vulvodynia, essential or dysesthetic vulvodynia, and burning vulva syndrome are used to describe a subtype where the pain is unprovoked, diffuse, and affects the entire vulva [8]. The neural distribution for the vulvar area is complex, ts innervation originates from branches of the iliohypogastric, ilioinguinal, genitofemoral, pudendal, posterior femoral cutaneous, and cluneal nerves which in turn arise from the lumbar and sacral plexuses (Table 12.3, Figure 12.1).

Vulvar pain can result from damage, inflammation, or entrapment of any of these nerves resulting in a complexity of overlapping pain dermatomes (Figure 12.2). Patients may present with local or generalized pain, and both subtypes may present with spontaneous or provoked pain. At this point it is not clear whether provoked, unprovoked, localized, or generalized vulvar pain has overlapping or distinct pathophysiology. Additionally, because of this anatomical location, women with vulvar pain may experience symptoms not only with intercourse but also with daily activities such as sitting and walking.

Pathophysiology

Vulvodynia is characterized by chronic vulvar or vaginal pain that is often described by patients as burning, stinging, irritation, or rawness [4, 8]. Vaginal mucosa changes, neuronal proliferation and hyperactivity, central nervous system processing abnormalities, muscular dysfunction, heightened inflammatory response, psychological conditions, and genetic polymorphisms are all thought to play a role in the development, maintenance, and progression of pain [26, 27].

Hypersensitivity of the vulvar vestibule is one of the defining characteristics of vulvodynia (especially PVD); however, the mechanisms for this hypersensitivity are not well understood. Studies show that women with localized vulvodynia exhibit abnormally low sensory thresholds and increased nerve fiber proliferation (particularly hyperexcitable nociceptors) in vestibular tissue resulting in allodynia (painful response to a nonpainful stimulus such as light touch with a cotton-swab) and peripheral sensitization [26, 28–32]. Interestingly, this increased pain sensitivity is also present at nongenital sites (e.g., forearm), suggesting that these women may also experience central nervous system sensitization (central sensitization), perhaps explaining the high

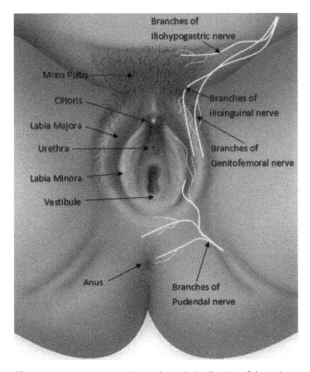

Figure 12.1 Anatomy and neurological distribution of the vulvar innervation.

Table 12.3 Abdominopelvic nerves and function

Nerve (root)	Motor innervation	Cutaneous innervation
Iliohypogastric (T12–L1)	Internal oblique	Lateral lower abdominal wall, suprapubic area, superior mons pubis, and lateral gluteal area
Ilioinguinal (T12–L1)	Internal oblique	Lateral lower abdominal wall, groin, mons of pubis, labia majora, scrotum
Genitofemoral (L1–L2)	Cremaster (males)	Groin, mons, labia majora, scrotum, upper anterior thigh
Obturator (L2–L3–L4)	Adductors, gracilis, and pectineal muscles, obturator externus	Superior inner thigh
Pudendal (S2–S3–S4)	Bulbospongiosus, ischiocavernosus, superficial and deep transverse of perineum, external sphincter of urethra, external anal sphincter	Clitoris, penis, labia majora and minora, vestibulum, perianal area, lower third of rectum
Posterior femoral cutaneous (S1, S2, S3)	n/a	Inferior buttocks, lateral perineum, proximal posteromedial thigh, posterolateral scrotum/labia majora, and part of penis/clitoris

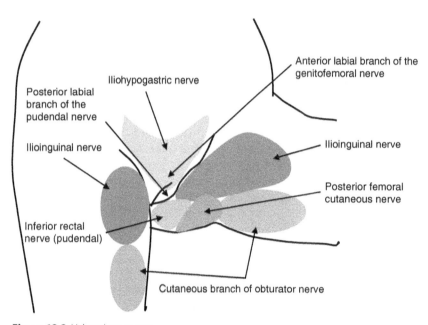

Figure 12.2 Vulvar dermatomes.

prevalence of comorbid nongenital pain syndromes, such as IBS, PBS, and fibromyalgia, found in vulvodynia patients [14, 32]. The concept of central sensitization playing a role in vulvodynia is additionally supported by several functional and structural brain imaging studies showing that women with a particular subtype of vulvodynia, PVD, demonstrate augmented neural activity in areas of the brain associated with increased perception to non-painful and painful stimulation of the vestibule [33].

Other imaging studies confirm heightened activation in areas of the brain involved in pain processing and changes in gray matter density in women with PVD compared to controls [32, 34]. Together, these findings are interpreted by scientists as evidence that augmented sensory processing [32] is an important pathophysiological process in vulvodynia.

Periodic swelling and erythema of the vestibule and vulva is another symptom commonly described by vulvodynia patients. Generally, erythema is recognized as an indicator of an underlying infectious process; however, in vulvodynia, erythema is not a reliable diagnostic marker for the presence of infection. Once acute infectious processes are ruled out, persistent erythema is thought to occur due to a persistent neuroinflammatory response, whereby an exaggerated inflammatory response, characterized by excess release of proinflammatory cytokines (e.g., interleukin [IL]-1β, IL-6, tumor necrosis factor [TNF]-α), leads proliferation of nociceptive fibers with lower thresholds, ensuing in pain and a process known as neurogenic inflammation [26, 35]. Histological studies show that evidence of neurogenic inflammation is not consistently identified in all cases of vulvodynia, leading researchers to question whether vulvodynia is an inflammatory condition at all [32].

Scientists speculate that the proinflammatory and hyperactive neuroendocrine histological markers found in women with chronic vulvar pain may be linked to specific genetic polymorphisms. To date, no single genetic marker for vulvodynia has been identified; however, genetic studies are focusing on (1) polymorphisms that increase the risks of candidiasis or other infections, (2) polymorphisms for an exaggerated inflammatory response, and (3) genetic markers for increased susceptibility to hormonal changes caused by oral contraceptives [32].

Although the role of hormones is well understood in the postmenopausal state, where hypoestrogenism is known to lead to vaginal atrophy and pain, the role of hormones and altered estrogen receptor function in promoting neurogenic inflammation or sensory abnormalities in premenopausal women is less well understood. Initial histological studies in reproductive aged women with vulvodynia identified vaginal samples containing "skip lesions" that lack estrogen receptors [36]. Other studies suggest that decreasing serum estradiol levels associated with use of oral combined hormonal contraceptives (CHCs) may lead to decreases in mechanical pain thresholds [32]. However, although some case-controlled studies suggest a link between CHCs and developing vulvodynia, this finding has not been consistently replicated in larger population based prospective studies [32].

Pelvic floor muscle dysfunction and pain are commonly found in women with vulvodynia; when using reliable methodology for examining the vaginal musculature, more than 90% of women enrolled in the National Vulvodynia Registry (NVR) had abnormal muscular exams [9]. Women with vulvodynia are reported to have lower pelvic muscle pressure pain thresholds, increased resting tone, impaired voluntary relaxation, and decreased voluntary muscle contractility [27]. In general, vulvodynia is associated with pelvic floor muscle overactivity and weakness. Chronic changes in muscle tissue can lead to hypoxia and perhaps neurogenic inflammation that can manifest as itching, burning, tingling, cold, or sharp and shooting pain in the vulvar and/or vaginal areas [32]. Changes in the biomechanics of the pelvic musculature can result from events such as acute infection, vaginal childbirth, and abdominal and pelvic surgery; thus in some cases, vulvodynia can result from deficiencies in the pelvic musculature that are due to a previous traumatic event [32]. In other cases, the muscular dysfunction is thought to be a secondary process, that is, the muscular dysfunction develops secondary to chronic mucosal inflammation and vulvar pain [37].

The brief review provided previously does not cover the extent of all vulvodynia research. Although the exact pathophysiology of vulvodynia is not yet understood, there is little doubt that it may involve multiple processes, that is, that women may develop the symptom of chronic vulvar pain via different mechanisms. Additionally, psychosocial factors such as depression, anxiety, physical and sexual abuse, sexual dysfunction, and partner and relationship influences have all been implicated in the development and maintenance of vulvar pain [32]. Hence a multifactorial/multidisciplinary approach is key to the diagnosis and treatment of this condition [7].

Clinical Presentation

Often the pain experienced by women is described as burning, stabbing, shooting pain, in the vulvar or vaginal area [4, 8]. Patients may also present with complaints of itching or a chronic (noninfectious) discharge. Although erythema and discharge may be present, it is important to remember that in vulvodynia, these symptoms are not reliably associated with infectious causes, despite studies suggesting that recurrent yeast infections and specially *Candida albicans* may predispose women to developing vulvodynia [27, 32].

The pain can be described as localized to a specific area or generalized; among women enrolled in the NVR, 10% presented with generalized vulvar pain and 90% presented with pain localized to the vestibule [9]. Pain during touch or intercourse (provoked pain) is reported by most women who are sexually active and some continue to be sexually active despite being in pain [9]. As previously stated, a substantial proportion of patients have signs of pelvic floor muscle dysfunction that often manifests as dyspareunia [14]. Approximately 20% of women will report comorbid pain conditions such as IBS, PBS, migraines, TMD, fibromyalgia, and chronic pelvic pain [9, 15] and nearly 40% will present with signs of distress such as anxiety, depression, and sexual dysfunction [9, 14]. Sometimes women are able to identify a specific trigger such as trauma (including surgical interventions), vaginal childbirth, recurrent vaginal or bladder infections, hormonal changes, and oral contraceptive use; however, in many of cases a specific trigger is not clearly identified [32].

Clinical Evaluation

Vulvodynia is a chronic pain syndrome; therefore, an extensive biopsychosocial assessment that begins with a history and physical exam is crucial to determining the source and impact of the pain [38]. The widespread impact and the high proportion of women who do not seek care emphasizes the need for screening, especially for women who present with other chronic pain syndromes [14]. Although validated screening questionnaires are available [22], screening can be easily done by asking women whether they experience pain with activities such as sitting, walking, or intercourse. Many women report being invalidated and dismissed [23, 39] by providers, family, and peers. Therefore, after screening, the next step in the evaluation should include establishing rapport and trust through validation of the patient's symptoms. In addition, it is important to remember that many women will not discuss symptoms related to sexuality or sexual pain, until they feel they can trust their healthcare provider. Overall, the goal of the initial (and subsequent) medical interviews should be to (1) validate the patient's symptoms, (2) gather relevant medical history that may help identify causes of pain, and (3) provide education and reassurance [13].

Classically vulvodynia has been described as a diagnosis of exclusion where clinicians are taught to first determine if there is an obvious cause for the pain. This task can be overwhelming because

comorbidities that may cause (or have been associated with) vulvodynia include vulvar/vaginal infection such as recurrent yeast or bacterial vaginosis, inflammation from vulvar dermatoses such as lichen sclerosus; neoplasm; trauma from life events such as childbirth; trauma from sexual abuse; iatrogenic trauma such as surgery; hormonal deficiencies that may or may not be associated with vaginal atrophy; neuropathies such as pudendal neuralgia, pelvic floor muscle dysfunction; structural defects; visceral pain syndromes such as IBS, PBS, and endometriosis, and psychosocial factors such as anxiety and sexual dysfunction [13, 14]. At minimum, a detailed history should review (1) a general medical, surgical, and obstetrical history; (2) pain characteristics (location, duration, exacerbating factors); (3) associated symptoms such as bowel, bladder, or musculoskeletal symptoms; (4) sexual behavior and sexuality; (5) psychological history; (6) comorbid medical problems; (7) previous treatments; and (8) physical or sexual abuse [13]. Before considering lengthy differential diagnoses, it may be more efficient for providers to categorize the patient's symptoms by organ systems, that is, urological, gastroenterological, reproductive, musculoskeletal, neurological, psychiatric. It is also important to note that this type of extensive history taking may require more than the time allotted to the first visit. Moreover, some patients may not disclose some information until they feel they can trust the provider; thus important elements of the history may not become evident until subsequent visits. Validated questionnaires such as the Female Sexual Function Index (FSFI), the McGill Pain Questionnaire (MPQ), or the PROMIS® vulvar discomfort scales, are more helpful than asking patients to rate their pain from 0 to 10 and allow patients to provide self-reported pain measures that give clinicians a better understanding of the quality, intensity, and impact of the pain on daily activities and quality of life. In addition, questionnaires are efficient and allow providers to collect a large amount of information in the limited clinical time available for face-to-face interaction [13].

Questions about the quality of pain, location, radiation pattern, intensity, factors that improve symptoms or worsen symptoms, and therapies tried previously and their impact on symptoms are essential and should be included in the history taking process. When painful intercourse is reported as a symptom, providers should clarify if the discomfort is perceived either upon entry or deep penetration, or both. The use of a pain map is useful to localize the pain and research has shown that patients with multiple pain areas (generalized pain) are more likely to exhibit signs of central sensitization [40], which has been associated with the need for multidisciplinary treatments [41]. Women may also use pain descriptors such as burning, stinging, hotness, rawness, and irritation, which have been associated with neuropathic pain [42]. Identifying such descriptors in combination with a specific neuralgia could lead the clinician to investigate a neuropathy as a cause of symptoms.

Research confirms that women want information about the examination process before, during, and after the physical evaluation [43]. Experts recommend the physical inspection start by first educating the patient about the examination; the anatomy that will be examined; and the reasons for performing the assessment, that is, what information will be obtained during the examination [8, 39, 44]. A strategy used to minimize anxiety and discomfort during the examination is the interactive educational pelvic examination, which includes (1) explanations to the patient while performing the assessment, (2) describing the specific actions during each step, and (3) using a mirror to enable the patient to visualize her anatomy and the examination [8, 45]. This allows the clinician to thoroughly evaluate the patient's pain, exclude diagnoses, educate the patient regarding normal anatomy and sexual function, and reassure the patient when no pathology is uncovered [46, 47].

In women with vulvodynia, the physical examination starts with a general assessment of the patient's mood, affect, and musculoskeletal status before proceeding to the pelvic evaluation. The nongenital musculoskeletal examination includes evaluation of the patient's gait; posture in standing and sitting positions; palpation of the back, abdominal, gluteal, and upper lower extremity muscles; palpation of the sacroiliac joints; and assessment of muscle strength, range of motion, sensation and reflexes. Palpation of these areas can identify areas of pain, hypercontractility, and instability [48].

The next step, the pelvic examination, begins with an external inspection of the vulvar and perineal areas to identify lesions, scars, or signs of trauma; dermatological changes; or signs of infection such as discharge. Vestibular erythema may be present; however, as previously stated, this is not consistently found in women with vulvodynia, and often, the external examination is normal. After visual inspection, providers should perform a neurosensory evaluation to identify areas of allodynia, a painful response to a nonpainful stimulation, such as light touch with the cotton end of a cotton-tipped applicator, or hyperalgesia, an excessively painful response to a painful stimulus such as the wooden end of a cotton-tipped applicator. Unilateral or bilateral allodynia and/or hyperalgesia in the S2–S4 neuronal distribution of the vulva and perineum, or absence of an anal wink reflex, may be indicators of neuropathies such as pudendal neuralgia that can also present as vulvodynia [49, 50]. Neuropathic pain can also be identified in nongenital areas, such as the abdomen and lower back, by using similar testing to identify allodynia and hyperalgesia. Neuropathies should be suspected in patients presenting with (1) pain that radiates along a particular dermatomal distribution and (2) risk factors such as a history of surgical interventions, trauma, childbirth, and repetitive activities such as long-distance cycling or prolonged sitting [51, 52].

Vulvodynia can also be characterized with a neurosensory exam of the vestibular area. The cotton swab test is performed by applying gentle pressure to six anatomical sites on the vestibule using the face of a clock for reference, where 12 o'clock and 6 o'clock correspond to the midline just below the urethra and midline at the level of the posterior fourchette that is just above the anus (Figure 12.3). This type of neurosensory testing can help localize areas of tenderness and distinguish localized from generalized pain. Branches of the ilioinguinal, iliohypogastric, and pudendal nerves all contribute to the sensory innervation of the vulva; thus the cotton-tipped evaluation can also identify neuropathies in these corresponding dermatomal distributions.

After inspection of the perineum, a single-digit examination can be used to assess the pelvic floor muscles for strength, tone, and pain. The internal musculoskeletal single-digit examination is the most reliable method for assessing pelvic muscle tenderness [48]. To perform this part of the examination, the examiner can gently and slowly insert a lubricated digit into the vagina and ask the patient to squeeze and relax around the digit. Next, the

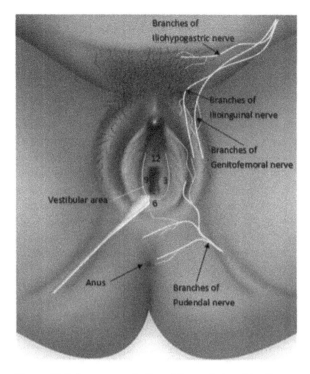

Branches of
Iliohypogastric nerve

Branches of
Ilioinguinal nerve

Branches of
Genitofemoral nerve

12

Vestibular area

6

Anus

Branches of
Pudendal nerve

Figure 12.3 Sensory examination of the vestibule to identify vestibular allodynia.

examiner can palpate the levator ani, piriformis, obturator, and coccygeus muscles by applying deep palpation to the lateral, anterior, and posterior vaginal walls. The Valliex's sign can be done by pressing medial to the ischial spine bilaterally, in order to stimulate the pudendal nerve at the point of nerve injury and identify radiation of pain or paresthesia along the course of the nerve [8]. Tenderness, high tone, and involuntary spasm with mild or moderate palpation of the muscles of the vaginal introitus and the pelvic floor is abnormal; pelvic floor muscles can normally tolerate as much as 2 kilograms of pressure without pain. Pain elicited during this portion of the examination can be indicative of myalgias and pelvic floor muscle dysfunction.

Cotton-tipped examination of the vestibule and the single-digit examination are considered essential to the diagnosis of vulvodynia; however, studies show there is little correspondence between higher levels of pain during daily activities such as intercourse and what providers can replicate with the cotton-tipped applicator test or the single-digit examination [13]. In fact, patients may demonstrate improvements in pain

during clinical evaluation without demonstrable improvement in pain or function outside clinical settings. In such cases, the "gold-standard" cotton-tipped test may underestimate the degree of pain and distress experienced by women in their daily lives [13] and it is recommended that providers follow patient reported outcomes instead.

If the patient can tolerate a single-digit muscular assessment, a bimanual evaluation of the uterus and adnexa can be completed before proceeding to the speculum examination. The speculum may cause extreme discomfort in patients with vulvodynia, as such it should be performed using lubrication and slow insertion that avoids touching the urethra or pinching the cervix. At this time, vaginal culture and swabs can be collected to rule out infections and dysplasia. For patients who cannot tolerate single-digit examination the speculum examination may be postponed to subsequent visits after treatment is initiated, unless concerning symptoms such as bleeding or discharge are reported by the patient.

The diagnosis of vulvodynia is based primarily on patient symptoms and clinical examination, including findings of the cotton swab test [53–56]. Additional diagnostic tests such as urinalysis, pelvic ultrasound, or CT scan are not necessary unless patients present with urinary or GI symptoms, pelvic pain, pelvic mass identified on examination, and bleeding abnormalities.

Treatments

Because vulvodynia is a chronic pain disorder and current treatment recommendations vary, treatment selection can be challenging. Therapies should be targeted if a specific cause for the pain is identified (e.g., antimicrobials for vaginal infections, physical therapy for pelvic myalgias). However, in most cases there are multiple factors contributing to pain and poor quality of life, requiring multiple treatments (physical, emotional, and behavioral) individualized to patient needs. This often involves a team approach with providers from fields such as gynecology, gastroenterology, urology, physical therapy, pain management, and mental health. Treatment should start with conservative, noninvasive approaches, as surgery is rarely necessary. Medical therapies for vulvodynia include education and life-style modification, physical therapy, topical anesthetics, tricyclic antidepressants (TCAs), oral or topical hormonal treatments, oral antiinflammatory agents, intramuscular Botox, trigger point injections, anesthetic blocks, physical therapy, cognitive behavioral therapy (and other types of brain-based therapies), and surgery.

The most recent evidence-based review of vulvodynia treatments was published by Goldstein et al. in 2016 [8]. Although all treatment options are described in this chapter, it is important to note that according to Goldstein and colleagues, the evidence supports the following recommendations:

- Psychological interventions and physical therapy are recommended (grade B) based on Level II and III evidence.
- Vestibulectomy is recommended with caution for PVD only, once less invasive treatments have been attempted (grade B) based on Level II and III evidence.
- Tricyclic antidepressants are *not* recommended for management of PVD alone (grade A) based on Level I evidence, although TCAs are recommended for the management of pain in patients with centralized pain syndromes.
- Topical corticosteroids are *not* recommended (grade C) based on Level III–V evidence.
- Lidocaine ointment is not recommended for long-term use for PVD (grade B) based on Level II and III evidence, although it may be beneficial for short-term use.
- There is not enough evidence to recommend antiinflammatory agents, anticonvulsants, hormonal treatments, capsaicin, and botulinum toxin A as first-line treatments.

Education

An understanding of what we currently know about vulvodynia could lead to decrease levels of anxiety and improve therapeutic response [54, 56, 57]; therefore, extensive education is recommended for all patients. Providers should review pelvic anatomy, physiology, lifestyle modifications, treatment options, and expectations.

Lifestyle modification based on recommendations by the National Vulvodynia Association and the American College of Obstetricians and Gynecologists [55] can be helpful. Gentle vulvar care or hygiene is recommended, including (1) avoiding potential irritants (such as soap, shampoo, scented toilet paper, menstrual pads or tampons, fabric softener on underwear); (2) avoiding excessive washing of the vagina; (3) avoiding tight fitting clothes; and (4) using soft white unscented toilet paper [58]. Women

should be instructed to use lubrication during sexual intercourse and to avoid contraceptive creams, spermicides, and daily activities that worsen the pain. Generally, it is also advisable to avoid activities that put constant pressure on the vulva, such as bicycle or horseback riding.

During the educational session, it is important to discuss realistic treatment expectations, acknowledging that treatment often involves multiple therapies at the same time, from multidisciplinary healthcare teams, sometimes over a prolonged period of time. As in other chronic pain syndromes, a "cure" may not be attainable; instead patients may experience improvements in pain and still require life-long changes in lifestyle and behavior. Lastly, providers must review treatment options in such a way that patients feel empowered to make informed medical decisions [13].

Physical Therapy

Physical therapy is useful in patients who demonstrate an abnormal musculoskeletal exam (internal and external) and the goal of physical therapy is to decrease muscle tone and tension, which leads to decreased pain and improved muscle function. Different strategies, internal and external, can be used to improve muscle function including education, pelvic floor exercises, manual therapy techniques, pelvic floor and girdle reeducation, and home exercises. Other modalities that can be used to improve muscle function and tone include vaginal dilators, ultrasound, electrical stimulation, or biofeedback [53, 55, 59].

In a recent systematic review performed by Morin et al. on the effectiveness of physical therapy modalities in women with provoked vestibulodynia, researchers found ample variation in modalities used and the duration of treatment, making it difficult to establish standardized guidelines for treating patients. Nonetheless, researchers concluded that biofeedback, dilators, electrical stimulation, education, and physical therapy is consistently effective for decreasing pain during intercourse and could improve sexual function [60]. Moreover, multimodal physical therapy showed consistent effectiveness across studies, with a significant improvement of pain in up to 80% of women with provoked vestibulodynia [60].

Psychological Interventions

In general depression, anxiety, catastrophization, and poor coping are conditions frequently encountered in chronic pain conditions, and there is enough evidence supporting the association of these conditions with vulvodynia as well. Elevated levels of emotional distress have been directly linked with higher levels of pain [61]. An abundance of research suggests that pain-related psychological distress is linked to sexual dysfunction, that is, pain and distress can lead to fear and avoidance of intercourse eventually affecting intimacy and the ability to maintain healthy relationships [62]. Pain, anxiety and fear of experiencing pain can also contribute to pelvic floor muscle hypertonicity and spasm, which in turn can contribute to a vicious cycle of worsening pain and sexual dysfunction that may include decreases in arousal, desire, satisfaction, and lubrication [63].

Psychological interventions aim to decrease pain, emotional distress, and sexual function. Cognitive-behavioral therapy (CBT) uses techniques that generally focus on behavior that decreases genital pain, reduces anticipatory fear of pain, and improves overall sexual function for patients and their partners. CBT is the most studied for the treatment of vulvodynia and has been shown in randomized controlled trials (RCTs) to be an effective modality for improving many aspects of genito-pelvic pain including catastrophizing, satisfaction with treatment, and improvements in sexual functioning compared with women who did not receive CBT [8, 63–65]. The results of these RCTs, the high prevalence of psychiatric distress and sexual dysfunction among women with vulvodynia, and the association of high levels of distress with high levels of pain lead us to recommend that women with vulvodynia should be:

1. Screened for emotional distress and psychiatric and sexual dysfunction
2. Referred for psychiatric interventions such as CBT and sexual and relationship therapy if needed
3. Referred for psychiatric intervention if they show signs of severe anxiety or depression
4. Treated with psychiatric interventions in conjunction with pain management using other medical, pharmacological, or surgical interventions

Other techniques such as mindfulness, meditation, and hypnosis have not been rigorously studied and thus evidence is lacking to support routine use of these techniques for the treatment of vulvodynia;

however, they are noninvasive and show promise in other chronic pain syndromes [62].

Topical Treatments Targeting Peripheral Nociceptors

Sodium channel blockade of peripheral nociceptors can block discharge and transmission pain signals from peripheral sensory nerves. Sensitization of peripheral nerves has been suggested as a potential mechanism for the development of provoked vestibulodynia [66]. Therefore, local anesthetics were thought to be possible inhibitors of pain and several studies report on the use of topical ointments and submucosal injections using lidocaine. Zolnoun and colleagues demonstrated that 5% topical lidocaine applied nightly can provide significant pain relief for up to 6 months [67]. However, this was an uncontrolled study and a subsequent double-blinded RCT using lidocaine failed to show any benefit [8]. Three case series reported that patients had pain relief after anesthetic injections (lidocaine, ropivacaine, and bupivacaine); unfortunately, these findings were never confirmed with larger controlled trials [8]. Therefore, at this time, topical lidocaine is recommended only in patients with PVD for short-term management (less than 6 months). It can be used nightly, during intercourse, or before physical therapy for limited comfort.

Capsaicin, which has been shown to produce desensitization of peripheral nociceptors that mediate burning and pain, and botulinum type A, which is hypothesized to also decrease peripheral and central sensitization, have been studied. Capsaicin was thought to be effective in small uncontrolled studies; however, in these studies it was coadministered with lidocaine because capsaicin can cause burning and irritation on application. Thus, capsaicin use is not recommended for the treatment of vulvodynia [8]. Botulinum toxin A, with doses ranging from 20 IU to 100 IU injected into superficial perineal muscles or the deep pelvic floor, has been studied in uncontrolled studies and one RCT with conflicting results; therefore there is not enough evidence to recommend its use as first-line treatment [8].

Topical Treatments Targeting Inflammation

Higher tissue levels of interleukin-B and cytokines, as well as increased mast cell activity, have all been demonstrated in patients with PVD compared to controls. As a result, antiinflammatory agents such as corticosteroids, interferon, and cromolyn have been studied as potential therapeutic agents for vulvodynia. Although data on these agents are still emerging, study results can be generalized as follows [8]:

- Topical low potency corticosteroids are minimally effective in PVD; additionally, there is not enough evidence to support use of low-potency steroids in anesthetic injections and the potential side effects of high-potency corticosteroids are significant enough to recommend against their use.
- Interferon, a potent mast cell inhibitor, may lead to modest improvements in pain when injected into the vestibular area; however, RCTs using this intervention are lacking and its use cannot be recommended as a first-line treatment.
- Cromolyn cream, a mast cell stabilizer, was shown to reduce pain in a very small double-blind, placebo-controlled RCT; there are no additional data to evaluate in order to recommend its use.
- Cell lysate of fetal fibroblasts, thought to contain different antiinflammatory cytokines, was shown in a small RCT to decrease vestibular pain and dyspareunia; however, there are no additional studies that replicate these results.
- Low-molecular-weight heparin injected into the vestibule was shown to decrease vestibular pain in a small RCT of 40 patients. These results have not been replicated in other studies.

Overall, although some of these therapies seem promising, there is not yet enough evidence to recommend their use except as experimental therapies.

Hormonal Treatments

Estrogen has been shown to restore normal vaginal pH and help thicken and revascularize the vaginal epithelium of postmenopausal women [68]. In cases in which vaginal pain and dryness are attributed to postmenopausal vaginal atrophy, vaginal estrogen is available in a variety of FDA-approved topical and oral formulations, including a selective estrogen receptor modulators (SERM). An RCT conducted by Foster et al. found that topical estradiol decreased pain sensitivity in postmenopausal women with mixed vulvovaginal pain [69].

However, the use of estrogen therapy in premenopausal women who have no visual evidence of vaginal atrophy and yet suffer with vulvodynia has been debated. In an uncontrolled series, Burrows and colleagues reported that topical estradiol (0.01%) combined with testosterone (0.1%) decreased pain in women with PVD who were thought to have developed pain from combined oral contraceptive use (which in itself is still being debated) [70]. At this time, the evidence supports the use of estrogen and SERM formulations in postmenopausal women with vaginal atrophy and pain; however there is not yet enough evidence to support the use of hormonal treatments in premenopausal women.

When using hormonal treatments care must be taken to limit use in women who do not have contraindications to estrogen use, such as a history of recent or active breast cancer, stroke, or cardiovascular disease. In addition, hormonal therapy may take as long as 4–8 weeks to provide symptomatic relief. Lastly, except for one uncontrolled study done in 1997 [71], topical testosterone has not been well studied for pain relief. Furthermore, the FDA approved testosterone use only for men and in addition issued an advisory highlighting the potentially increased risk of heart attack and stroke, risks that have not been well studied in women [72]. Given the lack of data confirming benefit for pain relief and the potential for significant risk, testosterone topical therapy should not be recommended to women with vulvodynia.

Systemic Oral Medications

TCAs such as amitriptyline have been shown to decrease peripheral nerve sensitization in patients with neuropathic pain. The use of TCAs for management of pain in women with vulvodynia was initially recommended as a treatment option by several treatment guidelines [4, 73]. This recommendation was based on several descriptive and uncontrolled studies and unsubstantiated by RCTs [74]. A more recent systematic review of the evidence on using antidepressant pharmacotherapy for the treatment of vulvodynia pain concluded that there is not enough evidence to support the use of antidepressants as a treatment option for providing pain relief in vulvodynia patients, although they may provide relief from other symptoms associated with vulvodynia such as depression, anxiety, and sleep deprivation [74]. When the decision is made to use TCA therapy, dose titration is recommended, as side effects may be difficult to tolerate and include constipation, dry mouth, sedation, cognitive impairment, and sexual dysfunction. Selective norepinephrine reuptake inhibitors (SNRIs) such as duloxetine or venlafaxine are used for treatment of pain and depression in patients with other chronic pain conditions and have a better side effect profile. However, there are no studies to evaluate the effect of these drugs on vulvodynia [8, 53, 74].

Calcium channel blockers such as gabapentin and pregabalin are membrane stabilizers that are beneficial for patients with chronic neuropathic pain and have been increasingly used for treatment of vulvodynia based on initial uncontrolled studies that reported gabapentin efficacy to range between 50% and 82% [8, 53, 54, 56]. However, a 2013 literature review by Leo and colleagues concluded that the evidence to support use of anticonvulsants, including gabapentin, was limited and based predominantly on descriptive reports [74]. Systematic RCTs on using anticonvulsants for the treatment of vulvodynia have not been successfully conducted. If this class of medication is used, dose titration and a discussion of common side effects (drowsiness, dizziness, nausea, vomiting, edema, headache) [75] are advised.

Surgical Treatment

Surgical excision of the posterior vestibule and hymeneal ring mucosa is a procedure offered to patients who fail to respond to conservative measures. This procedure, known as a vestibulectomy, was first performed in 1981 [76] and has since undergone several technical modifications. Currently the two most commonly used techniques involve a complete vulvar vestibulectomy or a modified partial vestibulectomy, both with a vaginal flap advancement.

Vulvar vestibulectomy is a procedure that is reportedly helpful in patients; low-quality research that suggests the overall success rate of vestibulectomy (in patients who have failed other therapies) ranges from 60% to 90%. However, this research is plagued by lack of standardization of the surgical techniques, patient selection that does not distinguish between various forms of vestibular pain (although most studies are limited to patients with localized pain and PVD), and variability in the length of follow-up. At this time, based on the limited data available, vestibulectomy should be reserved for patients with localized pain (PVD) after less invasive conservative treatments have failed. Patients should be educated that although the pain may improve, there is no evidence that this procedure improves long-term sexual well-being and function [8]. In addition, surgical intervention should not be offered to patients with generalized or unprovoked vulvodynia [8, 53, 56, 77–79].

Summary

Vulvodynia is a heterogeneous chronic pain disorder resulting from a complex interplay of biopsychosocial factors. An extensive history and physical examination are key to making the correct diagnosis and excluding acute and treatable causes for pain. Emphasis should be placed on screening for vaginal pain, pain during intercourse, other chronic pain disorders, and biopsychosocial factors that affect pain and well-being such as emotional distress, sleep disorders, and sexual dysfunction. Current vulvodynia treatment guidelines describe a variety of therapies that, except for physical therapy and psychological interventions, are not supported by convincing evidence. As a result, patients and providers are often left to experimenting with a variety of treatments for extended periods of time. A recent report from the National Vulvodynia Registry showed that in a cohort of approximately 300 women, providers prescribed 78 individual treatments [10]. Despite this wide variation in treatment selection, patients consistently reported improvements in quality of life, distress, and pain, regardless of the number of treatments prescribed at the first visit [10]. Surprisingly, the authors also found that sexual function continued to worsen over the course of treatment, leading to the recommendation that in addition to pain and distress, providers need to continuously screen women for sexual dysfunction, and sexual therapy should be incorporated into the treatment plan when necessary [10]. Despite wide variation in treatment selection and outcomes, experts recommend multimodal and interdisciplinary care that addresses all components of the patient's pain and dysfunction [8].

Five Things You Need to Know

- Vulvodynia is a common condition that is underreported issues of invalidation and social stigmatization.
- Vulvodynia has many elements in common with other chronic pain conditions; thus the biopsychosocial model of evaluation and treatment applies to vulvodynia, as it does in other chronic pain syndromes.
- In addition to pain, patients with this condition also report physical disability, psychological distress, and sexual dysfunction.

- The clinical evaluation should include a full internal and external musculoskeletal examination, as many patients with vulvar pain also have associated myalgias and pelvic floor muscle dysfunction.

- Although many treatments are described in the literature, the bulk of the evidence supports the use of pelvic floor physical therapy and cognitive behavioral interventions as primary treatments for this type of pain.

References

1. McElhiney J, Kelly S, Rosen R, Bachmann GA. Satyriasis: the antiquity term for vulvodynia? *J Sex Med.* 2006;3(1):161–3. DOI: 10.1111/j.1743-6109.2005.00171.x.

2. Friedrich EG Jr. The vulvar vestibule. *J Reprod Med.* 1983;28(11):773–7.

3. Moyal-Barracco M, Lynch PJ. 2003 ISSVD terminology and classification of vulvodynia. *J Reprod Med.* 2004;49(10):772–7. DOI: 10.3109/01443615.2015.1019437.

4. Haefner HK, Collins ME, Davis GD, et al. The vulvodynia guideline. *J Low Genit Tract Dis.* 2005;9:40–51. DOI: 10.1097/00128360-200501000-00009.

5. U.S. Department of Health and Human Services (DHHS), National Institutes of Health, and National Institute of Child Health and Human Development. The research plan on vulvodynia. 2012. www1.nichd.nih.gov/publications/pubs/documents/NIH_Vulvodynia_Plan_April2012.pdf

6. Bachmann G a, Rosen R, Pinn VW, et al. Vulvodynia: a state-of-the-art consensus on definitions, diagnosis and management. *J Reprod Med.* 2006;51(6):447–56.

7. Bornstein J, Goldstein AT, Stockdale CK, et al. 2015 ISSVD, ISSWSH, and IPPS consensus terminology and classification of persistent vulvar pain and vulvodynia. *J Sex Med.* 2016;20(2):126–30. DOI: 10.1097/AOG.0000000000001359.

8. Goldstein AT, Pukall CF, Brown C, Bergeron S, Stein A, Kellogg-Spadt S. Vulvodynia: assessment and treatment. *J Sex Med.* 2016;13(4):572–90. DOI: 10.1016/j.jsxm.2016.01.020.

9. Lamvu G, Nguyen RHN, Burrows LJ, et al. The evidence-based Vulvodynia Assessment Project: a national registry for the study of vulvodynia. *J Reprod Med.* 2015;60(5–6):223–35.

10. Lamvu G, Alappattu M, Witzeman K, Bishop M, Robinson M, Rapkin A. Patterns in vulvodynia treatments and 6-month outcomes for women enrolled in the National Vulvodynia Registry: an exploratory prospective study. *J Sex Med.* 2018;15(5):705–15.

11. Harlow BL, Stewart EG. A population-based assessment of chronic unexplained vulvar pain: have we underestimated the prevalence of vulvodynia? *J Am Med Womens Assoc.* 2003;58(2):82–8.

12. Harlow BL, Kunitz CG, Nguyen RHN, Rydell SA, Turner RM, Maclehose RF. Prevalence of symptoms consistent with a diagnosis of vulvodynia: population-based estimates from 2 geographic regions. *Am J Obstet Gynecol.* 2014;210(1):2–9. DOI: 10.1016/j.ajog.2013.09.033.

13. Sorensen J, Bautista K, Lamvu G, Feranec J. Evaluation and treatment of female sexual pain: a clinical review. *Cureus.* 2018;10(3):e2379. DOI: 10.7759/cureus.2379.

14. Lamvu G, Barron K. Vulvodynia: a prevalent yet underdiagnosed chronic pain syndrome. *PainWeek J.* 2015;3(Q1):14–21.

15. Arnold LD, Bachmann GA, Rosen R, Kelly S, Rhoads GG. Vulvodynia: characteristics and associations with comorbidities and quality of life. *Obstet Gynecol.* 2006;107(3):617–24. DOI: 10.1097/01.AOG.0000199951.26822.27.

16. Khandker M, Brady SS, Vitonis AF, MacLehose RF, Stewart EG, Harlow BL. The influence of depression and anxiety on risk of adult onset vulvodynia. *J Womens Health.* 2011;20(10):1445–51. DOI: 10.1089/jwh.2010.2661.

17. Reed BD, Harlow SD, Sen A, Edwards RM, Chen D, Haefner HK. Relationship between vulvodynia and chronic comorbid pain conditions. *Obstet Gynecol.* 2012;120(1):145–51. DOI: 10.1097/AOG.0b013e31825957cf.

18. Zolnoun DA, Rohl J, Moore CG, Perinetti-Liebert C, Lamvu GM, Maixner W. Overlap between orofacial pain and vulvar vestibulitis syndrome. *Clin J Pain.* 2008;24(3):187–91. DOI: 10.1097/AJP.0b013e318159f976.

19. Heddini U, Bohm-Starke N, Nilsson KW, Johannesson U. Provoked vestibulodynia-medical factors and comorbidity associated with treatment outcome. *J Sex Med.* 2012;9(5):1400–6. DOI: 10.1111/j.1743-6109.2012.02665.x.

20. Granot M, Zimmer EZ, Friedman M, Lowenstein L, Yarnitsky D. Association between quantitative sensory testing, treatment choice, and subsequent pain reduction in vulvar vestibulitis syndrome. *J Pain.* 2004;5(4):226–32. doi:10.1016/j.jpain.2004.03.005.

21. Xie Y, Shi L, Xiong X, Wu E, Veasley C, Dade C. Economic burden and quality of life of vulvodynia in

the United States. *Curr Med Res Opin*. 2012;**28**(4):601–8. DOId: 10.1185/03007995.2012.666963.

22. Thomas TG. *A Practical Treatise on the Diseases of Women*, 5th ed. Philadelphia: Henry C. Lea's Son & Co.

23. Nguyen RHN, Ecklund AM, MacLehose RF, Veasley C, Harlow BL. Co-morbid pain conditions and feelings of invalidation and isolation among women with vulvodynia. *Psychol Heal Med*. 2012;**17**(5):589–98. DOI: 10.1080/13548506.2011.647703.

24. Nguyen RHN, MacLehose RF, Veasley C, Turner RM, Harlow BL, Horvath KJ. Comfort in discussing vulvar pain in social relationships among women with vulvodynia. *J Reprod Med*. 2012;**57**(3–4):109–14.

25. Yeung J, Pauls RN. Anatomy of the vulva and the female sexual response. *Obstet Gynecol Clin North Am*. 2016;**43**(1):27–44. DOI: 10.1016/j.ogc.2015.10.011.

26. Zolnoun D, Hartmann K, Lamvu G, As-Sanie S, Maixner W, Steege J. A conceptual model for the pathophysiology of vulvar vestibulitis syndrome. *Obstet Gynecol Surv*. 2006;**61**(6):395–401. DOI: 10.1097/01.ogx.0000219814.40759.38.

27. Wesselmann U, Bonham A, Foster D. Vulvodynia: current state of the biological science. *Pain*. 2014;**155**(9):1696–701. DOI: 10.1016/j.pain.2014.05.010.

28. Bohm-Starke N, Hilliges M, Falconer C, Rylander E. Increased intraepithelial innervation in women with vulvar vestibulitis syndrome. *Gynecol Obstet Invest*. 1998;**46**(4):256–60. DOI: goi46256 [pii].

29. Tympanidis P, Terenghi G, Dowd P. Increased innervation of the vulval vestibule in patients with vulvodynia. *Br J Dermatol*. 2003;**148**(5):1021–7. doi:10.1046/j.1365-2133.2003.05308.x.

30. Zolnoun D, Bair E, Essick G, Gracely R, Goyal V, Maixner W. Reliability and reproducibility of novel methodology for assessment of pressure pain sensitivity in pelvis. *J Pain*. 2012;**13**(9):910–20. DOI: 10.1016/j.jpain.2012.06.006.

31. Bohm-Starke N, Hilliges M, Brodda-Jansen G, Rylander E, Torebjörk E. Psychophysical evidence of nociceptor sensitization in vulvar vestibulitis syndrome. *Pain*. 2001;**94**(2):177–83. DOI: 10.1016/S0304-3959(01)00352-9.

32. Pukall CF, Goldstein AT, Bergeron S, et al. Vulvodynia: definition, prevalence, impact, and pathophysiological factors. *J Sex Med*. 2016;**13**(3):291–304. DOI: 10.1016/j.jsxm.2015.12.021.

33. Pukall CF, Strigo IA, Binik YM, Amsel R, Khalifé S, Bushnell MC. Neural correlates of painful genital touch in women with vulvar vestibulitis syndrome. *Pain*. 2005;**115**(1–2):118–27. DOI: 10.1016/j.pain.2005.02.020.

34. Alagiri M, Chottiner S, Ratner V, Slade D, Hanno PM. Interstitial cystitis: unexplained associations with other chronic disease and pain syndromes. *Urology*. 1997;**49**(5 Suppl.):52–7. DOI: 10.1016/S0090-4295(99)80332-X.

35. Wesselmann U. Neurogenic inflammation and chronic pelvic pain. *World J Urol*. 2001;**19**(3):180–5. DOI: 10.1007/s003450100201.

36. Eva LJ, MacLean AB, Reid WM, et al. Estrogen receptor expression in vulvar vestibulitis syndrome. *Am J Obstet Gynecol*. 2003;**189**(2):458–61.

37. Reissing ED, Brown C, Lord MJ, Binik YM, Khalifé S. Pelvic floor muscle functioning in women with vulvar vestibulitis syndrome. *J Psychosom Obstet Gynecol*. 2005;**26**(2):107–13. DOI: 10.1080/01443610400023106.

38. Fillingim RB, Bruehl S, Dworkin RH, et al. The ACTTION-American Pain Society Pain Taxonomy (AAPT): an evidence-based and multidimensional approach to classifying chronic pain conditions. *J Pain*. 2014;**15**(3):241–9. DOI: 10.1016/j.jpain.2014.01.004.

39. Braksmajer A. Struggles for medical legitimacy among women experiencing sexual pain: a qualitative study. *Women Health*. 2018;**58**(4):419–33. DOI: 10.1080/03630242.2017.1306606.

40. Woolf CJ. Central sensitization: implications for the diagnosis and treatment of pain. *Pain*. 2011;**152**(Suppl. 3). DOI: 10.1016/j.pain.2010.09.030.

41. Maixner W, Williams DA, Smith SB, Slade GD. Overlapping chronic pain conditions: implications for diagnosis and classification. *J Pain*. 2016;**17**(9):T93–T107. DOI: 10.1016/j.jpain.2016.06.002.

42. Jensen M. Review of measures of neuropathic pain. *Curr Pain Headache Rep*. 2006;**10**(3):159–66. DOI: 10.1007/s11916-006-0041-z.

43. Larsen SB, Kragstrup J. Experiences of the first pelvic examination in a random sample of Danish teenagers. *Acta Obstet Gynecol Scand*. 1995;**74**(2):137–41. DOI: 10.3109/00016349509008923.

44. Flynn KE, Carter J, Lin L, et al. Assessment of vulvar discomfort with sexual activity among women in the United States. *Am J Obstet Gynecol*. 2017;**216**(4):391.e1–391.e8. DOI: 10.1016/j.ajog.2016.12.006.

45. Huber JD, Pukall CF, Boyer SC, Reissing ED, Chamberlain SM. "Just relax": physicians' experiences with women who are difficult or impossible to examine gynecologically. *J Sex Med*. 2009;**6**(3):791–9. DOI: 10.1111/j.1743-6109.2008.01139.x.

46. Oshinowo A, Ionescu A, Anim T, Lamvu G. Dyspareunia and vulvodynia. In Valovska A (ed), *Pelvic Pain Management*. Oxford: Oxford University

Press; 2016. DOI: 10.1093/med/9780199393039.003.0006.

47. Sadownik LA. Etiology, diagnosis, and clinical management of vulvodynia. *Int J Womens Health*. 2014;**6** .(1):437–49. DOI: 10.2147/IJWH.S37660.

48. Gyang A, Hartman M. Musculoskeletal causes of chronic pelvic pain: what a gynecologist should know. *Obstet Gynecol*. 2013;**121**(3):645–50.

49. Labat JJ, Riant T, Robert R, Amarenco G, Lefaucheur JP, Rigaud J. Diagnostic criteria for pudendal neuralgia by pudendal nerve entrapment (Nantes Criteria). *Neurourol Urodyn*. 2008;**27**(4):306–10. DOI: 10.1002/nau.20505.

50. Hibner M, Desai N, Robertson LJ, Nour M. Pudendal neuralgia. *J Minim Invasive Gynecol*. 2010;**17**(2):148–53. DOI: 10.1016/j.jmig.2009.11.003.

51. Cardosi RJ, Cox CS, Hoffman MS. Postoperative neuropathies after major pelvic surgery. *Obstet Gynecol*. 2002;**100**(2):240–4. DOI: 10.1016/S0029-7844(02)02052-5.

52. Possover M, Forman A. Neuropelveological assessment of neuropathic pelvic pain. *Gynecol Surg*. 2014;**11**(2):139–44. DOI: 10.1007/s10397-014-0838-4.

53. De Andres J, Sanchis-Lopez N, Asensio-Samper JM, et al. Vulvodynia: an evidence based literature review and proposed treatment algorithm. *Pain Pract*. 2015; online ahe(2):1–33. DOI: 10.1111/papr.12274.

54. Edwards L. Vulvodynia. *Clin Obstet Gynecol*. 2015;**58**(1):143–52. DOI: 10.1097/GRF.0000000000000093.

55. Nicolaides KH. Committee opinion 673: persistent vulvar pain. *Obstet*. 2016;**128**(654):1–4. DOI: 10.1016/S0140-6736(16)31898-0.

56. Henzell H, Berzins K, Langford JP. Provoked vestibulodynia: current perspectives. *Int J Womens Health*. 2017;**9**:631–42. DOI: 10.2147/IJWH.S113416.

57. Lindström S, Kvist LJ. Treatment of provoked vulvodynia in a Swedish cohort using desensitization exercises and cognitive behavioral therapy. BMC Womens Health. 2015;**15**:121. DOI: 10.1186/s12905-015-0265-3.

58. National Vulvodynia Association. Self-help tips. www.nva.org/for-patients/self-help-tips

59. Prendergast SA. Pelvic floor physical therapy for vulvodynia: a clinician's guide. *Obstet Gynecol Clin North Am*. 2017;**44**(3):509–22. DOI: 10.1016/j.ogc.2017.05.006.

60. Morin M, Carroll MS, Bergeron S. Systematic review of the effectiveness of physical therapy modalities in women with provoked vestibulodynia. *Sex Med Rev*. 2017;**5**(3):295–322. DOI: 10.1016/j.sxmr.2017.02.003.

61. Alappattu M, Lamvu G, Feranec J, et al. Vulvodynia is not created equally: empirical classification of women with vulvodynia. *J Pain Res*. 2017;**10**(1):509–22. DOI: 10.1016/j.ajog.2016.12.006.

62. Dunkley CR, Brotto LA. Psychological treatments for provoked vestibulodynia: integration of mindfulness-based and cognitive behavioral therapies. *J Clin Psychol*. 2016;**72**(7):637–50. DOI: 10.1002/jclp.22286.

63. Bergeron S, Morin M, Lord MJ. Integrating pelvic floor rehabilitation and cognitive-behavioural therapy for sexual pain: what have we learned and where do we go from here? *Sex Relatsh Ther*. 2010;**25**(3):289–98. DOI: 10.1080/14681994.2010.486398.

64. Bergeron S, Khalifé S, Dupuis MJ, McDuff P. A randomized clinical trial comparing group cognitive-behavioral therapy and a topical steroid for women with dyspareunia. *J Consult Clin Psychol*. 2016;**84**(3):259–68. DOI: 10.1037/ccp0000072.

65. Masheb RM, Kerns RD, Lozano C, Minkin MJ, Richman S. A randomized clinical trial for women with vulvodynia: cognitive-behavioral therapy vs. supportive psychotherapy. *Pain*. 2009;**141**(1–2):31–40. DOI: 10.1016/j.pain.2008.09.031.

66. Reed BD, Sen A, Harlow SD, Haefner HK, Gracely RH. Multimodal vulvar and peripheral sensitivity among women with vulvodynia: a case-control study. *J Low Genit Tract Dis*. 2017;**21**(1):78–84. DOI: 10.1097/LGT.0000000000000267.

67. Zolnoun DA, Hartmann KE, Steege JF. Overnight 5% lidocaine ointment for treatment of vulvar vestibulitis. *Obstet Gynecol*. 2003;**102**(1):84–7. DOI: 10.1016/S0029-7844(03)00368-5.

68. Kelley C. Estrogen and its effect on vaginal atrophy in post-menopausal women. *Urol Nurs Off J Am Urol Assoc Allied*. 2007;**27**(1):40–5.

69. Foster DC, Palmer M, Marks J. Effect of vulvovaginal estrogen on sensorimotor response of the lower genital tract: a randomized controlled trial. *Obstet Gynecol*. 1999;**94**(2):232–7. DOI: 10.1016/S0029-7844(99)00264-1.

70. Burrows LJ, Goldstein AT. The treatment of vestibulodynia with topical estradiol and testosterone. *Sex Med*. 2013;**1**(1):30–3. DOI: 10.1002/sm2.4.

71. Joura EA, Zeisler H, Bancher-Todesca D, Sator MO, Schneider B, Gitsch G. Short-term effects of topical testosterone in vulvar lichen sclerosus. *Obstet Gynecol*. 1997. DOI: 10.1016/S0029-7844(97)81071-X.

72. FDA. FDA drug safety communication, safety announcement. 2014.www.fda.gov/downloads/Drugs/DrugSafety/UCM436270.pdf

73. Basson R. Female sexual response: the role of drugs in the management of sexual dysfunction. *Obstet Gynecol.* 2001;**98**(2):350–3. DOI: 10.1016/S0029-7844(01)01452-1.

74. Leo RJ, Dewani S. A systematic review of the utility of antidepressant pharmacotherapy in the treatment of vulvodynia pain. *J Sex Med.* 2013;**10** (10):2497–505. DOI: 10.1111/j.1743-6109.2012.02915.x.

75. van Beekhuizen HJ, Oost J, van der Meijden WI. Generalized unprovoked vulvodynia: a retrospective study on the efficacy of treatment with amitriptyline, gabapentin or pregabalin. *Eur J Obstet Gynecol Reprod Biol.* 2018;**220**:118–21. DOI: 10.1016/j.ejogrb.2017.10.026.

76. Woodruff J, Genadry R, Polickoff S. Treatment of dyspareunia and vaginal outlet distortions by perineoplasty. *Obstet Gynecol.* 1981;**57**:750–4.

77. Stenson AL. Vulvodynia: diagnosis and management. *Obstet Gynecol Clin North Am.* 2017;**44**(3):493–508. DOI: 10.1016/j.ogc.2017.05.008.

78. Tommola P, Unkila-Kallio L, Paavonen J. Surgical treatment of vulvar vestibulitis: a review. *Acta Obstet Gynecol Scand.* 2010;**89**(11):1385–95. DOI: 10.3109/00016349.2010.512071.

79. Kliethermes CJ, Shah M, Hoffstetter S, Gavard JA, Steele A. Effect of vestibulectomy for intractable vulvodynia. *J Minim Invasive Gynecol.* 2016;**23**:1152–7. DOI: 10.1016/j.jmig.2016.08.822.

Chapter 13

Pelvic Pain Arising from Adhesive Disease

Joseph M. Maurice and Sheena Galhotra

Editor's Introduction

Treatment of pain caused by abdominal and pelvic adhesions is possibly one of the most controversial issues among physicians taking care of patients with pelvic pain, and science is not helpful. There are publications that show that adhesions do not cause pain and others that show they do. The same goes for usefulness of adhesiolysis to relieve that pain. This discrepancy may be due to the fact that some surgeons perform more complete adhesiolysis than others and that coexisting pain conditions may be an additional confounding factor. I believe that certain adhesions cause pain and, in many cases, adhesiolysis is helpful. Laparoscopic or robotic adhesiolysis is a preferred way because chances of recurrence of adhesions is decreased. This may be due to the fact that CO_2 prevents fibroblast migration. Risks of adhesiolyis including a risk of unrecognized bowel injury have to be very clearly explained to the patient and this procedure should be performed only by a skilled surgeon.

Etiology

Pelvic Adhesive Disease

Postoperative adhesion formation occurs virtually after every intraperitoneal surgery [1]. It is one of the most common findings in women with pelvic pain [2]. It is estimated to account for up to 50% of patients with pelvic pain [3]. Other causes of pelvic adhesive disease include the byproduct of infectious stimuli, for example, pelvic inflammatory disease (PID). The adhesive disease generated by PID acts in a protective manner by isolating the harmful microorganisms. Germ cell tumors, such as dermoid cysts, cause a chemical peritonitis and precipitate pelvic adhesion formation in a similar, isolating manner as seen with infectious etiologies. Other gynecological

conditions, especially endometriosis, produce and enrich pelvic adhesive disease.

The formation of pelvic adhesive disease follows a cascading process; it is subject to various physiological and pathological pathways depending upon the extent of the initial injury and the subsequent response. Pelvic adhesive disease formation starts with an injury to the peritoneum, most notably as a natural response to surgery. The pathological process develops mostly as a consequence of mechanical, thermal, or devascularization trauma during a surgical procedure [4]. Disruption of the peritoneal surface produces an inflammatory response [5]. Subsequently, the activation of white blood cells, macrophages, and platelets occurs [4]. As a protective measure, fibroblast recruitment produces fibrin deposition to the denuded surfaces, and, if not degraded, will ultimately result in collagen deposition with subsequent pelvic adhesion formation [4]. As a result of this peritoneal trauma, the cascade of inflammation, mesothelial repair, and incomplete fibrinolysis contributes to the development of pelvic adhesive disease [6]. The common denominator of pelvic adhesive disease formation, regardless of the etiology, is determined by the exaggerated inflammatory response, decreased fibrinolysis, extracellular matrix deposition, and incomplete remodeling [7]. Prostaglandin formation also is involved with adhesion formation in in vitro studies [8].

Pelvic Pain

Pelvic pain arising from pelvic adhesive disease is a complex, variable, and unpredictable condition that has plagued gynecological surgeons for centuries. The consequences of pelvic adhesive disease are many, but the most distressing sequela is the development of pain, especially pelvic pain, and has the potential to traumatize patients and frustrate gynecological surgeons. The etiology of this pain is unknown, but is thought to involve the disruption of normal organ mobility [9]. This mechanical cause of pelvic pain may be the direct consequence of excessive traction of the adhesive disease against well innervated viscous organs. As a result, this traction adversely stimulates visceral and parietal peritoneum, producing the noxious response [10, 11]. Pelvic adhesive disease is a significant contributor to chronic pelvic pain syndrome [10, 12]. This cause-and-effect theory makes logical sense, but the entire process may be more complicated. Debilitating pelvic pain resulting from pelvic adhesive disease can contribute to the central sensitization of pain, thus further complicating diagnostic and therapeutic interventions [13–15]. Correlation between the location of the pain symptoms and the commensurate anatomical site, unfortunately, is not clear. The anatomical site of adhesive disease is not necessarily associated with the amount of pain [16]. But the consistency and architecture of the tissue may guide gynecological surgeons [17]. Pain localized to the abdomen is usually associated with bowel and omental attachment to the lower portion of the abdominal wall. Dyspareunia as a result of pelvic adhesive disease can be the result of adhesions to the uterus, adnexa, and cul-de-sac [17]. While the anatomical site can provide the surgeon with some guidance into the areas of therapy, it is not foolproof. The etiology of pelvic pain may not be due to its anatomical site and may be due to the presence of the adhesion itself. This confounding factor may be due to the fact that adhesive disease itself contains de novo nerve tissue and may contribute to the clinical symptoms [18–20].

Concerns

In addition to pelvic pain, pelvic adhesive disease promotes infertility, dyspareunia, bowel obstruction, and increased risk of injury with subsequent surgical intervention. Cesarean section, myomectomy, and adnexal surgery are the three highest risk gynecological procedures that promote postoperative development of pelvic adhesive disease [21, 22]. The most devastating consequence of adhesive disease is the increased risk of postoperative bowel dysfunction and obstruction [1]. This is a critical consideration when planning operative removal of adhesions, and an important part of the preoperative informed consent.

Symptoms

Pelvic pain arising from pelvic adhesive disease may not have consistent symptomatology; in addition, its presentation can be confounded by other concomitant gynecological or nongynecological conditions. When pelvic adhesive disease constrains or restricts movement of viscous organs in the abdominal cavity, movement of the underlying encased tissue generates a pain response. In the case of adhesive disease to the bowel, the pain may be precipitated with ingestion of food, bowel movements, or normal gut motility. This type of pelvic pain is usually described as a pinpoint pain response. Adhesive disease to the female pelvic organs can manifest as dyspareunia or uterine or adnexal pain. Persistent pain at cesarean section scar is another example of localized pain and may be the result of adhesive disease. Dysmenorrhea is usually separate from pelvic pain arising from adhesive disease and its presence may help with deciphering the etiology. Documentation of pelvic pain is cumbersome and prone to nebulous descriptions because there are no standardized descriptors. Research examining this issue is difficult, and most studies are fatally flawed, as gynecologists are unable to reliably reproduce the symptoms. Additionally, validated scoring systems to accurately document the extent of disease and its clinical and research implications are not available [6].

Prevention

Prevention of postoperative adhesion formation is critical for all gynecological surgeons. This includes, but is not limited to, meticulous surgical technique with prevention of excessive tissue trauma [23]. Other preventative measures include minimization of tissue ischemia and desiccation, as well as prevention of infection and foreign body retention [3]. Postoperative adhesion formation produces adhesions for up to seven days after the procedure [3]. Ideally, administration of an adhesion blocking measure would have to be available for that amount of time. For a time, there was great promise with use of adhesion preventing measures, but unfortunately, use of adhesion barriers or intraperitoneal irrigates suggests a suboptimal, if any, response to combatting pelvic adhesive disease [3]. The authors cannot recommend any of these measures. Closure of the peritoneum, a long held paradigm in gynecological surgery, is no longer recommended as a way to prevent pelvic adhesive disease [24]. Use of nonsteroidal anti-inflammatory drugs (NSAIDs) or blood thinning medication lacks efficacy [3]. Use of laparoscopy over laparotomy appears to convey a benefit of decreasing adhesion formation [25].

Diagnosis

The preoperative workup includes a thorough history documenting symptoms and attempting to localize the pain. If the pain is isolated to a particular area, as opposed to a generalized complaint, then the surgeon may have a greater opportunity to address the issue. Generalized complaints of pain, while still important findings, may not be necessarily due to adhesive disease, and surgical exploration in these patients will yield less optimal intraoperative and postoperative results. A more structured assessment of pain via standardized pain score testing is limited, as it does not correlate well with degree of pain both preoperatively and postoperatively [26]. Standardized questionnaires, however, such as those produced from the International Pelvic Pain Society, may be useful [27]. Physical exam, especially abdominal and pelvic portions, may pinpoint the disease process. Adherent attachment of the uterus to the abdominal wall, tenderness at cesarean section site, fixed pelvis, decreased bladder capacity, and bowel complaints all may help pinpoint the affected area. Imaging modalities and laboratory assessment are not usually beneficial. Diagnosis of pelvic pain from adhesive disease is primarily made intraoperatively and remains the most accurate means of making the diagnosis [28].

Treatment

Surgical removal of adhesive disease is a major procedure in the United States, with 400,000 cases performed daily, costing in excess of $1.3 billion every year [3]. Surgical treatment options are wide, varied, and, unfortunately, weakly supported by academic studies. The only two randomized controlled trials examining the effect of adhesiolysis on pelvic pain each have serious methodological flaws [3, 29]. Despite the scarcity of convincing research, patients with pelvic pain arising from pelvic adhesive disease may benefit from adhesiolysis [17]. The authors of this publication concur. An existential question arises with patients afflicted by pelvic pain arising from adhesive disease: what can a gynecological surgeon do to help alleviate the suffering in these patients with pelvic pain? As surgeons, we must rely on sound clinical judgment when treating patients with pelvic adhesive disease, and advocate adhesiolysis as a treatment for pelvic adhesive disease in certain patients. The location and extent of adhesions must be considered when planning surgical approach. Laparoscopic adhesiolysis is preferred over an open approach because of decreased length of recovery and extent of adhesion recurrence [30]. If there is concern for adhesions at the umbilicus, initial trocar can be placed at the left upper quadrant to avoid unintended bowel injury [31]. During lysis of adhesions, it is important to maximize visualization and avoid injury to surrounding structures. Sharp dissection should be utilized when organs are nearby to avoid injury; cautery is especially useful on vascular tissue. The ultimate goal of adhesiolysis should be to resect the offending scar tissue and return structures back to their anatomical positions while minimizing the extent of dissection. Counseling and managing pain expectations preoperatively are important prior to adhesiolysis. Preoperative evaluation is also important. If patients complain of localized or pinpoint pain, suggesting adhesive disease encasing an organ, then removal of the offending tissue is warranted [17, 32]. Adhesiolysis is especially useful in patients with well vascularized adhesive disease to the bowel [29]. Direct visual inspection of tissue composition may also offer the surgeons some guidance. Thin, filmy adhesions are associated with the most pain, especially when tethered to visceral organs [33]. Removal of dense, adherent adhesive disease referred to as "abdominal cocoon" will less likely provide relief [1]. Adhesiolysis for generalized pelvic pain may be less successful, but may be an important adjunct of their diagnosis and therapeutic care. Even with detailed preoperative screening and meticulous intraoperative technique, the most devastating, and, at times, unpredictable postoperative consequence is the return of symptomatic pelvic adhesive disease [10, 25, 33]. Benefits of adhesiolysis are still murky, and until definitive studies come forth, adhesiolysis for pelvic pain secondary to pelvic adhesive disease can be used judiciously [20]. Noninvasive strategies such as humidified CO_2, human amniotic membrane, or pharmaceuticals to prevent adhesion formation generally deliver suboptimal results [7]. Additionally, adhesion barriers for pelvic pain secondary to pelvic adhesive disease are limited and are based on insufficient outcome analysis [34].

Conclusion

Performing adhesiolysis to relieve pain entangled viscous or vital organs, such as bowel, uterus, and adnexa, is a viable option. An attempt to localize a patient's area of pain preoperatively and confirm intraabdominally will yield the best postoperative results. Lysis of pelvic adhesions should be considered for symptomatic areas and avoided in nonsymptomatic areas. Adhesiolysis in patients with generalized pelvic pain complaints may not be as useful. It is appropriate to avoid innocuous-appearing adhesions, as their removal does not appear to affect the symptomatology. The principal harm of surgical intervention is recurrence. One should proceed with surgical intervention judiciously. Also, gynecological surgeons should be wary of the known postoperative placebo effect that can confound our interventions. As we have stated earlier, the research in this area of surgical management of pelvic adhesive disease is limited. Anecdotal case reports are especially limited in their external validity; we ask the reader to review the surgical management of one of our patients of a primary band of adhesive disease that developed de novo. She presented to many physicians describing an acutely accurate, reproducible set of symptoms of right-sided pelvic pain with athletic movement. After extensive preoperative counseling, the patient opted for an operative laparoscopic procedure. On laparoscopic entrance a small 4 × 1 cm adhesive band was attached from the right pelvic side wall and extended around the small bowel. Placing the patient in the Trendelenburg position did not reveal any abnormal impingement. Yet, when the patient was placed in a left-ward tilt, the surgeons noticed the small bowel kinking under the strain of the abnormal adhesive attachment with the subsequent transient cyanosis of the small bowel. Adhesiolysis commenced and proceeded to release the small bowel from its attachment and restored it to its normal anatomical position. The patient was postoperatively followed without recurrence of symptoms. To the nay-sayers who believe that the adhesions will recur, we say maybe, but not likely in the exact same area ensnaring the same organ. In conclusion, when surgically managing pelvic pain from adhesive disease, our recommendations are based on clinical judgment, as confounding factors, faulty studies, and the inability to standardize the categorization of pelvic adhesive disease make recommendations difficult [17]. But as surgeons practicing the art of medicine, it is our obligation to safely investigate potential therapies such as adhesiolysis.

Five Things You Need to Know

- Pelvic adhesions can form secondary to surgery, pelvic inflammatory disease, tumors, endometriosis, and a variety of other agents/diseases that irritate or injure to the peritoneum, triggering an inflammatory response.
- Prevention of adhesion formation includes meticulous surgical technique, avoidance of unnecessary tissue trauma, minimization of tissue ischemia and desiccation, and prevention of infection and foreign body retention.
- Despite the scarcity of convincing research, patients may benefit from surgical adhesiolysis. It is important to counsel and manage pain expectations preoperatively.
- Patients with symptoms that indicate a pinpoint or localized source of pain have better outcomes after surgical adhesiolysis than patients with generalized pain complaints. Removal of thin, filmy tissue provides more pain relief than removal of densely adhered tissue.
- The principal harm of surgical intervention is recurrence of adhesions. However, recurrence is unlikely to happen in the same area and may not produce the same symptoms, so consideration for surgery should happen on an individual case basis.

References

1. van Goor H. Consequences and complications of peritoneal adhesions. *Colorect Dis.* 2007;**9**(s2):25–34.
2. Howard FM. The role of laparoscopy as a diagnostic tool in chronic pelvic pain. *Best Pract Res Clin Obstet Gynaecol.* 2000;**14**(3):467–94.
3. González-Quintero VH, Cruz-Pachano FE. Preventing adhesions in obstetric and gynecologic surgical procedures. *Rev Obstet Gynecol.* 2009;**2**(1):38.
4. Holmdahl L, Ivarsson M. The role of cytokines, coagulation, and fibrinolysis in peritoneal tissue repair. *Eur J Surgery.* 1999;**165**(11):1012–19.
5. Weibel M-, Majno G. Peritoneal adhesions and their relation to abdominal surgery. *Am J Surg.* 1973;**126**(3):345–53.
6. Monk BJ, Berman ML, Montz FJ. Adhesions after extensive gynecologic surgery: clinical significance, etiology, and prevention. *Am J Obstet Gynecol.* 1994;**170**(5 Pt 1):1396–403.
7. Ward BC, Panitch A. Abdominal adhesions: current and novel therapies. *J Surg Res.* 2011;**165**(1):91–111.
8. Golan A, Bernstein T, Wexler S, Neuman M, Bukovsky I, David MP. The effect of prostaglandins and aspirin: an inhibitor of prostaglandin synthesis–on adhesion formation in rats. *Hum Reprod (Oxf).* 1991;**6**(2):251–4.
9. Kresch A, Seifer D, Sachs L, Barrese I. Laparoscopy in 100 women with chronic pelvic pain. *Obstet Gynecol.* 1984;**64**(5):672–4.

10. Stovall TG, Elder RF, Ling FW. Predictors of pelvic adhesions. *J Reprod Med.* 1989;**34**(5):345.

11. Keltz MD, Peck L, Liu S, Kim AH, Arici A, Olive DL. Large bowel-to-pelvic sidewall adhesions associated with chronic pelvic pain. *Am Assoc Gynecol Laparosc.* 1995;**3**(1):55–9.

12. Cunanan RG, Courey NG, Lippes J. Laparoscopic findings in patients with pelvic pain. *Am J Obstet Gynecol.* 1983;**146**(5):589–91.

13. Zondervan KT, Yudkin PL, Vessey MP, et al. Chronic pelvic pain in the community: symptoms, investigations, and diagnoses. *Am J Obstet Gynecol.* 2001;**184**(6):1149–55.

14. Mathias SD, Kuppermann M, Liberman RF, Lipschutz RC, Steege JF. Chronic pelvic pain: prevalence, health-related quality of life, and economic correlates. *Obstet Gynecol.* 1996;**87**(3):321–7.

15. Apte G, Nelson P, Brismée J, Dedrick G, Justiz R, Sizer PS. Chronic female pelvic pain-part 1: Clinical pathoanatomy and examination of the pelvic region. *Pain Pract.* 2012;**12**(2):88–110.

16. Steege JF, Stout AL. Resolution of chronic pelvic pain after laparoscopic lysis of adhesions. *Am J Obstet Gynecol.* 1991;**165**(2):278–83.

17. Hammoud A, Gago LA, Diamond MP. Adhesions in patients with chronic pelvic pain: a role for adhesiolysis? *Fertil Steril.* 2004;**82**(6):1483–91.

18. Tulandi T, Chen MF, Al-Took S, Watkin K. A study of nerve fibers and histopathology of postsurgical, postinfectious, and endometriosis-related adhesions. *Obstet Gynecol.* 1998;**92**(5):766–8.

19. Kligman I, Drachenberg C, Papadimitriou J, Katz E. Immunohistochemical demonstration of nerve fibers in pelvic adhesions. *Obstet Gynecol.* 1993;**82**(4):566–8.

20. Cheong Y, Stones RW. Chronic pelvic pain: aetiology and therapy. *Best Pract Res Clin Obstet Gynaecol.* 2006;**20**(5):695–711.

21. Steege J. Repeated clinic laparoscopy for the treatment of pelvic adhesions: a pilot study. *Obstet Gynecol.* 1994;**83**(2):276–279.

22. Tulandi T, Murray C, Guralnick M. Adhesion formation and reproductive outcome after myomectomy and second-look laparoscopy. *Obstet Gynecol.* 1993;**82**(2):213.

23. Gomel V. *Microsurgery in Female Infertility*, 1st ed. Boston: Little, Brown; 1983.

24. Tulandi T, Al-Jaroudi D. Nonclosure of peritoneum: a reappraisal. *Am J Obstet Gynecol.* 2003;**189**(2):609–12.

25. Diamond MP, Decherney AH. Pathogenesis of adhesion formation/reformation: application to reproductive pelvic surgery. *Microsurgery.* 1987;**8**(2):103–7.

26. Malik E, Berg C, Meyhöfer-Malik A, Haider S, Rossmanith W. Subjective evaluation of the therapeutic value of laparoscopic adhesiolysis. *Surg Endosc.* 2000;**14**(1):79–81.

27. The International Pelvic Pain Society. Pelvic pain assessment form. https://pelvicpain.org/IPPS/Profess ional/Documents-Forms/IPPS/Content/Professiona l-Patients/Documents_and_Forms.aspx?hkey=2597a b99-df83-40ee-89cd-7bd384efed19

28. Swank D, Swank-Bordewijk S, Hop W, et al. Laparoscopic adhesiolysis in patients with chronic abdominal pain: a blinded randomised controlled multi-centre trial. *Lancet.* 2003;**361**(9365):1247–51.

29. Peters AA, Trimbos-Kemper GC, Admiraal C, Trimbos JB, Hermans J. A randomized clinical trial on the benefit of adhesiolysis in patients with intraperitoneal adhesions and chronic pelvic pain. *Br J Obstet Gynaecol.* 1992;**99**(1):59–62.

30. Sallinen V, Di Saverio S, Haukijärvi E, et al. Laparoscopic versus open adhesiolysis for adhesive small bowel obstruction (LASSO): an international, multicentre, randomised, open-label trial. *Lancet Gastroenterol Hepatol.* 2019;**4**(4):278–86.

31. Pickett SD, Rodewald KJ, Billow MR, Giannios, Hurd, William W. Avoiding major vessel injury during laparoscopic instrument insertion. *Obstet Gynecol Clin.* 2010;**37**(3):387–97.

32. Senapati S, Atashroo D, Carey E, Dassel M, Tu FF. Surgical interventions for chronic pelvic pain. *Curr Opin Obstet Gynecol.* 2016;**28**:290–6.

33. Luciano DE, Luciano AA, Roy G. Adhesion reformation after laparoscopic adhesiolysis: where, what type, and in whom they are most likely to recur. *J Minim Invasive Gynecol.* 2008;**15**(1):44–8.

34. Ahmad G, O'Flynn H, Hindocha A, Watson A. Barrier agents for adhesion prevention after gynaecological surgery. *Cochrane Database Syst Rev.* 2015(4):CD000475.

Pelvic Pain Arising from Ovarian Remnant Syndrome

Mohammad R. Islam and Javier F. Magrina

Editor's Introduction

Ovarian remnant syndrome occurs in patients who have had attempted oophorectomy and part of the ovary was inadvertently left behind. It often happens in patients who are undergoing total abdominal hysterectomy with bilateral salpingo-oophorectomy in the setting of severe pelvic adhesions. In those cases, the surgeon, to avoid injury to the ureter, which is not well visible, clamps gonadal vessels too close to the ovary and some ovarian tissue remains in the patient. The patient often experience severe, sharp unilateral pelvic pain that is cyclical in nature. On the ultrasound there is often a cystic adnexal mass but lack of a mass does not rule out an ovarian remnant. Hormonal assays may also be helpful. Treatment is surgical but surgery for this condition may be overly difficult because the original surgery to remove the ovary was most likley difficult in the first place. Procedures to remove ovarian remnants should be performed only by highly qualified providers who are experienced in operating in the setting of severe adhesions. On a positive note, patients in whom ovarian remnant was successfully removed are almost always cured of their pain.

Introduction/Definition

Ovarian remnant syndrome (ORS) is defined as the presence of ovarian tissue after oophorectomy [1]. It typically presents with pelvic pain and/or a pelvic cystic lesion. Traditionally, ORS only included patients with a history of bilateral salpingo-oophorectomy (BSO). However, the definition has since been expanded to include patients with unilateral oophorectomy with residual ovarian tissue on the side of the previous resection [2]. It is also possible to have ectopic implantation of excised ovarian tissue, especially if the specimen is cut into pieces and removed uncontained at the time of extraction through laparoscopic trocar sites. There are reports of patients developing ovarian tissue at trocar sites from the removal of uncontained fragmented ovaries [3].

ORS was described in a study conducted in 1970 in which felines, after surgical excision of the ovaries, had portions of the ovarian cortex intentionally left in the abdominal cavity. These portions were able to reimplant and demonstrate ovarian function [4].

ORS should not be confused with supernumerary ovary syndrome or residual ovarian syndrome (ROS). Supernumerary ovary syndrome is a rare condition that refers to the development of extraovarian tissue during embryogenesis [5]. ROS, or retained ovary, refers to subsequent pelvic pain or pathology caused by an ovary that is intentionally left in place during surgery.

Incidence

The available data on the incidence of ORS is difficult to determine and limited to case reports and retrospective case series [4, 6]. A small cohort study looked at 119 symptomatic women who underwent operative laparoscopy after total hysterectomy and BSO. Five of the women were already diagnosed with ovarian remnant with at least one prior laparoscopic attempt at removal of tissue. Of the remaining 114 patients, 21 (18%) had ovarian remnant [7]. It is believed that the incidence may be increasing [8].

Risk Factors

Incomplete removal of ovarian tissue at the time of oophorectomy, regardless of route (vaginal, laparoscopy, or laparotomy), is the main risk factor for ORS, and typically is due to deficient surgical technique in a patient with adhesions. Factors that prevent complete removal of ovarian tissue include limited visualization due to adhesive disease, distorted anatomy, anatomical variations, and intraoperative bleeding [8]. Previous abdominal surgeries, history of appendicitis, and inflammatory pelvic (including endometriosis) or bowel disease increase the risk of adhesive disease and distorted anatomy. Endometriosis can increase the risk of functional ovarian tissue on nearby structures (i.e., pelvic peritoneum), thus making identification and complete ovarian removal challenging [9]. Interestingly, the majority of case reports since 2006 demonstrate that endometriosis is the most common reason for oophorectomy in those diagnosed with ORS [10].

Prevention

Incomplete ovarian tissue removal is almost always a result of deficient surgical technique. This includes improper dissection to gain adequate access to the infundibulopelvic ligament. The most commonly affected side for ORS is the left, where the sigmoid colon is frequently attached at the pelvic brim [10, 11]. A common technique for oophorectomy is placing traction on the ovary medially and ligating the infundibulopelvic ligament without opening the retroperitoneum. Ligating and excising too close to the ovary may leave ovarian tissue behind (Figure 14.1). Microscopic ovarian stroma has been noticed in the infundibulopelvic ligament within 0.2–1.4 centimeters of the proximal pole of the ovary in 14% of patients [12]. It is also believed that blunt dissection of ovarian adhesions instead of sharp dissection can risk tearing the ovarian cortex, leaving fragments in surrounding structures [8]. Failure to adequately remove ovarian tissue in this manner may increase the risk of ORS as well as ureteral injury. All ovarian adhesions and tissue must be removed with the ovary to prevent ORS (Figure 14.2).

Clinical Presentation

The most common complaints of ORS include chronic pelvic pain (84%), dyspareunia (26%), cyclic pelvic pain (9%), dysuria (7%), and tenesmus (6%). ORS may also present as a pelvic mass after oophorectomy, which may be accompanied by pain or be asymptomatic. In a study of 186 patients who had a history of BSO and were treated surgically for pathologically confirmed residual ovarian tissue, 56% presented with a pelvic cystic lesion. Symptoms will typically present within 5 years of oophorectomy; however, it has also been noted 20 years later [13, 14].

Pain can be cyclic or chronic, and can range from dull and achy to severe, sharp, and stabbing [15, 16]. The mechanism of pelvic pain for patients with endometriosis may include hormonal stimulation of endometriotic implants by remnant ovarian tissue, infiltration of nerves, or local inflammatory processes. In addition, in women without endometriosis, pain can be elicited due to cystic enlargement with compression of surrounding pelvic structures (i.e., ureteral compression) or the inability for expansion of ovarian volume within a fixed space due to adhesive disease (ovarian tissue entrapment) [15, 17, 18].

One should suspect ORS when there is an absence of menopausal symptoms after BSO in a premenopausal woman who has not received estrogen replacement therapy (ERT). These symptoms include lack of vasomotor symptoms, mood changes, and/or vaginal dryness. In women who are on ERT immediately following menopause, discontinuation and subsequent lack of menopausal symptoms may be helpful in diagnosing ORS [8].

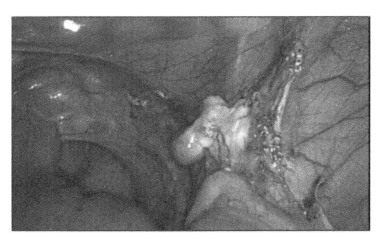

Figure 14.1 Right ovarian remnant. The numerous staples indicate the technique consisted in retracting the right ovary and tube medially and applying several stapling cartridges. This technique is at high risk of ovarian remnant, such as shown here, and it should be abandoned.

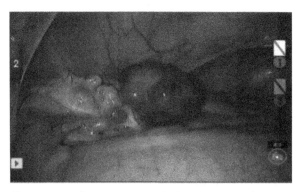

Figure 14.2 Left ovarian remnant. In this patient, the adhesions between the sigmoid and the left ovary present in her first surgery were left attached to the sigmoid and peritoneum, resulting in ovarian remnant.

Diagnosis

Clinical Suspicion

Usually there is a history of a difficult unilateral or bilateral oophorectomy. It is helpful to obtain operative and pathology reports to identify risk factors (i.e., dense ovarian adhesions from prior surgeries, other pathology such as endometriosis, poor surgical technique, etc.).

One should also ask about indicators, including the presence or absence of menopausal symptoms, in women with bilateral oophorectomy. In addition, asking about menstrual molimina or cyclical bleeding is helpful in determining if ovarian function is intact. Cyclic vaginal bleeding in a patient post-hysterectomy and post-BSO is indicative of ORS and endometriosis infiltrating the vaginal wall [19].

Laboratory Evaluation

In premenopausal women with a history of BSO, the use of serum follicle-stimulating hormone (FSH) levels (<30 UI/dL) and/or serum estradiol levels (>20 pg/mL) is useful but unreliable. Even then, these levels are not used to confirm menopausal status, but rather to test for any evidence of ovarian function. Pathologically confirmed ovarian remnants have been found in patients with menopausal hormone levels [8].

Unfortunately, a single test may be of little use, as women with ORS can have fluctuating FSH and estradiol levels, ranging from postmenopausal levels (high FSH, low estradiol) to premenopausal levels (low FSH, high estradiol).

Serum levels are also affected by women who are on ERT. Therefore, one should consider discontinuation of ERT for at least 10 days prior to obtaining serum FSH and estradiol [10].

Imaging

Imaging is necessary when suspecting ORS. A pelvic ultrasound is the imaging modality of choice and should be first in line for testing, as it appears to adequately identify the presence of cystic pelvic masses. In one study on excision of pathologically confirmed ovarian remnants, 89.6% had an adnexal mass detected by preoperative ultrasound [2]. Computed tomography (CT) and magnetic resonance imaging (MRI) are other options that can provide higher-resolution images (though they are more costly). In a series of 186 patients, complex pelvic masses related to ORS were seen in 93 of 100 (93%) patients by ultrasound, in 67 of 73 (92%) patients by CT, and in 7 of 9 (78%) patients by MRI [13].

Clomiphene Stimulation Test

In patients with negative imaging but high clinical suspicion, a stimulation test is mandatory. This entails the use of clomiphene citrate aimed to stimulate ovarian follicular development. Administering clomiphene citrate (100 mg daily for 10 days) followed by a pelvic ultrasound is highly effective to diagnose ORS. A study examined six patients with pelvic pain, a history of BSO, and a negative ultrasound. These patients received clomiphene citrate followed by repeat ultrasound. Four of the six patients developed cystic structures consistent with ovarian follicles [20]. Therefore, a positive provocation test with clomiphene citrate may potentially identify ORS and allow for a definite location of the remnant for surgical planning to expedite surgical removal. On the other hand, a negative provocation test does not necessarily exclude ORS, as some women may have a very small amount of unresponsive remnant tissue [10].

Gonadotropin-Releasing Hormone Analog Stimulation Test

With a negative clomiphene test, the next diagnostic step is an estrogen stimulation test. Gonadotropin-releasing hormone (GnRH) analog 1.75 mg intramuscularly daily for 5 days will stimulate the production of estradiol, raising its blood levels. A pre- and postinjection estradiol level will determine whether there is an ovarian remnant with negative imaging.

Patients with previous oophorectomy and pelvic pain with negative imaging, negative clomiphene test, and negative GnRH testing do not have ORS. In these patients, other causes of pain must be ruled out.

Ovarian Remnant Syndrome and Cancer

There are at least 12 cases of ovarian adenocarcinoma arising in an ovarian remnant described in the medical literature [15]. In one series, 2 of 20 women had malignancy in ovarian remnant tissue [14]. Additionally, a case of ovarian endometrioid carcinoma was noted in a patient with ORS 10 years after oophorectomy [21–23]. The mean time to development of adenocarcinoma in an ovarian remnant is 12.6 years after oophorectomy [15]. There is also an association between endometriosis and ovarian cancer, with studies suggesting a threefold increased risk for endometrioid and clear cell cancer in patients with ORS and endometriosis [24].

Management

Radical Surgery

The gold standard treatment for ORS is radical surgical resection, which always requires retroperitoneal dissection. This allows for complete removal and histological confirmation of ovarian tissue, whether it is benign or malignant.

Surgical resection can be performed via conventional laparoscopy, robot-assisted laparoscopy, or laparotomy. A minimally invasive approach is recommended to decrease morbidity as compared to laparotomy. Laparoscopy has been described with good outcomes. In a series of 20 patients with ORS, 19 patients (95%) underwent a minimally invasive approach with conventional laparoscopy or robot-assisted laparoscopy. There were no intraoperative complications and no conversion to laparotomy. One patient had postoperative pneumonia and required hospital admission [14].

Resection is always challenging and requires a retroperitoneal approach in all patients. Excellent understanding of intra- and retroperitoneal anatomy is crucial to avoid injury to surrounding structures such as the bowel, bladder, ureters, and vessels. In a retrospective cohort study of 30 patients, 29 (96.7%) required retroperitoneal dissection, 27 (90.0%) required enterolysis, 28 (93.3%) required ureterolysis, and 20 (66.7%) required ligation of the uterine artery at

its origin [2]. Additional surgical expertise is required for these types of surgeries due to the involvement of the ureters, bladder, and rectosigmoid region.

Ovarian remnant tissue can be located anywhere along the pelvic side wall [8]. Commonly, it involves the vaginal cuff. Surgery is further complicated by the extensive, dense fibrotic reaction surrounding the ovarian tissue (Figure 14.3). Our approach involves entering the pelvic retroperitoneum lateral and parallel to the infundibulopelvic ligament (ovarian vessels). This space is opened widely, identifying critical structures such as the iliac vessels and ureter, and opening up avascular spaces such as the paravesical and pararectal spaces. The ovarian vessels will be close to the ureter, so proper ureterolysis with lateral displacement is integral to achieving complete resection.

The ovarian vessels are transected above the pelvic brim. This is due to possible microscopic ovarian stroma existing at that level [12]. It is recommended that ligation and excision be done at or more than 2 centimeters above any visual ovarian tissue. As mentioned earlier, ovarian tissue may also be present on the pelvic peritoneum, especially in adhesions. It is recommended that the surrounding pelvic peritoneum of the remnant tissue be excised with a wide margin of 1–2 centimeters [8]. Sometimes it is necessary to perform segmental resection of the bladder, ureter, rectosigmoid, or upper vaginectomy. Frozen section may also be utilized intraoperatively to confirm ovarian remnant tissue and to obtain clear margins [14]. With surgical intervention, one study

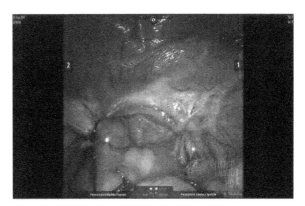

Figure 14.3 Bilateral retroperitoneal ovarian remnants. In the original surgery, this patient had both ovaries deeply adherent to the peritoneum and only the intraperitoneal portions of the ovaries were removed. The retroperitoneal portions of the ovaries were left intact. Her surgery was primarily retroperitoneal, with dense retroperitoneal adhesions to ureters, pelvic wall vessels, vaginal cuff, and rectum.

involving patients demonstrated a 95% improvement or resolution in symptoms with no recurrence of ORS at a mean follow-up of 30 months [14].

Nonsurgical Methods

Nonsurgical methods are used only in exceptional circumstances when adequately performed radical surgical excision failed and there is a persistent ovarian remnant in the same location. Focused radiotherapy may be used in such situations or in patients with severe comorbidities at high risk for surgical complications. However, it is not routinely recommended because of unreliable results, low usage data, risk of malignant transformation of ovarian remnant tissue, and adverse effects of radiation on surrounding tissues [8]. Therefore, it should be reserved only for highly selected patients.

Medical therapy involves the suppression of cyclic ovarian function using oral contraceptive pills, GnRH analogs, aromatase inhibitors, progestins, or danazol. There are limited data on the efficacy of pharmacologic medical therapy for ORS. In a series of 186 patients, 30 patients received prior medical management. Oral contraceptive agents were used in 6 (3%) patients, GnRH agonists were used in 17 (9%) patients, and danazol used in 7 (4%) patients. Although 18 (60%) of these patients experienced some symptomatic improvement, all ultimately continued to have significant symptoms warranting surgical intervention [8].

Embolization

A case report described the use of ovarian artery embolization for the management of symptomatic ORS after failed surgery. The patient subsequently underwent embolization, with follow-up arteriogram demonstrating complete occlusion of the ovarian artery, marked improvement in pelvic pain at 4-month follow-up, and CT demonstrating a substantial decrease in the size of the ovarian remnant volume (from 12.5 mL to 3.2 mL) [25]. However, the vast majority of patients with ORS do not have ovarian blood supply through the ovarian vessels.

Conclusion

ORS is an uncommon and challenging condition for gynecologists to treat. It is usually a result of poor surgical technique because of incomplete removal of ovarian tissue and surrounding adhesions. Prevention of ORS requires removal of all adhesions left attached to the ovary, not simply transection of the adhesions.

Radical surgical excision through a retroperitoneal approach is the only effective therapy and usually requires ureter, bladder, and rectosigmoid resection.

Five Things You Need to Know

- Ovarian remnant syndrome (ORS) is the presence of ovarian tissue after uni- or bilateral oophorectomy.
- Incomplete removal of ovarian tissue is due to deficient surgical technique and it is usually due to dense ovarian adhesions.
- The most common symptom is pelvic pain, cyclic or not, appearing a few months to years after oophorectomy.
- Diagnosis is established with pelvic ultrasound, CT, or MRI. If negative imaging but clinical suspicion is high, a clomiphene or GnRH stimulation test will identify patients with negative imaging. Follicle-stimulating hormone (FSH) and estradiol levels may be useful in the absence of hormonal replacement therapy but are unreliable.
- Treatment is radical surgical resection requiring a retroperitoneal approach including ureterolysis in almost all patients. Occasionally, segmental resection of ureter, bladder, or rectosigmoid is necessary.

References

1. Webb MJ. Ovarian remnant syndrome. *Aust N Z J Obstet Gynaecol.* 1989;**29**(4):433–5.

2. Arden D, Lee T. Laparoscopic excision of ovarian remnants: retrospective cohort study with long-term follow-up. *J Minim Invasive Gynecol.* 2011;**18** (2):194–9.

3. Chao HA. Ovarian remnant syndrome at the port site. *J Minim Invasive Gynecol.* 2008;**15**(4):505–7.

4. Shemwell RE, Weed JC. Ovarian remnant syndrome. *Obstet Gynecol.* 1970;**36**(2):299–303.

5. Cruikshank SH, Van Drie DM. Supernumerary ovaries: update and review. *Obstet Gynecol.* 1982;**60** (1):126–9.

6. Elkins TE, Stocker RJ, Key D, McGuire EJ, Roberts JA. Surgery for ovarian remnant syndrome: lessons learned from difficult cases. *J Reprod Med.* 1994;**39** (6):446–8.

7. Abu-Rafeh B, Vilos GA, Misra M. Frequency and laparoscopic management of ovarian remnant syndrome. *J Am Assoc Gynecol Laparosc.* 2003;**10** (1):33–7.

8. Magtibay PM, Magrina JF. Ovarian remnant syndrome. *Clin Obstet Gynecol.* 2006;**49**(3):526–34.

9. Podgaec S, Abrao MS, Dias JA Jr, Rizzo LV, de Oliveira RM, Baracat EC. Endometriosis: an inflammatory disease with a Th2 immune response component. *Hum Reprod.* 2007;**22**(5):1373–9.

10. Kho RM, Abrao MS. Ovarian remnant syndrome: etiology, diagnosis, treatment and impact of endometriosis. *Curr Opin Obstet Gynecol.* 2012;**24** (4):210–14.

11. Nezhat F, Nezhat C. Operative laparoscopy for the treatment of ovarian remnant syndrome. *Fertil Steril.* 1992;**57**(5):1003–7.

12. Fennimore IA, Simon NL, Bills G, Dryfhout VL, Schniederjan AM. Extension of ovarian tissue into the infundibulopelvic ligament beyond visual margins. *Gynecol Oncol.* 2009;**114**(1):61–3.

13. Magtibay PM, Nyholm JL, Hernandez JL, Podratz KC. Ovarian remnant syndrome. *Am J Obstet Gynecol.* 2005;**193**(6):2062–6.

14. Kho RM, Magrina JF, Magtibay PM. Pathologic findings and outcomes of a minimally invasive approach to ovarian remnant syndrome. *Fertil Steril.* 2007;**87**(5):1005–9.

15. Imai A, Matsunami K, Takagi H, Ichigo S. Malignant neoplasia arising from ovarian remnants following bilateral salpingo-oophorectomy (Review). *Oncol Lett.* 2014;**8**(1):3–6.

16. Johns DA, Diamond MP. Adequacy of laparoscopic oophorectomy. *J Am Assoc Gynecol Laparosc.* 1993;**1** (1):20–3.

17. Dmowski WP, Radwanska E, Rana N. Recurrent endometriosis following hysterectomy and oophorectomy: the role of residual ovarian fragments. *Int J Gynaecol Obstet.* 1988;**26**(1):93–103.

18. Fat BC, Terzibachian JJ, Bertrand V, Leung F, de Lapparent T, Grisey A, et al. Ovarian remnant syndrome: diagnostic difficulties and management. *Gynecol Obstet Fertil.* 2009;**37**(6):488–94.

19. Magrina JF, Lidner TK, Cornelia JL, Lee RA. Cyclic vaginal bleeding after total hysterectomy. *J Pelvic Surg.* 1998;**4**(2):62–6.

20. Kaminski PF, Meilstrup JW, Shackelford DP, Sorosky JI, Thieme GA. Ovarian remnant syndrome, a reappraisal: the usefulness of clomiphene citrate in stimulating and pelvic ultrasound in Locating Remnant Ovarian Tissue. *J Gynecol Surg.* 1995;**11** (1):33–9.

21. Narayansingh G, Cumming G, Parkin D, Miller I. Ovarian cancer developing in the ovarian remnant syndrome: a case report and literature review. *Aust N Z J Obstet Gynaecol.* 2000;**40**(2):221–3.

22. Mahdavi A, Kumtepe Y, Nezhat F. Laparoscopic management of benign serous neoplasia arising from persistent ovarian remnant. *J Minim Invasive Gynecol.* 2007;**14**(5):654–6.

23. Donnez O, Squifflet J, Marbaix E, Jadoul P, Donnez J. Primary ovarian adenocarcinoma developing in ovarian remnant tissue ten years after laparoscopic hysterectomy and bilateral salpingo-oophorectomy for endometriosis. *J Minim Invasive Gynecol.* 2007;**14** (6):752–7.

24. Rossing MA, Cushing-Haugen KL, Wicklund KG, Doherty JA, Weiss NS. Risk of epithelial ovarian cancer in relation to benign ovarian conditions and ovarian surgery. *Cancer Causes Control.* 2008;**19** (10):1357–64.

25. Chan TL, Singh H, Benton AS, Harkins GJ. Ovarian artery embolization as a treatment for persistent ovarian remnant syndrome. *Cardiovasc Intervent Radiol.* 2017;**40**(8):1278–80.

Pudendal Neuralgia

Mario E. Castellanos, Katherine de Souza, and Michael Hibner

Editor's Introduction

In our practice pudendal neuralgia is defined as pain in the area of innervation of pudendal nerve. Pudendal nerve entrapment is a compression of the nerve by scar tissue, ligaments, or surgical material. Pudendal neuralgia may be caused by pudendal nerve entrapment, but other conditions described in this manual may lead to pudendal neuralgia. Diagnosis of pudendal nerve entrapment is difficult, and it is often made by exclusion of other conditions leading to pudendal pain (pudendal neuralgia). Most patients with pudendal nerve entrapment have a traumatic event that caused the onset of pain. Pelvic MRI may be helpful in ruling out other conditions causing pain and CT-guided pudendal nerve blocks narrow down the diagnosis to the pudendal nerve. Conservative treatments include avoidance of nerve reinjury, physical therapy, nerve blocks, and oral medications such as gabapentin or pregabalin. Patients may also benefit from nerve ablation procedures (pulse radiofrequency and cryoablation) and nerve stimulators. For patients who have failed all the conservative treatments, surgical decompression is an option with good outcomes.

Introduction

Pudendal neuralgia is a severely painful and often disabling neuropathic condition in the dermatomal distribution of the pudendal nerve [1]. It can affect any individual, regardless of gender, leading to pain in the clitoris/penis, vagina/scrotum, perineum, and rectum. Pudendal neuralgia is caused by a direct or indirect injury of the pudendal nerve and is often seen in conjunction with other pelvic pain conditions such as irritable bowel syndrome (IBS), interstitial cystitis/bladder pain syndrome (IC/BPS), and pelvic floor tension myalgia. Since the genitals are primarily affected, pudendal neuralgia is often confused with IC/BPS, vulvodynia, vaginismus, and vestibulitis.

In this chapter, we will focus on pudendal neuralgia in patients with phenotypically female genitalia. The term *pudendal neuralgia* is defined as pain along the distribution of the pudendal nerve. In contrast, the term *pudendal nerve entrapment* is defined as compression of the pudendal nerve that is identified during surgical decompression.

Anatomy of the Pudendal Nerve

The pudendal nerve originates from the ventral rami of the second, third, and fourth sacral spinal nerves and carries motor, sensory, and autonomic fibers. Afferent fibers project onto thoracolumbar sympathetic and sacral parasympathetic systems, although exact pathways are not well understood. Effects are primarily inhibitory in the bladder, and thus suppress bladder overactivity [2]. In addition, the pudendal nerve is involved in physiological changes during sexual response through regulation of vaginal and clitoral blood flow [3]. The pudendal nerve carries motor innervation to the external anal sphincter, urethral sphincter, muscles of the urogenital triangle, and muscles of the pelvic floor. In 88% of cases, the levator ani muscles are primarily innervated by the pudendal nerve and often share innervation with nerves directly from the S3–S4 nerve roots [4]. Terminal branches of the pudendal nerve reach the skin of the clitoris, labia major/minora, vestibule, perineum, and anus. Therefore, neuralgia of the pudendal nerve may lead to burning/pain in these areas. It is important to note that many other nerves overlap with the pudendal nerve to innervate this dermatome, including the ilioinguinal nerve, genitofemoral nerve, and posterior femoral cutaneous nerve. (See Chapter 16.)

After the pudendal nerve arises from S2 to S4, it courses through the greater sciatic foramen ventral to the piriformis muscle and enters the interligamentous space, the area between the sacrotuberous ligament and sacrospinous ligament, where it is joined with the pudendal artery and vein. The nerve then bends around the sacrospinous ligament to enter the lesser sciatic foramen. At this point, it courses through Alcock's canal, a narrow canal that is formed by the fascia of the obturator internus muscle. The canal ends at the medial aspect of the ischial tuberosity where typically three branches emerge: the inferior rectal, perineal, and dorsalclitoral nerves. The inferior rectal nerve travels medially and terminates at the external anal sphincter. The perineal branch courses ventrally along the inferior aspect of the inferior pubic ramus and stays superficial and caudal to the perineal membrane. It innervates the superficial transverse perineal, bulbocavernosus, and ischiocavernosus muscles. The dorsal/clitoral branch travels along the inferior edge of the inferior pubic ramus and may pierce the perineal membrane. It crosses either cephalad or caudad to the crus of the clitoris and then enters the crura of the clitoris on the dorsomedial side.

Anatomical Variations and Implications

The trunk of the pudendal nerve at the sacrospinous ligament has variability within the interligamentous space relative to the ischial spine. At that point, the pudendal nerve is a single trunk in 61.5% of cases and is divided into multiple trunks in 27% of cases [5]. The pudendal nerve fixed to the sacrospinous ligament by connective tissue. When dissected in an unembalmed cadaver, the nerve is mobile with hyperflexion of the hip, causing a lateral deviation at the sacrospinous ligament of 4 millimeters [6]. The degree of pudendal nerve mobility may have implications for postoperative recovery from pudendal nerve decompression.

The pudendal nerve is typically found 14.5–37 millimeters medial to the ischial spine. Therefore, performing a sacrospinous ligament fixation or placement of transvaginal mesh 3–4 centimeters from the ischial spine, as traditionally instructed, may lead to direct injury of the nerve.

The interligamentous space is narrow, measuring 10 millimeters, and can be further constricted by the falciform process of the sacrotuberous ligament that may be attached to the sacrospinous ligament. The pudendal nerve has been observed to also pierce the sacrospinous ligament and sacrotuberous ligament

and its falciform process [7]. This narrow space and anatomical variance results in the interligamentous space to be the most common location of entrapment.

Alcock's canal is variable in length and typically formed by the aponeurosis of the internal oblique muscle. The falciform process of the sacrotuberous ligament has also been observed to form Alcock's canal by either terminating at the obturator fascia or extending along the ischial ramus, fusing with the obturator fascia and continuing toward the ischioanal fossa [8]. These findings have implications of the sacrotuberous ligament being involved in pudendal nerve entrapment.

The variability of the clitoral branch of the pudendal nerve along the inferior pubic ramus may be vulnerable to entrapment. The nerve may pierce the perineal membrane and is therefore susceptible to entrapment. Also, its proximity to the inferior pubic ramus may increase its susceptibility to injury against bone in the event of trauma.

Anatomical Considerations of Pudendal Nerve Entrapment

Along the course of pudendal nerve, entrapment may occur in areas of fixation, acute flexion, within narrow canals, and by dynamic forces. Common anatomical locations of compression listed from cephalad to caudad are

- The piriformis muscle
- Interligamentous space
- Alcock's canal
- Ischial tuberosity
- Inferior pubic ramus

The most common location of entrapment of the pudendal nerve is within the interligamentous space and Alcock's canal. Compression of the nerve occurs when there are repetitive impact forces, acute direct trauma, or dynamic factors. Repetitive impact forces affect patients who develop pudendal nerve entrapment from activities such as cycling, where pressure from the bicycle seat at the perineum can cause nerve compression. Direct trauma is seen in patients following vaginal surgery, especially in reconstructive pelvic surgery that utilizes the sacrospinous ligament. Muscle spasms and dysfunction of the piriformis muscles and obturator internus muscle can lead to narrowing of the course of the pudendal nerve, leading to compression. Compression along the course of the pudendal nerve causes a narrowing that leads to increased pressure. Increased pressure can cause arterial compression, leading to ischemia, and venous compression leading to edema or congestion. These events result in the formation of fibrosis and entrapment. Intraoperatively, the pudendal nerve is seen fixed to the sacrospinous ligament with connective tissue. This observation should not be confused with nerve impingement but is an example of a physiological fixation that increases the susceptibility to injury.

Epidemiology

The prevalence of neuropathic pelvic pain has not been well defined, but has been estimated as 3.3% to 8.2% of the general population. It has been published that the prevalence of pudendal neuralgia is 1 in 100,000, but this is an estimate and not substantiated by any study. The portal for rare diseases (orphan.net) reports that the incidence in France is 1 in 6,000 people, updated in 2014 by Jean Jaque Labat. Prevalence of pudendal neuralgia may be much higher if the definition of "pain in the dermatomal distribution of the pudendal nerve" is used. This definition could include diagnoses such as vulvodynia, vaginismus, perineal pain, clitoral pain, and persistent sexual arousal disorder. Gender distribution can be estimated in studies of the reported outcomes of pudendal decompression surgery and other treatments. In these studies, women accounted for 60%–72% and men for 28%–40% of the study populations [9, 10]. Women may be more susceptible to developing pudendal neuralgia because of potentially traumatic events such as vaginal deliveries and vaginal surgery.

Etiology

Pudendal neuralgia can have somatic, visceral, and neuropathic origins and can be divided into pudendal neuralgia with and without entrapment. Somatic causes of pudendal neuralgia cause pudendal neuralgias via three mechanisms.

1. Hypertonic pelvic floor disorders may lead to symptoms of pudendal neuralgia without any true neuropathy. For instance, tension of the puborectalis muscle may lead to pain in the vagina and rectum with sitting.
2. Persistent hypertonicity can lead to peripheral sensitization of the pudendal nerve and neuralgia, and thus pudendal neuralgia without entrapment.

3. Pudendal neuralgia with entrapment can occur by muscle compression such as within Alcock's canal by the obturator internus muscle or within the greater sciatic foramen by the piriformis muscle.

Visceral origins cause pudendal neuralgia via viscero-somatic convergence or referred pain. Patients with IBS, endometriosis, and IC/BPS have associated hypertonic pelvic floor disorders via viscero-somatic convergence. Hypertonic pelvic floor disorders can then lead to pudendal neuralgia as described earlier. Visceral pain or pathology of the cervix, lower uterine segment, and vagina may refer pain to the pudendal nerve from sympathetic splanchnic nerves and the superior hypogastric nerve plexus [11]. Indeed, the pudendal nerve also carries sympathetic fibers that are associated with bladder function, and therefore patients with IC/BPS may have associated pudendal neuralgia.

Neuropathic causes of pudendal neuralgia usually result from injury of the pudendal nerve. Peripheral nerve injuries from crushing, stretching, or infections can lead to neuropathy without entrapment. Entrapment can occur when injuries result in fibrosis or narrowing in the spaces along the course of the pudendal nerve. Nerve impingement can occur iatrogenically from surgery or from a mass effect. For example, impingement at the sacral nerve root from Tarlov cysts has also been described as a cause of pudendal neuralgia and persistent genital arousal disorders [12]. It is hypothesized that the hydrostatic pressure of the fluid within the cyst causes compression of the pudendal nerve root. Nevertheless, in a series of patients with pudendal neuralgia and MRI evidence of Tarlov cysts, location of the cyst did not correlate with laterality of symptoms.

Traumatic events are often associated with the onset of pudendal neuralgia. For example, cycling is a very well described mechanism of pudendal nerve injury via pressure from the narrow bicycle seat at the perineum. From a case series of more than 100 patients who underwent pudendal decompression, inciting events proposed by the authors were frequently related to repetitive activity or acute trauma. Repetitive activities, seen in 19% of patients, included prolonged sitting, new sedentary work, cycling, horseback riding, and other athletic/sports. Acute traumas were seen in 57% of patients and included vaginal surgery, vaginal deliveries, falls, and acute sports injuries. No inciting event was identified in 24% of cases.

Presentation

Pudendal neuralgia is characterized by a searing or burning sensation in the dermatomal distribution of the pudendal nerve. The hallmark symptom is neuropathic pain with sitting that is improved or alleviated by standing. Many patients have pain continuously, but sitting always exacerbates the pain. Pain may be bilateral or unilateral and may be localized to the clitoris, vagina, perineum, or rectum depending on which branch or branches are affected. Patients with pudendal nerve entrapment experience sharp stabbing pain in the vagina or rectum secondary to activation of the nervi nevorum (unmyelinated or poorly myelinated fibers that play a role in the transmission of evoked sensory information) of the pudendal nerve within the interligamentous space. Allodynia and hyperalgesia are common. This frequently leads to external pain with touch or pressure from clothing. Patients often experience an exaggerated pain response with exams or other touching. In rare cases, this sharp pain may be perceived in the right or left lower quadrant abdomen and be confused with visceral pathology.

Pudendal neuralgia has unique alleviating and aggravating factors. The pain is usually less severe in the morning and worse in the evening, but it does not wake up the patient at night. It is dependent on physical activity and sitting progressively worsen symptoms throughout the day. Sitting on a toilet seat alleviates the pain because pressure from the seat is focused the lateral aspects of the ischial tuberosities and allows for relaxation of the pelvic floor. Heat may improve somatic causes of pudendal neuralgia, while ice to the sacrum or vagina helps pain of neuropathic origin.

Associated symptoms include allotriesthesia, the sensation of a foreign object in the vagina or rectum, such as a ball. Some patients describe a sensation of a hot poker in those areas. Pudendal neuralgia prevents most patients from having sexual intercourse secondary to dyspareunia and postcoital pain that can persist for days. Bowel and bladder function may be affected, causing pain with a full bladder, urinary frequency and urgency, urinary hesitancy, dyschezia, and constipation.

Persistent genital arousal disorder (PGAD), sometimes referred to as restless genital syndrome, is one of the most vexing manifestations of pudendal neuralgia. Patients experience a physical sensation of arousal that is extremely unsettling and unrelenting. Masturbation and orgasm can temporarily alleviate symptoms, but, in some cases, these interventions can worsen the condition. It is not uncommon for patients with pudendal nerve entrapment to present with persistent genital arousal in the absence of pain. Therefore, patients with PGAD should be evaluated for possible pudendal neuralgia.

Without intervention, symptoms seem to worsen over time and patients begin to experience pain outside the dermatomal distribution of the pudendal nerve. Lower back, sacroiliac joints, lower abdomen, buttocks, and lower extremity are common areas of associated pain. Neuralgias may develop of the obturator, sciatic, posterior femoral cutaneous, and genitofemoral nerves. Pain outside of pudendal neuralgia in the setting of worsening pain may be a sign of central sensitization or complex regional pain syndrome. (See Chapter 2.)

This condition deeply affects patients' social interactions and personal relationships and can lead to isolation, anxiety, and depression. The authors have found that validated quality of life questionnaires such as SF-36 scores of their patients are low in comparison to the general population. Patients with pudendal neuralgia are often disabled and unable to work. They need to spend most of the day lying down because sitting and other simple physical activities such as prolonged standing severely exacerbates their pain. It is difficult for significant others, family members, physicians, and other healthcare providers to understand the immense impact of pudendal neuralgia and chronic neuropathic pain. As a result, patients often endure poor support from others.

Diagnosis

History

Pudendal neuralgia is largely a clinical diagnosis based on history. It may be challenging to diagnose because patients may not explain their pain as described in the preceding section. Therefore, it is very important to ascertain the exact location of the pain. If patients localize their pain to the dermatomal distribution of the pudendal nerve, then the following questions can be used to screen for possible pudendal neuralgia.

1. Is your pain worse with sitting?
2. Do you feel better when sitting on a toilet seat?
3. Does your pain awaken you from sleep?
4. Do you feel your pain more on one side? *
5. Did your pain start after an accident, surgery, or physical activity?

*Although a patient with pudendal neuralgia may have bilateral symptoms, unilateral symptoms are highly indicative of nerve injury or neuropathic origin of pudendal neuralgia.

It is important to elicit when and how the symptoms started. Onset of symptoms related to an event such as surgery or falls may lead to speedier diagnosis and management. For instance, if the pain started immediately following a sacrospinous ligament fixation, it raises suspicion that a suture is impinging the nerve. This guides the physical examination, counseling, and subsequent management. A comprehensive review of systems and validated pelvic pain questionnaires should also be used in patients with pudendal neuralgia to identify associated conditions.

Physical Examination

The purpose of the physical examination is to [1] localize the pain to the distribution of the pudendal nerve [2], assess the pelvic floor muscles, and [3] refine the differential diagnosis.

Examination starts with general inspection, especially patient position, during history-taking. Patients often prefer to stand and may refuse to sit. Patients who are sitting may be leaning to their unaffected side or relieving pressure from their affected side by crossing their legs or sitting on their feet. Patients may sit on a cushion brought by them from home or may lie down throughout the interview.

Examination of the pudendal nerve is performed in the lithotomy position. First, the external genitalia are inspected and sensory testing should be performed. A cotton swab can be used to evaluate for allodynia and a filament used to evaluate for hyperalgesia. Sensory testing should include the entire vulva, perineum, anus, buttocks, thighs, groin, and mons pubis. A pain map can be drawn to identify the affected nerve (Figure 15.1). Unlike other peripheral nerve injuries, pudendal neuralgia rarely is associated with sensory deficit or numbness. Motor defects are similarly uncommon. Anal wink reflect should be elicited and sphincter tone noted. Pudendal neuralgia may cause autonomic dysfunction resulting in dryness of the skin and decreased sweat. Next, a single digit is introduced vaginally or rectally and the pudendal nerve is palpated at the sacrospinous ligament, along the obturator internus muscles, and along the inferior pubic ramus. Digital compression of the nerve at these sites may elicit a Tinel's sign – pain at the site of examination with possible radiation of pain along the distribution of the nerve. Palpation of the nerve may reproduce symptoms such as genital arousal or foreign body sensation. Pelvic floor muscles should be palpated and muscle tension and tenderness noted. Reproducing pain with palpation of the muscle but not the nerve would suggest a pure muscle problem. Lastly, a full examination as discussed in [3] should be performed to develop a comprehensive differential diagnosis (Table 15.1). A particular focus on the musculoskeletal examination should be taken.

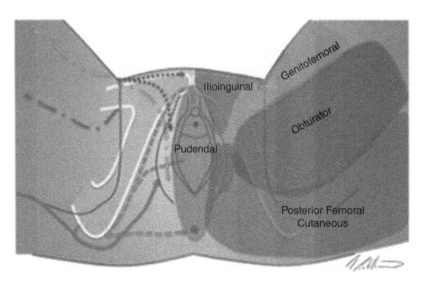

Figure 15.1 Innervation of the perineal area.

Table 15.1 Differential diagnosis of pudendal neuralgia

Musculoskeletal

Pelvic floor tension myalgia
Piriformis syndrome
Obturator internus syndrome
Labrum tear
Sacroiliac joint dysfunction
Coccydynia
Adductor myalgia
Hamstring tendinosis
Osteitis of the ischial tuberosity

Neuropathic

Ilioinguinal neuralgia
Genitofemoral neuralgia
Posterior femoral cutaneous neuralgia
Obturator neuralgia
Herpes
Varicella zoster
Diabetic neuropathy
Spinal nerve stenosis
Complex regional pain syndrome type 1

Dermatological

Vestibulitis
Lichen sclerosis
Lichen planus
Atrophic vaginitis

Vascular

Vulvar varicosities
Pelvic congestion syndrome

Visceral

Endometriosis
Pelvic adhesions
Adenomyosis
Interstitial cystitis/bladder pain syndrome

Testing

Pudendal Nerve Block A successful anesthetic block of the pudendal nerve confirms the diagnosis of pudendal neuralgia. A pudendal nerve block is diagnostic only if the block results both numbness exclusively along the distribution of the pudendal nerve and complete relief of pudendal pain symptoms. When interpreting the results of a nerve block, one must keep in mind that the anesthetic effect may be brief and therefore interpretation should be done quickly. Patients may have pain outside the distribution of the pudendal nerve and therefore may still report pain outside of the pudendal dermatome after a diagnostic block. Blocks that result in numbness

of the legs or buttocks are unreliable because the anesthetic agent has affected the sciatic nerve and/ or the posterior femoral cutaneous nerve. A successful diagnostic pudendal nerve block does not confirm pudendal nerve entrapment or a neuropathic cause of pudendal neuralgia. Patient with referred pain from visceral origins or who have muscle spasms such as levator ani syndrome may still report complete pain relief from a pudendal nerve block. Diagnostic block may be performed with or without image guidance.

Pudendal Nerve Block Without Image Guidance Without image guidance, a pudendal nerve block is performed transvaginally as traditionally practiced in obstetrics. This method results in anesthesia of the clitoris, vagina, perineum, and rectum. The injection is performed by palpating the ischial spine and injecting through or inferior to the sacrospinous ligament at a point that is 2 centimeters medial to the ischial spine. The anesthetic agent infiltrates the interligamentous space, affecting the trunk of the pudendal nerve. Advantages of this block is that it can be easily performed in the office and, if practiced consistently, has good precision. On the other hand, a vaginal block may result in infiltration of the coccygeus muscle instead of the interligamentous space if injected too superficially. Leakage of local anesthetic into the greater sciatic foramen can affect the sciatic or posterior femoral cutaneous nerves and therefore not provide diagnostic information. Thus, results of a transvaginal pudendal nerve block should be interpreted with caution [13].

Pudendal Nerve Block with Image Guidance CT guidance is the preferred image modality and the most studied technique for performing a pudendal nerve block. The injection is transgluteal with the patient in a prone position. The needle is guided into Alcock's canal through the interligamentous space. Injection of local contrast confirms accurate placement within the canal and images can be evaluated for malpositioning. Thus, the CT-guided pudendal nerve block is highly reproducible. The main disadvantage to this technique is its inability to block the inferior rectal nerve if it branches before the pudendal nerve enters Alcock's canal. Therefore, all patients should undergo sensory testing post procedure to confirm complete pudendal nerve block. If the rectum is unaffected, then the block can be repeated and the needle adjusted target the interligamentous space at

Alcock's canal. Other modalities using fluoroscopy or ultrasound have also been described, but those techniques have not been well studied.

Pudendal Nerve Motor Terminal Latency Testing A test of motor conduction, pudendal nerve motor terminal latency measures the velocity of impulses traveling along the pudendal nerve. Nerve injury or compression can result in slow conduction and prolonged latency. Measurements are obtained using a St. Mark's electrode placed on a gloved finger that is introduced into the vagina or rectum with the tip of the finger on the ischial spine. Transvaginally, the base of the finger is in contact with the bulbospongiosus muscles; transrectally, the base of the finger is in contact with the external anal sphincter. The electrical impulse causes a contraction in these terminal muscles and the time from impulse initiation to contraction is recorded. This test is useful in identifying pudendal nerve injury in patients with anal incontinence and other motor deficiencies. Since the vast majority of patients with pudendal neuralgia do not have signs of sphincter denervation, this test is infrequently useful. Testing is often normal in patients who have pain as their only symptom and therefore cannot be used to diagnose or exclude pudendal neuralgia. Furthermore, women with a history of vaginal deliveries are more likely to have abnormal testing. More frequently, sensory testing using two-point discrimination, warmth detection threshold test, and vibration test are used to assess nerve integrity. Again, these tests are less useful because most patients do not have sensory deficiencies.

Magnetic Resonance Imaging MRI of the pelvis is a promising technique for evaluation of the pudendal nerve. Using magnetic resonance neurography and anatomical protocols, the pudendal nerve can be visualized throughout its course and evaluated for abnormalities. The course of the pudendal nerve is visualized and evaluated for perineural scarring visualized as strand-like hypointensities. The vein is compared with its contralateral side and assessed for varicosities and engorgement. Vascular edema can lead to compression, mostly within Alcock's canal, causing compression and eventually fibrosis. The obturator internus muscle and muscle of the levator ani are evaluated for atrophy and signs of denervation. Along its course, mass effect may be noted from tumors, schwannomas, or endometriomas. Lastly, the sacral nerve roots are evaluated for

Table 15.2 Nantes Criteria (inclusion)

- Pain in the distribution of the pudendal nerve
- Pain predominately with sitting
- Pain does not wake the patient at night
- No objective sensory deficit on clinical exam
- Pain relieved by diagnostic pudendal nerve block

possible compression. MRI is a useful tool to rule out other causes of symptoms of pudendal neuralgia and help guide management. At this point, there are no studies that correlate findings of perineural scarring with intraoperative findings or with outcomes. In a study of our patients undergoing surgical decompression, the presence or absence of perineural scarring on MRI did not correlate with intraoperative findings.

Nantes Criteria In 2008, Prof. Roger Robert developed Nantes Criteria for the diagnosis of pudendal nerve entrapment (Table 15.2). Based on symptoms, clinical findings, and response to pudendal nerve block, he proposed inclusionary and exclusionary criteria to predict pudendal nerve entrapment. These criteria remain the best way to diagnose pudendal neuralgia from possible pudendal nerve entrapment.

Currently, pudendal nerve entrapment can be definitively diagnosed only through surgical evaluation demonstrating compression of the pudendal nerve. Therefore, Nantes Criteria can help predict only patients who may benefit for surgical intervention.

Treatment

Clinical Approach Because pudendal neuralgia may have multiple etiologies and presentations, a stepwise approach should be taken in formulating a treatment plan. After thoroughly evaluating the patient and performing a pudendal nerve block, the treatment options will depend on the (1) inciting event, (2) location of pain, (3) presence of pelvic floor muscle spasms, (4) response to pudendal nerve block, and (5) presence of associated chronic pain conditions.

Initial Measures for All Patients

Patient Education and Expectations The first step to management of pudendal neuralgia is to provide education and expectations. Many patients have gone through a long diagnostic process and may have seen multiple physicians who were unable to provide insight into their condition. Thus, giving the patient a diagnosis is the first therapeutic step; it provides emotional relief and validates their symptoms. Providers should also educate patients about the pudendal nerve and pelvic floor anatomy. This information further validates their condition by explaining how injury or dysfunction of the pudendal nerve and pelvic floor muscles can lead to the symptoms they are experiencing.

After providing education, it is important to establish expectations. A patient who has been in chronic pain will likely have a prolonged therapeutic course and experience incremental improvement of her symptoms. In addition, patients should understand that response to treatment is variable.

Behavior Modification Changes in behavior can have a significant impact on symptoms of pudendal neuralgia. Changes include (1) avoiding the activity that led to injury and (2) avoiding direct pressure on the perineum with sitting. If a particular activity is identified as the cause of pudendal neuralgia the patient should stop that activity. Additionally, any activity that worsens symptoms such as prolonged standing and sitting, bending, and squatting should be avoided.

Because sitting often worsens symptoms, modifications should be made to limit sitting time and to help alleviate pressure on the perineum when sitting is necessary. If their jobs permit it, patients can use a standing workstation and arrange for accommodations to rest and lie down during work. If the patient can tolerate sitting, breaks should be taken and the patient should always avoid sitting in uncomfortable conditions. Frequently, patients find relief by sitting on a cushion with a middle section cut out. This modification causes pressure to be applied lateral to the ischial tuberosities and avoids direct pressure on the pudendal nerve. Zero gravity chairs or lounge chairs can also be useful.

Behavior modifications should never be the sole treatment but should be used as a strategy to prevent further injury and give patients some measures to help prevent or minimize symptoms. However, it is imperative that additional treatments to address the root problem be utilized.

Medications The goal of medication is to reduce the pain experience. There are no FDA-approved medications for these patients and no single medication that works best [Table 15.3]. Pelvic floor muscle spasms can be treated with muscle relaxers in oral or

Table 15.3 Medications used in treatment of pudendal neuralgia

Medication	Dose	Side effects
Suppositories (vaginal/ rectal)		
Belladonna/ opium	16.2 mg/20–70 mg bid prn	Constipation, drowsiness
Valium/ baclofen	5–10 mg/4–8 mg bid prn	Drowsiness
Ketamine	15–60 mg bid prn	Nightmares, hallucinations
Neuroleptic		
Gabapentin	300–1,200 mg tid	Drowsiness, confusion
Pregabaline	75–150 mg bid	

suppository form. Neuropathic pain can be treated with antiepileptic γ-aminobutyric acid (GABA) analogs such as gabapentin and pregabalin. It is important to note that opioids have not been shown to provide effective neuropathic pain relief in chronic pain patients, and therefore providers should be cautious about starting these medications.

Physical Therapy All patients with pudendal neuralgia should be referred to pelvic floor physical therapy for evaluation and treatment of the pelvic musculature. The pelvic floor physical therapist should be knowledgeable about treating patients with pudendal neuralgia and pelvic pain. Therapy focuses on alleviating the pelvic floor spasms and addressing associated conditions such as sacroiliac joint dysfunction and adductor hypertonicity. There are also specific manual treatments to the pudendal nerve that can provide relief. Physical therapy should occur concurrently with other treatment. Progress should be monitored with regular office visits and there should be close communication with the physical therapist. Please refer to Chapter 20 for more information.

Addressing Associated Chronic Pain Conditions After a thorough history and physical examination, other painful chronic conditions may be identified such as IC/PBS, IBS, endometriosis, and/or fibromyalgia. Treatment should be started to address these conditions in conjunction with treatments for pudendal neuralgia. If the patient is diagnosed with complex regional pain syndrome, then this should be treated separately. Please see Chapters 2, 6, and 20.

Interventional Procedures

Pudendal Nerve Blocks A series of pudendal nerve blocks may be an effective treatment for pudendal neuralgia [14, 15]. From 75% to 88% of patients have shown improvement following a series of three pudendal nerve blocks. Traditionally, nerve blocks are performed with steroids to reduce perineural inflammation and ectopic activity. This practice has recently been challenged specifically for pudendal neuralgia in a randomized double blinded controlled trial of patients undergoing CT-guided pudendal nerve blocks with local anesthetic alone versus local anesthetic with corticosteroids. The study found that both groups had similar response rate at 3 months post injection, 11.8% versus 14.3% [16]. Nevertheless, the study only followed patients after one injection and it was not compared to the traditional treatment of a series of injections.

Our protocol is to perform a series of three CT-guided pudendal nerve blocks 6 weeks apart using bupivacaine 0.5% mixed with 40 mg of Kenalog. The injection is placed within Alcock's canal for a total volume of 10 mL.

We prefer CT guidance because it allows for visual confirmation of placement and is therefore reproducible. Also, it can be adjusted to target the interligamentous space to have more effect on the inferior rectal branch if needed.

Alternatively, a vaginal pudendal nerve block can be performed if image guidance is not available. To improve the technical success of a vaginal pudendal block, care must be taken to ensure that the pudendal needle transverses the sacrospinous ligament so that the block infiltrates the interligamentous space. The spacer from the pudendal block kit needle should be removed and the injection should have very little to no resistance. Aspiration should be performed prior to injection to minimize risk of intravascular injection.

Patients should be followed after every injection to ascertain effectiveness, side effects, and complications. Common side effects include numbness in the distribution of the sciatic nerve, pain at the injection site, bleeding, hematoma formation, nerve injury, and worsening of symptoms. Although concerning, worsening of symptoms is usually temporary and may be a result from muscles spasms or from needle trauma.

Botulinum Toxin Injections Injections of botulinum toxin can be beneficial in patients with persistent pelvic floor muscle spasms that have been refractory to physical therapy. Botulinum toxin inhibits muscle contraction by inhibiting neuropeptide release and blocking acetylcholine at the synapse, thus decreasing muscle spasms. In a recent meta-analysis this procedure has been shown to be effective for the treatment of chronic pelvic pain due to tension of the pelvic floor muscles [17]. In this study, botulinum toxin reduced pain scores by an average of 2.8.

In patients with pudendal neuralgia, botulinum toxin injections are indicated in patients who have hypertonic pelvic floor disorders and (1) persistent muscle tension despite physical therapy, (2) cannot tolerate physical therapy or physical examination, or (3) have localized trigger point/tender point of a muscle.

The procedure is performed under general anesthesia to minimize the pain response, as most patients have a component of peripheral and central sensitization. Prior to the procedure, the patient is examined and tender points/muscle spasms are identified along the levator ani and obturator internus muscles. A bilateral pudendal nerve block is performed using 10 mL of 0.5% bupivacaine to provide postoperative pain relief and decrease muscular activity of the levator ani. Onabotulinumtoxin A is diluted to 10 units/mL by mixing 200 units of onabotulinum toxin A with 20 mL of injectable 0.9% saline. Using a pudendal nerve block kit needle with trumpet, injections are performed transvaginally in 1-mL aliquots along the entire belly of the muscle or concentrated along the tender points. We find that 200 units of onabotulinum toxin A at this concentration allows for global coverage of the levator ani and obturator internus muscles in patients with bilateral involvement.

Effects of Botox are seen in 5–10 days, and patients usually report improvement of symptoms at 2 weeks post procedure. The chemical effects of the Botox can last up to 4 months, after which the patient may need repetitive injections or ongoing pelvic floor physical therapy. In our experience, repetitive injections are safe and there is no decrease is effectiveness over time. Side effects and complications of these injections include constipation, urinary urgency, worsening of pain, and rarely urinary or fecal incontinence. Care should be taken to not inject near the urethral sphincter or external anal sphincter to minimize risk of incontinence.

Other Described Procedures Other treatment options that have been reported include pulsed radiofrequency ablation, cryoablation, neuromodulation, and spinal cord stimulators. These techniques are still being studied and currently not recommended outside of clinical trials.

Surgery Surgical decompression of the pudendal nerve is the only treatment option that has been shown effective in a randomized controlled trial [9]. It is reserved for patients who have a high suspicion of pudendal nerve entrapment as the cause of pudendal neuralgia. A patient must meet Nantes Criteria and undergo extensive evaluation for other causes of pelvic pain prior to being a candidate for surgery. In addition, surgery may be recommended for patients who have not responded to previously described conservative treatments. True pudendal nerve entrapment can be confirmed only during surgery, and therefore, success of the surgery strongly depends on appropriate patient selection.

Patients who have high index of suspicion for pudendal nerve entrapment

1. Meet Nantes Criteria
2. Have onset associated with trauma or surgery
3. Have unilateral symptoms

Transgluteal Decompression of the Pudendal Nerve Transgluteal pudendal neurolysis and transposition is the most successful approach to surgical decompression of the pudendal nerve. It was first described by neurosurgeon Roger Robert in 1989 and has since been modified by the authors to improve visualization. This approach to pudendal neurolysis gives access to the nerve from just inferior to the piriformis muscle to the distal end of Alcock's canal at the ischial tuberosity. The surgery has two objectives: (1) to release the nerve from fibrosis and (2) to alleviate impingement. By achieving these two objectives, the nerve can begin to heal and regenerate. Over a follow-up period of 12 months, 71.4% of patients show improvement of symptoms including complete resolution of symptoms. In our experience, one third of patients are pain free, one third of patients are improved, and one third of patients show no improvement. About 1% of patient report worse symptoms after the surgery.

The procedure begins with the patient in a prone jack-knife position and the skin overlying the sacrotuberous ligament is marked (Figure 15.2). A transgluteal incision is made and the sacrotuberous ligament is exposed. At this point, a surgical microscope is used for adequate visualization. A Z-plasty incision is made over the sacrotuberous ligament, allowing for repair of the ligament at the end of the surgery. The interligamentous space is exposed (Figure 15.3). The nerve is identified using a Nerve Integrity Monitoring System and secured with a vessel loop. The falciform process of the sacrotuberous ligament is resected and the nerve is freed from any surrounding fibrosis. Next, the sacrospinous ligament is transected and the ischial spine is blunted if prominent. The nerve may be wrapped in a protective sheet at this point. We prefer an amniotic membrane wrap, as it is not permanent and helps reduce formation of adhesions. The nerve is then transposed anteriorly medial to the ischial spine. The catheter of an On-Q pain pump containing 0.5% bupivacaine is introduced through the skin and placed along the pudendal nerve. The sacrotuberous ligament is repaired with

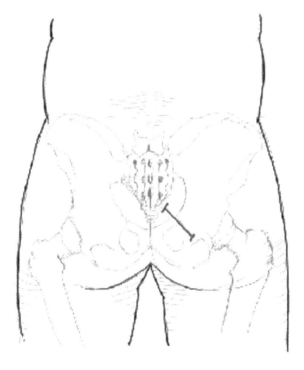

Figure 15.2 Location on the incision for transgluteal pudendal neurolysis.

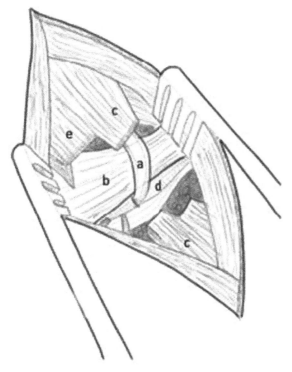

Figure 15.3 View through the right transgluteal incision. Skin, fat, and gluteus muscle are incised. (a) Pudendal neurovascular bundle. (b) Sacrospinous ligament. (c) Cut edges of sacrotuberous ligament. (d) Piriformis muscle. (e) Gluteus muscle.

Prolene sutures and the skin is closed. We place a negative-pressure wound dressing over the skin to help minimize infection.

Postoperatively, the On-Q pain pump is typically set to 2 mL/hour and removed when empty, about 10 days. Patients should work with a physical therapist immediately to help with mobility, particularly of the hip. For 2 months postoperatively, patients are restricted to not bend the hip on the operated side more than 90 degrees relative to the torso. Bending more than 90 degrees may cause excessive strain on the repaired sacrotuberous ligament and lead to injury. Patient may notice improvement of symptoms at 6 months with maximal improvement at 18 months. Risks of the procedure include bleeding, infection, hematoma, nerve injury, and worsening of symptoms.

Minimal or no improvement following surgery may be secondary to (1) incorrect diagnosis, (2) persistence of pelvic floor muscle spasms, (3) permanent nerve injury, or (4) central sensitization. Management strategies for these patients include revising the diagnosis,

treating pelvic floor muscles, and medical management for central sensitization (See chapters 2, 6, and 20.)

There is a small subset of patients who show initial improvement at 12 months, but their symptoms then worsen over time. A gradual regression of symptoms may be secondary to reformation of fibrosis. Acute recurrence of symptoms may be secondary to reinjury. In these patients, the treatment algorithm is the same as outlined in this chapter. If conservative management fails, reoperation and decompression of the pudendal nerve can be performed, with up to 80% of patients achieving pain reduction or cure [13].

Five Things You Need to Know

- Suspect pudendal neuralgia in patients who present with pain in the clitoris, vagina, perineum, and/or rectum when sitting.
- Vaginal palpation of the sacrospinous ligament will elicit a Tinel's sign in patients with pudendal neuralgia.
- An image-guided pudendal nerve block must be performed to confirm the diagnosis.
- Pudendal neuralgia is not equivalent to pudendal nerve entrapment.
- Transgluteal decompression of the pudendal nerve is reserved for patients who have a high index of suspicion for pudendal nerve entrapment and who have failed conservative treatments.

References

1. Hibner M, Desai N, Robertson LJ, Nour M. Pudendal neuralgia. *J Minim Invasive Gynecol.* 2010;**17**(2):148–53.

2. Reitz A, Schmid DM, Curt A, Knapp PA, Schurch B. Afferent fibers of the pudendal nerve modulate sympathetic neurons controlling the bladder neck. *Neurourol Urodyn.* 2003;**601**:597–601.

3. Connell K, Guess MK, Combe J La, et al. Evaluation of the role of pudendal nerve integrity in female sexual function using noninvasive techniques. *Am J Obstet Gynecol.* 2005;**192**(5):1712–7.

4. Grigorescu BA, Lazarou G, Olson TR, et al. Innervation of the levator ani muscles: description of the nerve branches to the pubococcygeus, iliococcygeus, and puborectalis muscles. *Int Urogynecol J Pelvic Floor Dysfunct.* 2008;**19**(1):107–16.

5. Maldonado PA, Chin K, Garcia AA, Corton MM. Anatomic variations of pudendal nerve within pelvis and pudendal canal: clinical applications. *Am J Obstet Gynecol.* 2015;**213**(5):727.e1–727.e6.

6. Brandon K, Robertson L, Castellanos M, Atashroo D, Chen A, Hibner M. Excursion of the pudendal nerve and change in distance between the sacrospinous and sacrotuberous ligaments. In International Pelvic Pain Society Annual Meeting; 2012, 75–6.

7. Labat JJ, Robert R, Bensignor M, Buzelin JM. [Neuralgia of the pudendal nerve: anatomo-clinical considerations and therapeutical approach] (in French). *J Urol (Paris)*. 1990;**96**(5):239–44.

8. Loukas M, Louis RG, Hallner B, Gupta AA, White D. Anatomical and surgical considerations of the sacrotuberous ligament and its relevance in pudendal nerve entrapment syndrome. *Surg Radiol Anat.* 2006;**28**(2):163–9.

9. Robert R, Labat J, Bensignor M, et al. Decompression and transposition of the pudendal nerve in pudendal neuralgia: a randomized controlled trial and long-term evaluation. *Eur Urol.* 2005;**47**(3):403–8.

10. Masala S, Calabria E, Cuzzolino A, Raguso M, Morini M, Simonetti G. CT-guided percutaneous pulse-dose radiofrequency for pudendal neuralgia. *Cardiovasc Intervent Radiol.* 2014;**37**(2):476–81.

11. Perry CP. Peripheral neuropathies and pelvic pain: diagnosis and management. *Clin Obstet Gynecol.* 2003;**46**(4):789–96.

12. Komisaruk BR, Lee H-J. Prevalence of sacral spinal (Tarlov) cysts in persistent genital arousal disorder. *J Sex Med.* 2012;**9**:2047–56.

13. Hibner M, Castellanos ME, Drachman D, Balducci J. Repeat operation for treatment of persistent pudendal nerve entrapment after pudendal neurolysis. *J Minim Invasive Gynecol.* 2012;**19**(3):325–30.

14. McDonald JS, Spigos DG. Computed tomography-guided pudendal block for treatment of pelvic pain due to pudendal neuropathy. *Obstet Gynecol.* 2000;**95**(2):306–9.

15. Fanucci E, Manenti G, Ursone A, et al. Ruolo della radiologia interventistica nella nevralgia del nervo pudendo: descrizione della tecnica e revisione della letteratura. *Radiol Medica.* 2009;**114**(3):425–36.

16. Labat JJ, Riant T, Lassaux A, et al. Adding corticosteroids to the pudendal nerve block for pudendal neuralgia: a randomised, double-blind, controlled trial. *BJOG.* 2017;**124**(2):251–60.

17. Meister M, Brubaker A, Sutcliffe S, Lowder J. Effectiveness of botulinum toxin injection to the pelvic floor for treatment of pelvic floor myofascial pain in women: a systematic review and meta-analysis. *Am J Obstet Gynecol.* 2019;**220**(3):S754.

Chapter 16

Other Peripheral Pelvic Neuralgias

Mario E. Castellanos and Katherine de Souza

Epidemiology

The incidence of neuropathic pelvic pain from peripheral nerves, other than the pudendal nerve is unknown. In a systematic review of epidemiological studies, it was estimated that 6.9% to 10% of patients with chronic pain have neuropathic pain symptoms [1]. Peripheral neuropathies may result after major gynecological surgery in 1.9% of patients. Affected nerves included the obturator (39%), iliohypogastric/ilioinguinal (21%), genitofemoral (17%), femoral (7.5%), and lumbosacral plexus (0.2%) [2].

Etiology

Neuropathic pain often arises as a direct consequence of a lesion or disease that affects the sensory component of the nervous system [3]. Peripheral nerves may be injured as a result of direct trauma, stretch, crush, fibrosis with entrapment, suture ligation, and repetitive low-impact forces. Patients may also develop

peripheral neuralgias from peripheral sensitization from repetitive painful stimuli or from central sensitization. In addition, a referral pattern from visceral pain via visceral somatic convergence can lead to pain along certain dermatomes [4] (Table 16.1).

Therefore, it is important to consider visceral etiologies when diagnosing a patient with peripheral neuralgias. Other causes of specific peripheral nerve injuries are organized by nerve later in this chapter.

History and Physical Examination

Patients with peripheral neuropathic pain may associate the start of their pain with a specific event such as blunt trauma, a fall, surgery, obstetrical procedure, or radiation. Repetitive activities such as sitting, exercising, and sports may also cause nerve injury. Pain is experienced either as dysesthetic pain or nerve trunk pain. Dysesthetic pain is usually described as a constant or intermittent searing, burning, or icy-cold pain. Skin and subcutaneous structures along the distribution of the nerve are affected. On the other hand, nerve trunk pain is experienced as a constant or paroxysmal deep-seated, sharp, knife-like pain. It is well localized at a specific point along the nerve, usually at the site of injury or impingement. Nerve trunk pain improves with rest or optimal position and is aggravated by movement. Symptoms may be localized in the lower abdomen, thighs, genitoanal region, and buttocks. Asking the patient to demonstrate or verbalize the location of the pain is the first step to identifying the affected nerve. In patients with pain in the genitoanal region, peripheral nerves other than the pudendal nerve should be considered. The ilioinguinal, genitofemoral, obturator, and posterior femoral cutaneous nerves may supply innervation of the skin of the vulva, perineum, and anus (Figure 16.1).

The goal of clinical examination is to discriminate between visceral and somatic pain and to localize the pain anatomically to a specific dermatome. Pain can

Table 16.1 Viscero-somatic convergence

Peripheral nerve	Visceral field
Ilioinguinal	Fallopian tube: Proximal Uterus: Fundus
Genitofemoral	Fallopian tube: Proximal Uterus: Fundus Ureter: Proximal
Lateral femoral cutaneous	Uterus: Lower segment
Pudendal	Cervix Bladder Ureter: Distal Vagina: Upper Rectum

be localized by testing the patient's response to light touch with a cotton swab. Sites where pain is produced either on the abdomen or perineal region should be documented and can be marked on the skin. A trigger point may be identified in the muscles within or surrounding the affected area. Indeed, the presence of allodynia and trigger points greatly increases the probability of neuropathic pain [5]. Special attention should be placed on scars and prior surgical incisions, as these may be sites of nerve injury. Please refer to Chapter 3 on physical examination.

Diagnostic Procedures

To diagnose peripheral neuralgia as a cause of chronic pelvic pain, alleviation of pain must be demonstrated

by a nerve block. There are two objectives when performing a nerve block: confirm the diagnosis and manage pain. It is important that the patient understands that the primary objective is diagnostic and that the procedure may not yield long-term pain relief. To accurately perform a nerve block, image guidance should be used to localize the nerve and to demonstrate site-specific infiltration of the analgesia.

In this chapter, we focus on the technique of performing ultrasound-guided nerve blocks. Some descriptions of how to perform selective nerve blocks are based on the authors' experiences and have not been published in peer-reviewed journals. References are given when available.

For a nerve block to provide diagnostic information, pain must be present at the time of the procedure. Evaluation of the analgesic effect should take place immediately following the block to allow for accurate interpretation of the results. Prior to performing a nerve block, informed consent should be obtained. Contraindications include coagulopathy, allergies to analgesic agent, and infection at the site of the injection. Patients with severe allodynia and/or central sensitization may require general anesthesia or conscious sedation, but this may complicate the interpretation of the results. Pain may be measured by a visual analog scale (VAS) or numerical rating before the injection and used to compare post procedure. If patients are not having any pain, the injection will not be useful for diagnosis, and patients should return when they are having pain. If pain results from

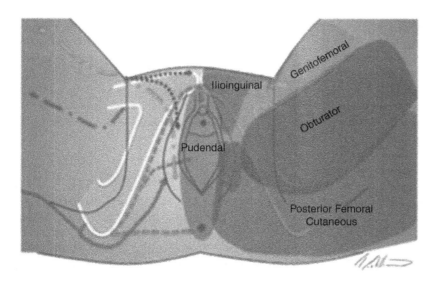

Figure 16.1 Innervation of the perineal area.

a specific activity or position, patients may induce pain in order to proceed with the block [6, 7].

The neurovascular bundle of peripheral nerves can be effectively visualized via ultrasound. Clinicians must understand the physics of ultrasounds in order to select the most effective ultrasound probe to visualize specific anatomical locations. For instance, to visualize the abdominal wall and the ilioinguinal nerve, a 14 MHz linear probe may provide appropriate penetration and resolution of superficial structures in a thin patient. However, in obese patients, a 9 MHz or lower probe may be required for deep penetration to visualize the same structures at a cost of resolution. When performing ultrasound-guided blocks, it is best to work with an ultrasonographer who is skilled in musculoskeletal imaging.

After the probe is selected, the procedure begins by visualizing the neurovascular bundle in the expected anatomical location. Color flow can be used to help visualize the artery and the vein. Next, a needle is advanced under ultrasound guidance and is placed adjacent to the neurovascular bundle within the fascial plane. It is important not to place the needle within the vessel, as this can lead to vascular or neurological injury if infiltration is performed within the nerve. The needle needed to perform the block should be long enough to reach the target and may be "etched" to help visualization on ultrasound. Twenty-two-gauge needles are useful because they are small, yet still provide the haptic feedback that aids in identification of fascial planes and muscles. It is best to use an in-plane technique when advancing the needle under ultrasound guidance so that the needle can be completely visualized throughout its path. The clinician must be aware of surrounding anatomy, particularly vascular structures, through which the needle may be traveling. Once the needle is at its target, a small volume of local anesthetic (1–3 mL) should be used to minimize spread of analgesia to surrounding structures and to specifically select for the nerve. Separation of the fascial plane should be visualized; infiltration of the anesthetic into the muscle should be avoided. Lidocaine and bupivacaine are popular choices, but any local anesthetic can be used. Clinicians must be familiar with the time of onset and duration of the anesthetic used so that patients are evaluated in the appropriate timeframe post procedure.

After the injection, a technical evaluation should be performed while the anesthetic is in effect. Analgesic effect should be demonstrated in the distribution of the target nerve. A cotton swab or alcohol swab can be used to demonstrate decreased sensation along the specific dermatome. If the analgesic effect is localized beyond the dermatome of the target nerve, then the block is not diagnostic and should be repeated. Absence of analgesia may be secondary to technical difficulty and the area surrounding the nerve may have not been infiltrated correctly.

If the block was technically successful, pain level is next evaluated. Absence of pain or reduction in pain by more than 50% is diagnostic. Patients with pain provoked by specific activity should be asked to perform the task that triggers their pain, such as sitting, bending, and stretching. In patients for whom the block improved but did not eliminate pain, clinicians should evaluate for other sources of pain such as a visceral component to pain or involvement of additional peripheral nerves. If patients have no reduction of pain but are experiencing numbness in the targeted dermatome, it is unlikely that the target nerve is causing their pain. Repeat examination for other visceral or somatic sources of pain post procedure may help in the diagnostic process.

There are important limitations to ultrasound-guided nerve blocks. Patients with visceral-somatic convergence may respond well to a nerve block even though their pain is secondary to underlying pathology. Local infiltration may relieve pain from muscular trigger points and not from neuralgias. Patients who receive sedation or general anesthesia may be responding to systemic medications and would have both numbness in the distribution of the targeted nerve and pain relief. Lastly, patients may experience a placebo effect or have a strong psychological need for the procedure to work. Complications are rare and include nerve or vascular injury, infection, bleeding, pain at the site of injection, and exacerbation of chronic pain.

Nerve Blocks as Treatment

The mechanism of how nerve blocks may provide long-term relief is poorly understood [8]. Nerve blocks may provide suppression of ectopic discharge in the neural membranes and have an antiinflammatory reaction. It may interrupt the "vicious cycle" of self-sustaining pain and central sensitization. No quality randomized studies exist for the evaluation of nerve blocks in long-term relief, but on average, about 30%–60% of patients can be helped with repetitive nerve blocks [8]. Addition of corticosteroids may have added benefits, but this has not been clearly demonstrated in prospective studies. Addition of dexamethasone or other corticosteroids can prolong the analgesic effect of regional anesthesia; however, it is unknown whether this positively impacts long-term outcomes. In the experience of these authors, a series of nerve blocks can reduce or eliminate pain in select patients. Performing a nerve block three to four times a year is a low-risk intervention that can effectively reduce pain and the need for medications.

Ablation, Neurectomy, and Decompression

Surgical management may be considered in patients with confirmed peripheral nerve injury who have not responded to medical management or nerve blocks. Peripheral neuralgias may be treated by nerve ablation, neurectomy, and/or decompression.

Nerve ablations disrupt signaling by producing a lesion along the path of the nerve via chemical ablation, radiofrequency ablation, or cryoablation. The effectiveness of these techniques has not been well studied for the treatment of chronic pelvic pain. Chemical ablation is performed by infiltrating the nerve with 100% ethanol or phenol. Radiofrequency ablation induces necrosis of the nerve by high alternating current that produces a coagulation effect. Cryoablation generates ice crystal around the nerve that results in lysis of the Schwan cells. Ablations effectively produce a long-term analgesic effect distal to the site of treatment. Anesthesia dolorosa, that is, pain and numbness, is a possible complicating factor of these procedures, as is neuroma formation. Patients who obtain pain relief may require repeat treatments.

Surgical resection of the nerve results in numbness in the dermatome of the affected nerve. A segment of the nerve is removed and the proximal end is usually implanted in muscles or bone to prevent neuroma formation. If a nerve is compressed either by suture ligation or fibrosis, decompression of the nerve can be performed. This is especially important in nerves with motor function, such as the obturator nerve, to avoid muscular weakness. Limited studies have evaluated the effectiveness of neurectomy and decompression and will be discussed in the text that follows.

Iliohypogastric and Ilioinguinal Nerves

The iliohypogastric nerve arises from T12–L1 and shares dorsal horn dermatomes with the ovary and the fallopian tubes; the ilioinguinal nerve arises from L1–L2 and shares the viscerotome with the fallopian tube and fundus. Both nerves course over the quadratis lumborum toward the abdominal wall after piercing the psoas muscle. Since they course through the psoas muscles, patients with hypertonicity or injury to this muscle may develop symptoms of iliohypogastric or ilioinguinal neuralgia. The nerves travel on the transverse abdominus along the border of the iliac crest and then pierce the muscles roughly 2 centimeters anterior and medial to the anterior superior iliac spine. Here they travel between the obturator internus and transverse abdominus muscles. The cutaneous branch of the iliohypogastric nerve supplies sensation of the lower abdomen, and mons. It also provides motor innervation to the internal oblique and transverse abdominus muscles. The inguinal branch of the ilioinguinal nerve courses through the inguinal canal and terminates at the labium majus. This provides sensation to the groin, labia majora, mons, and inner thigh.

These nerves may be injured during surgery, especially by Pfannenstiel incisions. At a level 2 centimeters superior to the pubic symphysis, the iliohypogastric and ilioinguinal nerves may course as close as 3.5 centimeters and 5.5 centimeters from the midline, respectively [9]. Suture ligation or transection of the nerves during an abdominal hysterectomy or cesarean section may result in pain along the distribution of the nerves or nerve trunk pain at the corners of the incision [10]. In fact, the Pfannenstiel incision may result in chronic pain in 7% of patients following cesarean sections. Risk factors for developing pain include cesarean section of emergent indication, more than two cesarean sections, and numbness. In addition, laparoscopic ports placed inferior to the anterior superior iliac spine have a risk of causing a nerve injury, especially if a large trocar is used or if the fascia is closed [11]. Repetitive injury to the abdomen or stretch injury to the abdominal wall may result in groin pain from entrapment of these nerves within the aponeurosis of the oblique muscles. The nerves may also be injured during an appendectomy or inguinal hernia repair.

Because their sensory distributions overlap, it may be difficult to determine which nerve is affected. The neurovascular bundle can be visualized with ultrasound to perform a targeted nerve block. The ilioinguinal and iliohypogastric nerves may be visualized on the abdominal wall at the level of the anterior superior iliac spine between the internal oblique and transverse abdominus muscle. The ilioinguinal nerve is usually lateral to the iliohypogastric nerve. Differentiation may be difficult at this level, as only one structure may be visualized. The nerve should be followed laterally and superiorly to allow for differentiation and to select a specific nerve for the block.

One study evaluated the effectiveness of radiofrequency ablation and found it to be superior to nerve blocks in duration of pain relief, 12.5 months versus 1.6 months [12]. In a study of patients with pain associated with Pfannestiel incisions, 5 out of 27 patients had long-term relief with a single nerve block. In the same study, Ilioinguinal/iliohypogastric neurectomy was performed in the patients who did not respond to nerve blocks, and pain relief was achieved in 73% of patients [13].

Genitofemoral Nerve

The genitofemoral nerve arises from L1–L2 and shares dorsal horn innervation with the proximal fallopian tube and fundus. The nerve courses retroperitoneally along the psoas muscle and then pierces the muscle approximately at the level of the L4 vertebrae. As with the ilioinguinal/iliohypogastric nerve, the genitofemoral nerve can be affected by hypertonicity or movement of the psoas muscle. The nerve divides into its genital and femoral branches with great anatomical variability. The femoral branch courses posterior to the inguinal canal and arises to supply sensation to the anterior thigh. The genital branch courses through the inguinal ring and terminates at the labia majora, where it gives sensation to the mons, groin, and labia major. This is an area of overlapping sensory innervation with the ilioinguinal and iliohypogastric nerves.

Injuries to the genitofemoral nerve during surgery most commonly occur due to self-retaining retractors. Improperly positioned lateral arms of retractors may apply pressure to the psoas muscle and result in a crush injury of the genitofemoral nerve. Improper positioning can also play a role; extreme flexion or extension of the thigh in lithotomy position may cause a stretch injury to the femoral branch resulting in parethesias of the anterior thigh. Psoas abscess or pathology of the appendix can also affect the nerve. The nerve may be inadvertently injured during an appendectomy, inguinal hernia repair, and psoas hitch after a ureteral reimplantation. Therefore, a detailed surgical history is important in the evaluation of patients with symptoms suggestive of genitofemoral neuralgia.

The nerve can be localized by ultrasound as it courses on the psoas muscles at the iliacus at inferior to the anterior superior iliac spine. In thin patients, the nerve may be visualized superior to this point with an ultrasound probe that allows for deeper penetration. Color flow is used to localize the neurovascular bundle. Alternatively, the nerve can be accessed within the inguinal canal. The probe is positioned over the inguinal ligament and the external iliac/femoral artery is identified. The inguinal canal is identified lateral to the artery and can be infiltrated to perform a block of the genital branch of the genitofemoral nerve. When evaluating a patient with groin and labial pain, it is vital to perform an ilioinguinal nerve block first to differentiate ilioinguinal neuralgia from genitofemoral neuralgia because a blockade performed within the canal would affect both nerves. Patients who have pain relief with an ilioinguinal nerve block are less likely to have a genitofemoral neuralgia.

Small studies have evaluated the effectiveness of radiofrequency ablation and cryoablation of the genitofemoral nerve with variable results. Genitofemoral neurectomy has been more extensively studied and may result in pain relief in 67%– 100% of patients [14, 15]. Neurectomy may be approached laparoscopically or preperitoneally and consists for resection of a portion of the nerve followed by implantation of the proximal end into the psoas muscle.

Lateral Femoral Cutaneous Nerve

The lateral femoral cutaneous nerve arises from L2–L3 and supplies sensation to the lateral thigh. It is lateral to the iliacus muscles before traveling posteriorly to the inguinal canal. It may pierce the inguinal ligament, which is a potential site of injury. It then terminates cutaneously on the lateral thigh. Pain in this area is called *meralgia paraesthetica* and may be misdiagnosed as hip pain or pain not addressed by the gynecologist. Injury to this nerve may result from a pelvic mass, tight belts or abdominal binders, pregnancy, obesity, or hip hyperextension in the lithotomy position during surgeries. Treatment consists of decompression at the inguinal canal or neurectomy.

The nerve can be localized by ultrasound immediately inferior and medial to the anterior superior iliac spine at the level of the thigh. A high-megahertz linear probe will allow for visualization of the sartorius overlapping the iliacus muscle. The lateral femoral cutaneous nerve can be identified superior to this junction approximately 1–2 centimeters medial to the anterior superior iliac spine.

Obturator Nerve

The obturator nerve emerges from L2–L4 and courses posterior to the psoas muscles. It travels lateral to the external iliac artery and courses along the obturator internus muscles before exiting the pelvis at the obturator canal. It then divides into anterior and posterior branches that innervate the obturator externus and adductor muscles of the thighs. Symptoms usually consist of dysesthetic pain of the groin and inner thigh or sharp groin pain.

The obturator nerve may be injured during the second stage of labor, during pelvic lymph node dissection, or with external rotation of the thigh in the lithotomy position. Direct injury to the nerve can occur during placement of transobturator slings. These injuries can occur within the obturator foramen or at the level of the thigh. Transobturator (TVT-O) sling placement can injure this nerve within the retropubic space.

The nerve can be localized with ultrasound lateral to the labia majora at the level of thigh. Using a linear probe, the adductor longus, adductor brevis, and pectineus muscles can be identified; the neurovascular bundle is located within the fascia where all three muscles meet. Transabdominally, it can also be visualized immediately superior to the pubic symphysis before it enters the obturator canal. Variation of the obturator artery and depth of the nerve makes a transabdominal approach more difficult. However, blockade via both approaches must be performed in order to evaluate for nerve entrapment at the obturator canal. Entrapment at the obturator canal is suspected when patients obtain pain relief from a block proximal to the obturator canal but not distal to the obturator canal.

If impingement is present, surgical decompression of the obturator can be performed laparoscopically [16]. If entrapment via vaginal mesh or slings is suspected, then complete excision of the mesh should be performed. Approach is via groin incision with exposure of the adductor muscles and obturator foramen. The obturator nerve is found on the lateral superior boarder of the obturator foramen.

Posterior Femoral Cutaneous Nerve

The posterior femoral cutaneous nerve emerges from S1–S4 and courses parallel to the pudendal nerve through the greater sciatic foramen, where it courses lateral to the ischial spine and ventral to the sacrospinous ligament until it reaches the ischial tuberosity. The nerve runs inferior to the ischial tuberosity and divides into anterior and posterior branches, the perineal nerve, and the inferior cluneal nerve. The inferior cluneal nerve gives sensory innervation to the inferior buttock and posterior thigh, while the perineal branch supplies sensation to the perineum, proximal medial thigh, posterior/lateral labia majora, and the periclitoral area.

Symptoms consist of a superficial burning/searing pain along the skin. Patients may also describe a sharp stabbing pain at the ischial tuberosity. Pain is provoked by sitting while standing alleviates the pain. In this way, neuralgia of the posterior femoral cutaneous nerve resembles the pudendal neuralgia. Distinguishing characteristics include superficial pain, lateral genital pain, and symptoms in the posterior thigh.

Neuralgia may develop from direct injury of the nerve at the ischial tuberosity. Since it courses over the bony prominence within adipose tissue, it is susceptible to impingement from trauma due to falls or from hard sitting surfaces.

The posterior femoral cutaneous nerve can be blocked via ultrasound guidance by visualizing the inferior edge of the ischial tuberosity using a linear probe. The nerve courses through adipose tissue that overlies the tuberosity of the hamstring muscles. The gluteus maximus can be visualized superiorly.

Surgical treatment consists of either decompression or neurectomy. There is wide anatomical variation of this nerve. Because it closely follows the course of the pudendal nerve, it may be entrapped within the interligamentous space or where it pierces through the sacrotuberous ligament. If entrapment or injury is at the ischial tuberosity, neurectomy should be performed via incision at the ischium. There are no quality studies evaluating the efficacy of this treatment option.

Implications in Vulvodynia

It is clear that the pelvis is richly innervated by a series somatic nerves with overlapping distributions. The ilioinguinal, genitofemoral, pudendal, and posterior femoral cutaneous nerves are the main nerves that supply sensation to the clitoris, vulva, perineum, and anus. Thus, neuralgias or injury of these nerves may manifest as vulvar pain and should be considered when assessing patients with vulvodynia. Indeed, visceral-somatic convergence and the observation that vulvodynia is common in patients with irritable bowel syndrome, interstitial cystitis/bladder pain syndrome, and endometriosis further supports that neuropathic etiologies of vulvar pain may be more common than previously thought.

Summary

Neuropathic chronic pelvic pain may be secondary to injury or sensitization of the somatic nervous system that includes the ilioinguinal, iliohypogastric, genitofemoral, lateral femoral cutaneous, posterior femoral cutaneous, obturator, and pudendal nerves. Diagnosis is confirmed by neuropathic pain and demonstrating allodynia in the distribution of the effected nerve. Image-guided selective nerve block confirms the diagnosis. A series of nerve blocks may be an effective treatment. Surgical decompression or neurectomy is considered definitive treatment.

Five Things You Need to Know

- Neuropathic pelvic pain may arise from peripheral neuropathy of the somatic nervous system.
- Primary somatic nerves of the pelvis include
  a. Iliohypogastric
  b. Ilioinguinal
  c. Lateral femoral cutaneous
  d. Genitofemoral
  e. Obturator
  f. Posterior femoral cutaneous
- Injury to these nerves may result in neuropathic pain in the distribution of the affected nerve.
- Diagnosis is confirmed by history and physical examination and via image-guided nerve block.
- Treatment is often surgical in conjunction with medical management.

References

1. van Hecke O, Austin SK, Khan RA, Smith BH, Torrance N. Neuropathic pain in the general population: a systematic review of epidemiological studies. *Pain.* 2014;**155**(4):654–62.

2. Cardosi RJ, Cox CS, Hoffman MS. Postoperative neuropathies after major pelvic surgery. *Obstet Gynecol.* 2002;**100**(2):240–4.

3. Treede R-D, Jensen TS, Campbell JN, et al. Neuropathic pain: redefinition and a grading system for clinical and research purposes. *Neurology.* 2008;**70**(18):1630–5.

4. Perry CP. Peripheral neuropathies and pelvic pain: diagnosis and management. *Clin Obstet Gynecol.* 2003;**46**(4):789–96.

5. Jarrell J, Giamberardino MA, Robert M, Nasr-Esfahani M. Bedside testing for chronic pelvic pain: discriminating visceral from somatic pain. *Pain Res Treat.* 2011;**2011**:692102.

6. Rigaud J, Riant T, Delavierre D, Sibert L, Labat J-J. [Somatic nerve block in the management of chronic pelvic and perineal pain] (in French). *Prog Urol.* 2010;**20**(12):1072–83.

7. Rigaud J, Riant T, Delavierre D, Sibert L, Labat J-J. Les infiltrations des nerfs somatiques dans la prise en charge thérapeutique des douleurs pelvipérinéales chroniques. *Progrès Urol.* 2010;**20**(12):1072–83.

8. Vlassakov K V., Narang S, Kissin I. Local anesthetic blockade of peripheral nerves for treatment of neuralgias: systematic analysis. *Anesth Analg.* 2011;**112**(6):1487–93.

9. Rahn DD, Phelan JN, Roshanravan SM, White AB, Corton MM. Anterior abdominal wall nerve and vessel anatomy: clinical implications for gynecologic surgery. *Am J Obstet Gynecol.* 2010;**202**(3):234.e1–5.

10. Loos MJ, Scheltinga MR, Mulders LG, Roumen RM. The Pfannenstiel incision as a source of chronic pain. *Obstet Gynecol.* 2008;**111**(4):839–46.

11. Shin JH, Howard FM. Abdominal wall nerve injury during laparoscopic gynecologic surgery: incidence, risk factors, and treatment outcomes. *J Minim Invasive Gynecol.* 2012;**19**(4):448–53.

12. Kastler A, Aubry S, Piccand V, Hadjidekov G, Tiberghien F, Kastler B. Radiofrequency neurolysis versus local nerve infiltration in 42 patients with refractory chronic inguinal neuralgia. *Pain Physician.* 2012;**15**(3):237–44.

13. Loos MJA, Scheltinga MRM, Roumen RMH. Surgical management of inguinal neuralgia after a low transverse Pfannenstiel incision. *Ann Surg.* 2008;**248**(5):880–5.

14. Murovic J a., Kim DH, Tiel RL, Kline DG. Surgical management of 10 genitofemoral neuralgias at the Louisiana State University Health Sciences Center. *Neurosurgery.* 2005;**56**(2):298–302.

15. Cesmebasi A, Yadav A, Gielecki J, Tubbs RS, Loukas M. Genitofemoral neuralgia: a review. *Clin Anat.* 2015;**28**(1):128–35.

16. Rigaud J, Labat J-J, Riant T, Hamel O, Bouchot O, Robert R. Treatment of obturator neuralgia with laparoscopic neurolysis. *J Urol.* 2008;**179**(2):5904-5.

Chronic Pain After Gynecological Surgery

Anna Reinert and Michael Hibner

Editor's Introduction

Postoperative pain is a common problem in gynecology and other surgical specialties. The risk of postsurgical pain is higher in patients undergoing surgery for pain conditions or who have pain elsewhere in the body. Patients need to be appropriately counseled and prepared for surgery. Using an enhanced recovery after surgery (ERAS) protocol, preoperative gabapentin as well as regional blocks for anesthesia and postoperative pain control may minimize the risk of postsurgical pain. One of the most devastating problems after surgery is onset of central sensitization and complex regional pain syndrome that may be caused by inadequate postoperative pain management, and pain management is becoming more and more difficult because of changing laws regarding opioid prescription administration.

Introduction

Chronic postsurgical pain (CPSP), or pain that persists after surgery, is an underrecognized cause of chronic pain and disability. CPSP has been defined as pain of at least 3 months duration with a significant negative effect on the quality of life, that developed or increased in intensity after a surgical procedure, for which other causes of pain such as infection have been excluded, which may be either a continuation of acute postoperative pain or develop after an asymptomatic period, that is localized to the surgical field or a referred area, and that does not appear to be attributable to a preexisting pain condition [1, 2]. Risk factors for CPSP include high preoperative pain levels, younger age, genetic predisposition, and psychological traits of catastrophizing and high anxiety or fear related to surgery [3].

It has been proposed that the majority of CPSP is neuropathic, due to damage to major nerves within the surgical field; genetic predisposition and mechanisms of chronic inflammation and central sensitization may also contribute to the etiology of CPSP [4]. Pain following gynecological surgery may also relate to muscle spasm, presence of intraperitoneal adhesions, incisional hernia, or scar endometrioma. Within gynecology, there are additionally several recognized iatrogenic postsurgical pain syndromes with unique mechanisms for generating chronic pain [5]. This chapter will review the phenomena of CPSP, its incidence following common gynecological procedures, and strategies for its prevention and management.

Causes of Pain Following Gynecological Surgery

Musculoskeletal pain is a common cause of CPSP. Myofascial pain syndrome, or pain originating from trigger points in skeletal muscle, is a poorly recognized and undertreated cause of acute and chronic pain [6], and may be a source of postoperative pain among gynecological patients, even following nonabdominal surgery [7]. Examination of the patient's abdomen in the office, using one finger to palpate muscles, and assessing for an increase in pain with increased muscular tension induced through patient effort (a positive Carnett's sign), can help to isolate musculoskeletal causes of abdominal pain. Surgery may also irritate and result in hypertonus of skeletal muscles of the pelvic floor, resulting in chronic pain and voiding dysfunction; this is especially a risk of gynecological surgeries that involve fixation of these muscles, such as sacrospinous vaginal vault suspension or mesh kits that employ muscular anchor sites [8]. Screening for symptoms of pelvic floor tension myalgia and performing an examination of pelvic floor muscle activity will confirm this etiology for postsurgical pelvic pain [9].

Incisional hernia should be considered for pain localized to an incision site, especially if a fascial defect or bulge is palpable at that site. CT imaging may be helpful in confirming suspected hernia, especially if the physical exam is equivocal [7]. Incarceration of omentum at a hernia site may cause severe pain without causing bowel obstruction [10].

Cyclical incisional pain and presence of a palpable mass that increases in size at the time of menstruation may be suggestive of scar endometrioma. Abdominal wall scars are the most common site of extrapelvic endometriosis, with only a minority of patients (approx. 14%) having associated pelvic endometriosis [11]. Accurate diagnosis of this condition can be challenging, requiring a high level of suspicion; for this reason the condition is not diagnosed until an average of 3.6–4.2 years following surgery [11, 12]. Imaging, such as MRI, may be helpful in diagnosis and perioperative planning; if possible, surgery should be scheduled to coincide with the time of menses, when the mass is at its largest.

Intraabdominal adhesions are considered a common cause of abdominopelvic pain, with 47% of adhesions shown to be a source of pain at the time of conscious laparoscopy [13]. Adhesions are thought to form in more than 70% of patients following abdominal or pelvic surgery, regardless of open or minimally invasive surgical approach [14]. Pain from adhesions is visceral in nature but may be referred to muscles and nerves of the abdominal wall, pelvis, or lower back through mechanisms of viscerosomatic convergence.

Nerve injury from stretching, ischemic compression, transection, blunt trauma, fibrosis with entrapment, or suture ligation may be a cause of postoperative pain. Nerve pain often has a burning quality, is aggravated by physical activity, and may arise anywhere from immediately postsurgery to several years after the surgery [15]. Familiarity with pelvic and abdominal wall neuroanatomy may help prevent nerve injury at the time of surgery and can assist in the accurate diagnose of nerve injury as a cause of postoperative pain.

Within the abdominal wall, the ilioinguinal, iliohypogastric, and genitofemoral nerves may be affected by transection, suture ligation, or fibrosis entrapment at the lateral margins of a low-transverse skin incision or lateral trocar sites [7], and have an overlapping sensory distribution in the vicinity of the groin and pubic symphysis. Cadaveric studies have demonstrated that the ilioinguinal nerve emerges from the transverse abdominal plane through the internal oblique muscle at an average of 2.5 cm, but up to 5.1 cm medial and at an average of 2.4 cm, but ranging from 0 to 5.3 cm inferior to the anterior superior iliac spine (ASIS); the iliohypogastric nerve similarly emerges at an average of 2.5 cm, but up to 4.6 cm and at an average of 2.0 cm, but ranging from 0 to 4.6 cm inferior to the ASIS [16]. The genital branch of the genitofemoral nerve passes through the inguinal canal and supplies the skin of the mons pubis and labium majus; the femoral branch passes lateral to the external iliac artery, behind the inguinal ligament, and throughout the fascia lata into the femoral sheath, where it supplies the skin of the femoral triangle; injury may occur from postappendectomy fibrosis overlying the psoas muscle, or from hernia repair [15]. The lateral femoral cutaneous nerve similarly passes under the inguinal ligament to supply the skin of the lateral upper thigh, and is susceptible to compression injury that can occur from a variety of causes, including surgery; this neuropathic syndrome is termed meralgia paresthetica [15].

The pudendal nerve enters the pelvis through the lesser sciatic foramen and wraps superior to the ischial spine, passing through Alcock's canal; in this area, it may undergo constriction between the sacrotuberous and sacrospinous ligaments that results in chronic pelvic pain [17]. Pudendal nerve injury may be caused by surgery, such as sacrospinous vaginal vault suspension or mesh kit placement, or following vaginal delivery [15]. Pudendal neuralgia should be suspected in patients with burning pain of the vulva, vagina, clitoris, perineum, or rectum, who report pain with sitting that is relieved with standing; onset of symptoms may be immediate following vaginal surgery [18]. Table 17.1 summarizes chronic pain after surgery by etiology.

When postoperative nerve injury is suspected, nerve blocks may be both diagnostic and therapeutic, and should be performed several times prior to proceeding with surgical management such as nerve transection or neuroma resection [15]. Abdominal wall nerve blocks can be performed under ultrasound guidance; pudendal nerve block can be performed transvaginally or via a transgluteal route under CT guidance [19]. Relief of pain with local anesthetic injection implicates the nerve as a cause of pain; lasting benefit may derive from steroid injection in the vicinity of the nerve.

Table 17.1 Chronic pain after surgery by etiology

Musculoskeletal	Abdominal wall muscle spasm
	Pelvic floor tension myalgia
Structural	Incisional hernia
	Scar endometrioma
	Intraabdominal adhesions
Neuropathic	Ilioinguinal/iliohypogastric neuropathy
	Genitofemoral neuropathy
	Lateral femoral cutaneous neuropathy (meralgia paresthetica)
	Pudendal neuralgia

Incidence of Chronic Postsurgical Pain Within Gynecology

There are limited studies assessing the incidence of persistent postoperative pain following laparoscopy for gynecological surgery, with a significant confounding factor being that laparoscopy is often performed to assess and treat causes of chronic pelvic pain, so that presence of pain at several months postsurgery may be due to persistence or recurrence of the preoperative pain etiology. One study compared 61 women undergoing laparoscopy for evaluation of nonacute pelvic pain to 16 women undergoing laparoscopy for tubal ligation, and found that women undergoing laparoscopy for tubal ligation had low preoperative pain scores (average 0.5) as well as no pain at 6 months postsurgery (average 0.0); this was in contrast to patients undergoing laparoscopy for evaluation of chronic pain, who exhibited an average decrease in pain from 5 to 3 (mean −1.8, $p < 0.001$), with 10 of 61 women (16%) reporting increased pain at 6 months postsurgery [20]; presence of pain at 6 months postsurgery was predicted by preoperative factors of pain levels, catastrophizing, and presence of cutaneous allodynia. Small sample sizes from this study impair conclusions about frequency of CPSP following laparoscopy for tubal ligation or assessment of chronic pain. A study comparing outcomes among women undergoing hysteroscopic sterilization versus laparoscopic tubal ligation reported an incidence of chronic pelvic pain of 26.8% at 24 months among the tubal ligation group; propensity score matching to control patient variables between the two groups had led to a study population with a baseline pelvic pain rate of 18.9%, although the initial patient population reported baseline chronic pelvic pain among 25.7% of women [21]; the presence of baseline pain was highly predictive of CPSP (odds ratio

[OR] 2.59, $p < 0.001$). A retrospective study of 8,051 women undergoing laparoscopic sterilization reported a diagnosis of chronic pelvic pain within 2 years post procedure among 11.4% of women who did not have a preexisting pain condition, compared to 23.8% of women who did have a preexisting pain condition (OR 2.3, $p < 0.001$) [22]. Overall, these studies suggest a new diagnosis of chronic pelvic pain among 7.9%–11.4% of women following laparoscopic tubal ligation.

Hysteroscopic sterilization with the Essure® device has been reported to result in cases of post-procedure chronic pain, often due to complicated placement such as device malposition or corneal perforation; a retrospective study of 458 patients showed persistent pain at more than 3 months post procedure in 4.2% of patients, with a previous chronic pain diagnosis such as chronic pelvic pain, fibromyalgia, chronic low back pain, or headaches significantly increasing one's risk for chronic post-procedure pain (OR 6.15, 95% confidence interval [CI] 2.09–18.05) [23]. A case series study of 4,274 patients undergoing Essure® microinsert placement reported chronic pain among 7 women (0.16%)[24]. Overall, these studies suggest an incidence of chronic pelvic pain of 0.16%–4.2% following hysteroscopic tubal occlusion with Essure®.

Assessment of chronic pain following hysterectomy has been thoroughly studied, with a range of frequencies reported from 10% to 50%, with severe pain reported by 1%–7% of women, and pain that has a significant effect on daily activities reported among 17%–18% of women [25]. Among women with CPSP following hysterectomy, 17%–52% describe symptoms suggestive of neuropathic pain. Incidence of CPSP after hysterectomy varies by surgical approach, with incidence after open abdominal hysterectomy of 25%–26%, compared to 12%–18% after vaginal hysterectomy, and 20%–31% after laparoscopic hysterectomy [26]. As with gynecological laparoscopy, a confounding factor for CPSP is the present of preoperative pelvic pain, which is a common cause for hysterectomy; one reason for decreased incidence of CPSP following vaginal hysterectomy compared to abdominal or laparoscopic approaches may be that patients selected to undergo vaginal hysterectomy are less likely to have preexisting pelvic pain conditions that would benefit from abdominal/intraperitoneal assessment.

Assessment of chronic pain following cesarean section has also been studied through a variety of clinical trials. A meta-analysis of chronic postsurgical pain following cesarean section included 38 trials; CPSP at 3–6 months ranged from 0% to 56%, with most studies reporting 26% or less, CPSP at 6–12 months ranged from 4% to 19%, and CPSP at 12+ months ranged from 2% to 35% [26]. One of the studies included in the meta-analysis was a retrospective survey of 220 patients at an average of 10.8 months following cesarean section; they showed chronic intermittent pain in 12.3% of patients, with 5.9% having daily or almost daily pain symptoms; patients with chronic postsurgical pain were more likely to have undergone general anesthesia and not spinal anesthesia, and were more likely to recall severe acute postoperative pain [27]. A prospective study too recent to be included within the meta-analysis followed 527 women undergoing cesarean section, and showed CPSP rates of 18.3%, 11.3%, and 6.8% at 3, 6, and 12 months, respectively; risk factors for CPSP included intensity of pain with movement in the immediate postoperative period, preoperative depression, and longer surgical time [28].

Chronic pain following global endometrial ablation most likely relates to persistent or recurrent endometrium in the uterine cornua that leads to hematometra. This condition is thought to be more prevalent in women who have also undergone tubal ligation, due to obstruction of retrograde menstruation, and has led to the identification of a "postablation tubal sterilization syndrome"; however, painful hematometra may occur following endometrial ablation in the absence of tubal ligation [5]. A retrospective cohort study of 270 women undergoing endometrial ablation showed new or worsening postprocedure pain in 23%, with history of tubal sterilization doubling one's risk for postprocedure pain (OR 2.06, 95% CI 1.14–3.70); a history of preprocedure dysmenorrhea was also a risk factor for pain after ablation (OR 1.74, 95% CI 1.06–2.87) [29]. Similar results were seen in a retrospective cohort study of 437 women following endometrial ablation, in which 20.8% of women reported postprocedure chronic pain, with history of dysmenorrhea (OR 1.73) and prior tubal ligation (OR 1.68) both associated with increased risk for pain; age less than 40 years (OR 1.90) and smoking status (OR 2.31) were additional risk factors for CPSP [30]. Hysterectomy is considered curative for pain of this etiology, but does not appear to be pursued by most affected patients; a retrospective study of 553 women undergoing endometrial ablation demonstrated similar rates of subsequent hysterectomy between women with prior tubal

Table 17.2 Incidence of chronic postoperative pain by surgery

Laparoscopic tubal ligation	11.4%–26.8%
Hysteroscopic tubal ligation	0.16%–4.2%
Endometrial ablation	20.8%–23%
Abdominal hysterectomy	25%–26%
Vaginal hysterectomy	12%–18%
Laparoscopic hysterectomy	20%–31%
Cesarean section	2%–35%

sterilization and those without (16.5% vs. 11.3%, χ^2 = 2.95, $p = 0.09$) [31].

History of synthetic vaginal mesh placement in pelvic reconstructive surgery for pelvic organ prolapse and/or stress urinary incontinence is addressed in Chapter 18 in this book but is worth mentioning here as a syndrome of iatrogenic chronic postsurgical pelvic pain. Pain may relate to mesh contraction as well as mesh erosion and may include musculoskeletal as well as neuropathic pain symptoms. Table 17.2 summarizes the incidence of chronic postoperative pain by surgery.

Prevention of Chronic Postsurgical Pain

Surgical techniques that avoid nerve damage, including minimally invasive surgery, may help reduce incidence of CPSP, and should be pursued whenever possible. Improved control of acute postoperative pain through multimodal pain management including perioperative ketamine, gabapentinoids, antidepressants, COX inhibitors, steroids, and afferent neural blockade with regional anesthesia has been proposed as a strategy to prevent central sensitization and thus decrease incidence of CPSP [4]. An early meta-analysis of the use of perioperative gabapentinoids concluded that there is evidence for moderate-to-large reduction in incidence of development of CPSP with use of preoperative gabapentinoids, with greatest benefit resulting from a high dose of gabapentin (i.e., 1,200 mg) at 2 hours presurgery [32]. Subsequent meta-analysis including data from unpublished clinical trials had a contrary conclusion, that there was no evidence to support a decreased in CPSP with use of perioperative pregabalin [33]. A Cochrane review evaluated the efficacy of diverse systemic medications for prevention of chronic pain after surgery, with conclusions as follows [34]. For gabapentin, no significant difference over placebo was seen at 3 or 6 months postsurgery. For pregabalin, studies were heterogeneous, but overall meta-analysis showed a significant benefit over placebo at 3 months postsurgery (OR 0.60, 95% CI 0.39–0.93), and benefit at 6 months from a single unpublished study. For ketamine, meta-analysis was performed for trials with similar postoperative timeframes with no meta-analysis showing superiority to placebo, but subgroup analyses showed a trend toward significance for reduction of pain at 3 months postsurgery when ketamine was used for greater than 24 hours (OR 0.37, 95% CI 0.14–0.98), and a significant effect of reduction of pain at 6 months when ketamine was used for less than 24 hours (OR 0.45, 95% CI 0.26–0.78). For corticosteroids and for nonsteroidal anti-inflammatory drugs (NSAIDs), meta-analysis was not possible because of trial heterogeneity, and trials showed mixed results.

Regional anesthesia has been proposed to protect against development of chronic postsurgical pain through mechanisms of decreasing pain sensitization from surgery, and by decreasing opioid requirements and therefore risk of opioid-induced hyperalgesia [35]. A Cochrane review of regional and local anesthesia for preventing chronic postsurgical pain concluded a reduced incidence of CPSP at 6 months following thoracotomy when regional anesthesia was used (OR 0.33, 95% CI 0.14–0.95) [36]. A study of 141 patients undergoing laparotomy for major gynecological surgery compared general anesthesia plus epidural fentanyl and lidocaine before or after incision, to general anesthesia with a sham epidural, and showed improved pain outcomes at 3 weeks postsurgery for both epidural groups, but not at 6 months (OR 0.81 but CI crossing the midline 95% CI 0.35--1.88) [37]. A study of 370 women undergoing primary cesarean section compared intraperitoneal instillation of 200 milligrams of lidocaine versus sterile saline and showed lower persistent postoperative pain at 8 months among the lidocaine group (10.8% vs. 20.8%, $p < 0.001$) [38]. More studies are indicated to delineate the precise benefits of regional anesthesia for prevention of chronic postoperative pain, but the advantages of regional anesthesia for acute postoperative pain control have led our practice to incorporate transverse abdominal plane block for laparoscopic surgery and spinal analgesia for cystoscopy with bladder overdistension, whenever possible.

Clinical pointer: Consider the addition of regional anesthesia when performing surgery on patients with chronic pain, high preoperative pain levels, or anxiety.

Five Things You Need to Know

- Chronic pain after gynecological surgery is common, affecting up to one quarter of women who undergo cesarean section, abdominal hysterectomy, laparoscopic hysterectomy, laparoscopic tubal ligation, or endometrial ablation.
- Chronic postsurgical pain (CPSP) may have diverse causes; common causes include neuropathic or musculoskeletal pain, intraabdominal adhesions, and incisional hernia.
- When postoperative nerve injury is suspected, a nerve block may be both diagnostic and therapeutic: relief of pain with local anesthetic injection implicates the nerve as a cause of pain, while steroid injection may result long-lasting pain relief.
- Risk factors for development of CPSP include high preoperative pain levels, younger age, genetic predisposition, and psychological traits of catastrophizing and high anxiety or fear related to surgery.
- Risk of developing CPSP may be reduced through the use of regional anesthesia and perioperative gabapentinoids.

References

1. Macrae WA. Chronic pain after surgery. *Br J Anaesth.* 2001;**87**(1):88–98.

2. Werner MU, Kongsgaard UE. Defining persistent post-surgical pain: is an update required? *Br J Anaesth.* 2014;**113**(1):1–4.

3. Bruce J, Quinlan J. Chronic post surgical pain. *Rev Pain.* 2011;**5**(3):23–9.

4. Kehlet H, Jensen TS, Woolf CJ. Persistent postsurgical pain: risk factors and prevention. *Lancet.* 2006;**367** (9522):1618–25.

5. Senapati S, Atashroo D, Carey E, Dassel M, Tu MFF. Surgical interventions for chronic pelvic pain. *Curr Opin Obstet Gynecol.* 2016;**28**(4):290–6.

6. Sharp HT. Myofascial pain syndrome of the abdominal wall for the busy clinician. *Clin Obstet Gynecol.* 2003;**46** (4):783–8.

7. Sharp HT. Management of postoperative abdominal wall pain. *Clin Obstet Gynecol.* 2015;**58**(4):798–804.

8. Butrick CW. Pathophysiology of pelvic floor hypertonic disorders. *Obstet Gynecol Clin North Am.* 2009a;**36**(3):699–705.

9. Butrick CW. Pelvic floor hypertonic disorders: identification and management. *Obstet Gynecol Clin North Am.* 2009b; **36**(3):707–22.

10. Suleiman S, Johnston DE. The abdominal wall: an overlooked source of pain. *Am Fam Physician.* 2001;**64**(3):431–8.

11. Vellido-Cotelo R, Muñoz-González JL, Oliver-Pérez MR, et al. Endometriosis node in gynaecologic scars: a study of 17 patients and the diagnostic considerations in clinical experience in tertiary care center. *BMC Womens Health.* 2015;**15**(1).

12. Horton JD, DeZee KJ, Ahnfeldt EP, Wagner M. Abdominal wall endometriosis: a surgeon's perspective and review of 445 cases. *Am J Surg.* 2008;**196**(2):207–12.

13. Howard FM, El-Minawi AM, Sanchez RA. Conscious pain mapping by laparoscopy in women with chronic pelvic pain. *Obstet Gynecol.* 2000;**96**(6):934–9.

14. Koninckx PR, Gomel V. Introduction: Quality of pelvic surgery and postoperative adhesions. *Fertil Steril.* 2016;**106**(5):991–3.

15. Perry CP. Peripheral neuropathies causing chronic pelvic pain. *J Am Assoc Gynecol Laparosc.* 2000;**7**(2):281–7.

16. Rahn DD, Phelan JN, Roshanravan SM, White AB, Corton MM. Anterior abdominal wall nerve and vessel anatomy: clinical implications for gynecologic surgery. *Am J Obstet Gynecol.* 2010;**202**(3):234.e1–234.e5.

17. Robert R, Prat-Pradal D, Labat JJ, Bensignor M, Raoul S, Rebai R, Leborgne J. Anatomic basis of chronic perineal pain: role of the pudendal nerve. *Surg Radiol Anat: SRA.* 1998;**20**(2):93–8.

18. Hibner M, Desai N, Robertson LJ, Nour M. Pudendal neuralgia. *J Minim Invasive Gynecol.* 2010;**17**(2):148–53.

19. McDonald JS, Spigos DG. Computed tomography-guided pudendal block for treatment of pelvic pain due to pudendal neuropathy. *Obstet Gynecol.* 2000;**95**(2):306–9.

20. Jarrell J, Ross S, Robert M, Wood S, Tang S, Stephanson K, Giamberardino MA. Prediction of postoperative pain after gynecologic laparoscopy for nonacute pelvic pain. *Am J Obstet Gynecol.* 2014;**211**(4):360.e1–360.e8.

21. Steward R, Carney P, Law A, Xie L, Wang Y, Yuce H. Long-term outcomes after elective sterilization procedures: a comparative retrospective cohort study of Medicaid patients. *Contraception.* 2018.

22. Carney PI, Yao J, Lin J, Law A. Occurrence of chronic pelvic pain, abnormal uterine bleeding, and hysterectomy postprocedure among women who have undergone female sterilization procedures: a retrospective claims analysis of commercially insured women in the US. *J Minim Invasive Gynecol.* 2017;**25**(4):651–60.

23. Yunker AC, Ritch JMB, Robinson EF, Golish CT. Incidence and risk factors for chronic pelvic pain after hysteroscopic sterilization. *J Minim Invasive Gynecol.* 2015;**22**(3):390–4.

24. Arjona Berral J, Rodríguez Jiménez B, Velasco Sánchez E, et al. Essure® and chronic pelvic pain: a population-based cohort. *J Obstet Gynaecol.* 2014;**34**(8):712–13.

25. Brandsborg B, Nikolajsen L, Kehlet H, Jensen TS. Chronic pain after hysterectomy. *Acta Anaesth Scand.* 2008;**52**(3):327–31.

26. Weibel S, Neubert K, Jelting Y, Meissner W, Wöckel A, Roewer N, Kranke P. Incidence and severity of chronic pain after caesarean section: a systematic review with meta-analysis. *Eur J Anaesthesiol.* 2016;**33**(11):853–65.

27. Nikolajsen L, Sorensen HC, Jensen TS, Kehlet H. Chronic pain following Caesarean section. *Acta Anaesthiol Scand.* 2004;**48**(1):111–16.

28. Jin J, Peng L, Chen Q, Zhang D, Ren L, Qin P, Min S. Prevalence and risk factors for chronic pain following cesarean section: a prospective study. *BMC Anesthesiol.* 2016;**16**(1):1–12.

29. Wishall KM, Price J, Pereira N, Butts SM, Badia CRD. Postablation risk factors for pain and subsequent hysterectomy. *Obstet Gynecol.* 2014;**124**(5):904–10.

30. Thomassee MS, Curlin H, Yunker A, Anderson TL. Predicting pelvic pain after endometrial ablation: which preoperative patient characteristics are associated? *J Minim Invasive Gynecol.* 2013;**20**(5):642–7.

31. Kreider SE, Starcher R, Hoppe J, Nelson K, Salas N. Endometrial ablation: is tubal ligation a risk factor for hysterectomy? *J Minim Invasive Gynecol.* 2013;**20**(5):616–19.

32. Clarke H, Bonin RP, Orser BA, Englesakis M, Wijeysundera DN, Katz J. The prevention of chronic postsurgical pain using gabapentin and pregabalin: a combined systematic review and meta-analysis. *Anesth Analg.* 2012;**115**(2):428–42.

33. Martinez V, Pichard X, Fletcher D. Perioperative pregabalin administration does not prevent chronic postoperative pain: systematic review with a meta-analysis of randomized trials. *Pain.* 2017;**158**(5):775–83.

34. Chaparro LE, Smith SA, Moore RA, Wiffen PJ, Gilron I. Pharmacotherapy for the prevention of chronic pain after surgery in adults (Review). *Cochrane Database Syst Rev.* 2013;(7): CD008307.

35. Rivat C, Bollag L, Richebé P. Mechanisms of regional anaesthesia protection against hyperalgesia and pain chronicization. *Curr Opin Anaesthesiol.* 2013;**26** (5):621–5.

36. Andreae M, Andreae D. Local anaesthetics and regional anaesthesia for preventing chronic pain after surgery. *Cochrane Database Syst Rev.* 2012; (10):1–77.

37. Katz J, Cohen L. Preventive analgesia is associated with reduced pain disability 3 weeks but not 6 months after major gynecologic surgery by laparotomy. *Anesthesiology.* 2004;**101**(1):169–74.

38. Shahin AY, Osman AM. Intraperitoneal lidocaine instillation and postcesarean pain after parietal peritoneal closure: a randomized double blind placebo-controlled trial. *Clin J Pain.* 2010;**26** (2):121–7.

Pain Arising from Pelvic Mesh Implants

Ashley L. Gubbels and Michael Hibner

Editor's Introduction

Polypropylene mesh implants have been widely used for treatment of urinary incontinence and pelvic organ prolapse. Although they have been shown to be effective in the treatment of these conditions, they also have considerable cost complications including significant and long-lasting pain. These mesh products were allowed to the market by the FDA without proper research and recently mesh for treatment of pelvic organ prolapse has been taken off the market. In my opinion, the part of the mesh that causes pain is the part that attaches to muscles or pierces through them; therefore it is important to remove that part when treating patients with pain resulting from mesh implants. This is especially important in transobturator meshes where the groin part has to be removed. Meshes that attach to the sacrospinous ligament have a risk of injuring the pudendal nerve, and patients who have developed pain after placement of such a mesh should be treated like patients with pudendal nerve entrapment.

Introduction

At one point up to 300,000 surgical procedures were performed annually in the United States for pelvic organ prolapse. It has most recently been estimated that women have a 20% estimated lifetime risk of surgery for stress urinary incontinence (SUI) or pelvic organ prolapse (POP)[1]. This had previously been estimated at 11.1% based on a small 1995 study in the Northwest region of the United States. A large percentage (6%–29%) of these women will require additional surgeries for recurrence. The evolution of midurethral slings and vaginal prolapse kits in the early 2000s may have contributed to this rise in surgical management, as more gynecologists could offer these procedures.

History and Development of Pelvic Mesh Implants

The first modern sling procedure evolved from a 1907 procedure by Giordano involving the use of gracilis muscle flaps. A permutation followed in 1917 by Goebell, Frankenheim, and Stoeckel using the pyramidalis muscle and rectus fascia. Over the 1930s and 1940s musculofascial slings began to fall out of favor and pure fascial slings became preferred. Procedures such as the Marshall–Marchetti–Kranz procedure and the Burch colposuspension soon followed [2]. Both were invasive, requiring an abdominal approach, and researchers began looking for less invasive alternatives. In 1986 it was discovered that pressure applied unilaterally to the mid-urethra could control urinary leakage during cough. A separate, and at the time unrelated, discovery revealed that implanted Teflon caused a collagenous tissue reaction. Experiments first began in dogs in 1987, where Mersilene tape was implanted retropubically in 13 large breed dogs with the goal of synthetically recreating the pubourethral ligament by placing and then removing the tape after 6 weeks. The goal was that fibrosis would reinforce the pubourethral ligament, leading to continence. Human testing began in 1988 on a total of 30 women. Results were very reassuring, with 100% cure of stress and mixed incontinence but unfortunately 50% had recurrence upon removal [3]. In 1990, Ulf Ulmsten of Sweden and Peter Petros of the United States collaborated and determined that a permanently implanted option was required. They theorized that stress incontinence resulted from a weakened pubococcygeus muscle that was unable to lift the urethra against the pubourethral ligament and compress it during times of increased intraabdominal pressure. The midurethral sling served to recreate this ligament and restore normal urethral coaptation [4]. Mersilene tape was eventually found to have a high rate of erosion and fistula formation therefore other materials were investigated and polypropylene was found to be a more ideal substance. Amid type 1 mesh (a macroporous mesh with pores >75 μm) was found to be ideal, as it facilitated infiltration of the mesh by macrophages, fibroblasts, and blood vessels. The promotion of tissue ingrowth resulted in improved support with decreased risk of infection.

In 2001 initial five-year data from Sweden, Finland, and France showed an 85% cure rate. Finland published a nationwide analysis in 2002 with data from 38 hospitals. This included 1,455 tension-free vaginal tape (TVT) procedures performed from 1997 to 1999. Rates of operative complications included bladder injury 3.8%; active bleeding (>200 mL) 1.9%; and injury to major nerve, artery, or urethra 0.07%. Postoperative complication rates included retropubic hematoma 1.9%, minor voiding difficulty 7.6%, urinary retention 2.3%, urinary tract infection 4.1%, and defect in vaginal healing 0.7% [5]. When evaluating these rates, it is important to understand the training required in Finland before surgeons were allowed to place these devices. Providers desiring to perform these procedures had to go through training at the University Hospital of Helinski beginning with theoretical training regarding a focus on the midurethra rather than bladder neck. They then had to attend and observe two to eight procedures, assist with two to four, and perform two or three under supervision. They obtained a certificate of completion at the conclusion of the training. Only certified surgeons could obtain TVT kits for clinical use. A follow-up program also called for registration of any intra- or postoperative complications. Given the extent of this training the early reported complication rates were low and not representative.

Development of Midurethral Sling Systems

In 1996, Boston Scientific released the ProteGen Sling. This sling was approved by the FDA on a 510(k) process. A 510(k) is a premarket submission for medical devices in which the device must demonstrate that it is substantially equivalent (i.e., at least as safe and effective) as a legally marketed device. This process allows for fast-track approval without a more rigorous premarket approval process or clinical testing. The approval of the ProteGen sling was based on the Ethicon Mersilene mesh created in the 1950s for repair of hernias. Multiple other companies followed suit: Ethicon's TVT sling (1997–98), Influence Inc's IN-SLING (1997) and TriAngle (1998), and the Mentor Suspend Sling (1998). The Ethicon Gynecare division began an aggressive marketing campaign and within years revolutionized the treatment of stress incontinence. Burch colposuspension quickly became a historic procedure. In the early 2000s companies marketed various retropubic slings such as American Medical Systems (AMS) SPARC and Boston Scientific's Advantage and Lynx systems. Unfortunately, at this point the story regarding mesh takes a downward turn. Complications began to appear relating both to the mesh itself as well as incorrect use. In January 1999 Boston Scientific submitted a voluntary recall of ProteGen to the FDA due to a higher than expected rate of vaginal erosion and dehiscence. It stated the device did not appear to function as anticipated. Despite this many other companies had already achieved approval through the 510 (k) process and had products on the market. Multiple different modifications and techniques were touted to be safer and easier. AMS developed SPARC (Suprapubic Arc system), which was inserted in a top-down approach. The theoretical benefit was that the most control occurred during initial insertion through the retropubic space when the device passed close to pelvic viscera and vasculature. Second-generation slings utilized the transobturator approach. This approach was touted as a safer option, as it did not traverse the retropubic space and risk of bladder and vascular injury was significantly decreased. In 2001, French surgeon Emanual Delorm introduced an outside-in technique through the transobturator membrane. The Belgian surgeon Jane De Leval followed with a description of an inside-out technique in 2003. Companies soon produced various transobturator slings such as Ethicon TVT-O, AMS Monarc, Boston Scientific ObTryx, and Coloplast Aris. While the transobturator approach had decreased rates of pelvic hematoma, bladder injury, and voiding dysfunction, it had its own unique complications such as groin pain and obturator neurovascular injury. Third-generation slings were aimed at becoming even less invasive. A single-incision approach called TVT-Secure was developed by Ethicon and approved by the FDA in 2006. Single-incision slings were placed through a vaginal incision with fixation to the pubic ramus typically through the obturator internus muscle. This

Table 18.1 Sling manufacturers and approaches

Name	Manufacturer	Approach	Technique
TVT	Ethicon	Retropubic	Bottom to top
TVT Exact	Ethicon	Retropubic	Bottom to top
SPARC	AMS	Retropubic	Top to bottom
Advantage	Boston Scientific	Retropubic	Bottom to top
Lynx	Boston Scientific	Retropubic	Top to bottom
TVT-O	Ethicon	Trans-obturator	Inside to out
TVT Abbrevo	Ethicon	Trans-obturator	Inside to out
Monarc	AMS	Trans-obturator	Outside to in
ObTryx	Boston Scientific	Trans-obturator	Outside to in
Aris	Coloplast	Trans-obturator	Outside to in
Align	C. R. Bard	Trans-obturator	Outside to in
TVT-Secur	Ethicon	Single Incision	
Solyx	Boston Scientific	Single Incision	
MiniArc	AMS	Single Incision	
Ajust	Bard	Single incision	Adjustable
Prefyx	Boston Scientific	Pre-pubic	

generation of slings had a lower complication rate with quicker recovery but was not immune to issues such as erosion, urinary retention, and pain. As was typical, AMS MiniArc, Boston Scientific Solyx, and Bard Adjust soon followed. In 2003, Daher described a new prepubic approach where vaginal placement exits anterior to the pubic bone. This avoided deep vascular and visceral structures but uniquely placed the clitoral neurovascular supply at risk. Boston Scientific released the Prefyx PPS based on this technique. The various slings, manufactures, and approaches are listed in Table 18.1.

Development of Mesh for Prolapse Repair

As previously mentioned, multiple studies have shown that women have a 30%–50% risk of pelvic organ prolapse and 20% will undergo surgery for pelvic organ prolapse (POP) or stress urinary incontinence (SUI). Based on the initial approval of mesh for midurethral slings, the FDA approved mesh specifically indicated for POP as well. Use of an abdominal hernia mesh had been used by gynecologists for POP repair but required surgeons to cut the mesh to the desired shape and size. Companies began designing and manufacturing products specific to POP based on the increase in this clinical practice. The FDA approved more than 60 different mesh products for POP under the 510(k) process. These mesh products were also made from Amid type 1 polypropylene mesh [6]. The first mesh kits were released in the United States in 2004. These kits were much larger, with more attachment points than the midurethral slings. The first kits released were the AMS Apogee and Perigee systems followed by the Ethicon Anterior/Posterior Prolift and the C. R. Bard Anterior/Posterior Avaulta. Table 18.2 summarizes the indications and attachment sites for these various mesh kits, as it is now very difficult to find this information following device withdrawal from the market. Mesh kits were likely produced, in part, to market to the masses, including lower volume surgeons. The marketing campaigns were aggressive. It has been suggested that surgeons were not provided appropriate training by the manufacturers. Company representatives could frequently be found in the operating room walking surgeons through the procedure.

From 2005 to 2007 there were increasing medical device reports (MDRs) of adverse events related to gynecological mesh products. These reports are maintained in the MAUDE (Manufacturer and User Facility Device Experience) Database, which houses MDRs submitted to the FDA [7]. The increasing frequency led to a review by the FDA and the release of a Public Health Notification informing providers and patients of increased complication rates.

Table 18.2 Prolapse mesh manufacturer and attachments

Name	Manufacturer	Indication	Attachments	Framework
Perigee	AMS	Cystocele	Transobturator arms ×4 with distal arms inserted in ATFP 1–2 cm medial to the ischial spine near SSL	Polypropylene + biological coating
Apogee	AMS	Rectocele, enterocele, apical prolapse	Transobturator arms ×2 with distal arms inserted 1–2 cm distal to ischial spine with exit through ischiorectal fossa	Polypropylene type 1 macroporous monofilament
Elevate	AMS	Cystocele and apical prolapse	Transobturator anchor and plastic bands through SSL	
Prolift-Anterior	Ethicon	Cystocele	Transobturator arms ×4 with distal arms inserted in ATFP 1–2 cm medial to the ischial spine in the coccygeus/SSL complex	Polypropylene + poliglecaprone
Prolift-Posterior	Ethicon	Rectocele, enterocele, apical prolapse	Through SSL and iliococcygeus exiting through ischiorectal fossa Deviates axis of vagina on tension	Soft type 1 macroporous monofilament
Avaulta-Anterior	C. R. Bard	Cystocele	Transobturator arms ×4 with distal arms inserted in ATFP 1–2 cm medial to the ischial spine near SSL	Porcine-collagen coated macro-porous mesh (stiff/dense)
Avaulta-Posterior	C. R. Bard	Rectocele, enterocele, apical prolapse	Perineal body attachment, distal arms through iliococcygeus near ischial spine with exit through ischiorectal fossa	Porcine-collagen coated macro-porous mesh (stiff/dense)
Uphold (anterior)	Boston Scientific	Cystocele, apical prolapse	Suture fixation to SSL using Capio suture device	
Pinnacle (posterior)	Boston Scientific	Rectocele, enterocele, apical prolapse	Suture fixation to SSL using Capio suture device	

SSL, sacrospinous ligament.

Summarized from Moore and Miklos [6].

Timeline of the Pelvic Floor Disorders Registry

1996: Protagen (Boston Scientific) first introduced for SUI.

1998: TVT (Ethicon) released.

2001: IVS Tunneler (Covidien) introduced as the first POP kit worldwide.

2004: Perigee (AMS) introduced in the United States

First study completed in 2004 and first randomized controlled trial (RCT) in 2008

2005: Prolift (Ethicon) released in the United States

First study completed in 2006 and first RTC in 2009

2005–2007: Increasing MDRs submitted to MAUDE database prompt FDA review

2008: Elevate (AMS) and Uphold (Boston Scientific) introduced in the United States

First study completed in 2012

2008: First FDA Public Health Notification released

2008–2010: Second review of MAUDE Database by FDA

2011:

July: FDA released an updated safety communication concluding that "serious adverse events associated with mesh use are not rare" and that "transvaginal mesh placement in pelvic organ prolapse repair does not conclusively improve clinical outcomes over traditional non-mesh repair." Findings are limited to mesh for POP repair but not SUI.

September: FDA convened a meeting of the Obstetrics-Gynecology Devices Panel of the Medical Devices Advisory Committee to review the safety of mesh for POP and SUI.

December: Committee Opinion on Vaginal Placement of Synthetic Mesh for POP was published and the American College of Obstetricians and Gynecologists (ACOG) and the American Urogynecologic Society (AUGS) published recommendations strongly supporting development of a postmarket surveillance registry.

2012:

January: FDA ordered manufacturers of POP mesh products to conduct prospective postmarket surveillance (522 order).

March: AUGS began a collaboration with industry, FDA, and additional organizations to create a registry designed to meet both the 522 requirement and aid practitioners.

June: Johnson & Johnson (Ethicon/Gynecare) removed Prolift and all mesh products from the market.

2013: The FDA issued 95 postmarket study orders to 34 manufacturers of POP mesh and 14 postmarket study orders to seven manufactures of single-incision slings for SUI.

2014: FDA recommended reclassification of POP mesh from a class II to a class III device (from moderate to high risk). Reclassification required any new devices or alterations of current devices to undergo preclinical testing. Devices were allowed to remain on the market as long as the company complied with the 522 order.

Manufacturers are also required to submit a premarket approval (PMA) application to support the safety and efficacy of mesh for POP repair. PMA was required within 30 months for devices already on the market and new devices required a PMA before they were approved for marketing.

Future Design

Ongoing research has aimed to produce alternative materials that may be better suited for use within the pelvic floor. The University of Sheffield in England recently published evidence supporting use of an estrogen-releasing polyurethane mesh that is more flexible and stimulates cells to produce tissue regeneration [8]. Studies have only been performed in ex vivo models to date. Other companies are evaluating titanium-coated polypropylene mesh as a biocompatible option with less inflammatory response and shrinkage [9]. Boston Scientific elected to modify their current mesh products with blue dye to make visibility during placement, and potential removal, easier.

Legal Status of Mesh

Over time it became clear that mesh complications were not rare and eventually lawsuits against physicians and manufacturers began to be filed [10]. Huge volumes of cases threatened to overwhelm the judicial system if tried individually. In January 2012, several different multidistrict litigations (MDLs) were established in Charleston, West Virginia, to consolidate and manage the vast numbers of similar federal claims. Given the large number of cases, bellwether trials were completed. These are test cases representative of the cases as a whole and are meant to ascertain liability and value for settlement purposes. Bellwether trials are commonly used in MDLs to ascertain what the likely outcomes will be and may lead plaintiff attorneys to pursue or abandon remaining suits based on the outcome. Some of the notable outcomes include:

1. *Scott v. C. R. Bard* (July 2012): $5.5 million to plaintiff

---

2. *Gross v. Ethicon/J&J* (February 2013): $11.11 million to plaintiff
3. *Lewis v. Ethicon/J&J* (February 2014): $0
4. Boston Scientific
   a. Pinnacle (July 2014) in favor of defendant
   b. Obtryx (August 2014) in favor of defendant in first two cases; however, a third case, *Salazar v. Boston Scientific*, resulted in $73.5 million to plaintiff

As of October 2015, more than 104,749 complaints had been filed through the federal court system.

In February 2017 Judge Joseph Goodwin, the judge overseeing all 104,000+ mesh cases, announced orders to expedite proceedings. Subsequently between August and November 2017 an additional 800 cases were added to the various MDLs. Table 18.3 provides a breakdown of the total complaints per company as of November 2017.

Ethicon (MDL 2327) was ordered to trial for 13,200 cases by September 2018. C. R. Bard's (MDL 2187) 2,876 cases were ordered to trial by October 2018. AMS (MDL 2325) never had a trial and was ordered to trial by October 2018 for 21,165 cases but in August 2017 the company announced settlement for all cases totaling $4.2 billion. This settlement agreement required lawyers to agree not to bring any additional cases against AMS. Boston Scientific (MDL 2326) was ordered to trial for 6,174 cases by October 2018. Coloplast has yet to be assigned and Cook was no longer referring cases into MDL, with 632 remaining cases as of September 2017. Cook, along with Neomedic, have aimed to resolve cases outside of court. At the time of this writing, these MDLs are still active.

The largest settlements at the time of publication include $73.5 million in favor of the plaintiffs in

Table 18.3 Cases in transvaginal mesh MDLs as of November 2017

Company	Pending actions	Total actions
C. R. Bard	3,621	15,568
American Medical Systems	1,264	21,180
Boston Scientific	8,603	25,334
Ethicon	26,393	39,442
Coloplast	145	2,620
Cook Medical	186	635

Data from Judicial Panel on Multidistrict Litigation [10].

Salazaar v. Boston Scientific in 2014 and $100 million in *Barba v. Boston Scientific* in 2015. While not every trial resulted in a judgment for the plaintiff, companies began to settle cases more frequently in response to some of these large payouts. Ethicon paid $120 million to resolve as many as 3,000 cases. Boston Scientific spent an additional $89 million on settlements for approximately 44,000 cases. C. R. Bard paid $319 million for 6,000 cases and Endo Pharmaceuticals (formerly AMS) paid $1.3 billion to settle 30,000 cases.

Given the aforementioned judgments some companies such as AMS (company acquired by Endo Pharmaceuticals in February 2016) went out of business and others (C. R. Bard, Covidien) decided to remove mesh products from the market. In November and December 2017, Australia, New Zealand, and the United Kingdom all issued bans on transvaginal meshes. Refer to Table 18.4 for mesh kits still available on the US market.

On July 13, 2018, the FDA ordered mesh products for transvaginal posterior compartment repair to be removed from the market. On April 16, 2019, the FDA ordered all manufacturers of vaginal mesh for anterior compartment prolapse to be removed from the market after the remaining manufacturers (Boston Scientific and Coloplast) had not demonstrated the appropriate safety and effectiveness of these devices. The order did not apply to transvaginal mesh for stress urinary incontinence or mesh placed abdominally for sacro-colpopexy.

Mesh Complications

Over time it became clear that complications from transvaginal mesh were not rare. The main risk factor for mesh complication is the surgical indication for placement with higher risk in mesh placed for pelvic organ prolapse than for stress incontinence. A systematic review published in 2014 showed risk factors for complications include surgeon experience, operative technique, concomitant hysterectomy, total mesh repair, young age, sexual activity, and smoking. The complication rate following midurethral slings has been estimated between 0 and 15% based on a meta-analysis involving 11 trials and 5 additional studies [11]. In a review of POP-related complications, rates were 27% in the anterior department, 20% in the posterior department, and 40% in combined anterior and posterior repairs [12]. Complications from mesh can occur at any time. A retrospective cohort study by Welk et al. showed

Table 18.4 Mesh manufacturers and products (italicized products no longer available)

Mesh manufacturers and products

American Medical Systems (AMS) (company acquired by Endo Pharmaceuticals February 2016)

- Apogee
- BioArc SP
- BioArc TO
- Elevate
- In-Fast Ultra Transvaginal Sling
- Mini-Arc Precise Single-Incision Sling
- Monarc Sling System
- Monarc Subfascial Hammock
- Perigee Pelvic Floor Repair System
- SPARC
- SPARC Self fixating
- Straight In

Boston Scientific

- Advantage Fit System
- Advantage Sling System
- Arise
- Lynx Suprapubic Mid-Urethral Sling System
- Obtryx I/II Systems
- Solyx SIS System
- Pinnacle Pelvic Floor Repair Kit I/II
- Prefyx Mid U Mesh Sling System
- Prefyx PPS System
- Uphold LTE Vaginal Support System
- Upsylon Y-Mesh
- Solyx

Covidien (all products removed from market)

- Duo
- IVS Tunneler Intra-Vaginal Sling
- IVS Tunneler Placement Device
- Parietene Polypropylene Mesh
- Surgipro Polypropylene Surgical Mesh

C. R. Bard (all products removed from market June 2017)

- Align
- Avaulta
- Avaulta Biosynthetic Support System
- Avaulta Plus Biosynthetic Support System
- Avaulta Solo Support System

Table 18.4 (cont.)

C. R. Bard (all products removed from market June 2017)

- Avaulta Solo Synthetic Support System
- CollaMend Implant
- Faslata Allograft
- Pelvicol Tissue
- Pelvilace
- PelviSoft Biomesh
- Pelvitex Polypropylene Mesh
- Ugytex
- Ugytex Dual Mesh Kit
- Uretex
- Uretex TO
- Uretex TOO2
- Uretex TOO3

Coloplast

- Minitape
- Omnisure
- Smartmesh
- Restorelle Y
- Restorelle Direct Fix
- T-Sling Universal Polypropylene Sling System
- Aris Transobturator Sling System
- Altris Single Incision Sling System
- Supris-Suprapubic Sling System

Cook Medical

- Surgis Biodesign
- Surgis Biodesign Tension Free Urethral Sling
- Surgis Biodesign Anterior Pelvic Floor Graft
- Surgis Biodesign Posterior Pelvic Floor Graft
- Urological Stratsis Tension-Free Urethral Sling

Ethicon (Gynecare/Johnson & Johnson)

- Artysin Y-Shaped Mesh
- Prosima
- Gynemesh PS
- Gynemesh PS Prolene Soft Mesh
- Gynemesh Prolene Mesh
- Gynemesh Prolift Mesh
- Prolene Polypropylene Mesh Patch Secur
- Prolift
- Total, Anterior, and Posterior Pelvic Floor Repair Systems
- Prolift+M

Table 18.4 (cont.)

Ethicon (Gynecare/Johnson & Johnson)

- Total, Anterior, and Posterior Pelvic Floor Repair Systems
- TVT Sling
- TVT Abbrevo
- TVT Exact
- TVT Obturator (TVT-O)
- TVT Retropubic System
- TVT Secur

Mentor Corporation (acquired by Johnson & Johnson in 2009)

- ObTape

Caldera

- Desara
- Desara SL
- Desara Blue
- Desara TV
- Vertessa

Neomedic

- KIM Sling
- Single Incision TOT
- TRT Reemex System
- Anchosure System
- Surelift System
- MIPS System
- Uplift System
- MRS II Reemex system (male sling)

Generic Medical Device Company

- Universal Sling System

that 1.2% of patients at 1 year will require a procedure for revision or removal and this increases up to 3.3% at 10 years [13]. It is important to identify modifiable risk factors prior to deciding to place mesh such as smoking, nutritional deficiencies, and vaginal atrophy. It has also been shown that abdominal and pelvic pain prior to surgery is independently associated with pain after surgery. A study looking specifically at this complication showed rates of dyspareunia following surgery in up to 45% of patients, with 26% of these being new in onset [14]. It may be that patients who receive mesh for incontinence or prolapse have increased pelvic floor muscle spasm, as the pelvic floor naturally has increased tone in an attempt to maintain continence. Mesh placed through these muscles can then further aggravate the already high muscle tone.

Surgical technique is important in avoiding complications. As with any procedure, the more experienced the surgeon the fewer complications and this is particularly true for vaginal mesh. A study of 198 patients revealed 14 with mesh erosion and on further evaluation experienced surgeons had fewer mesh exposures than inexperienced surgeons (2.9% vs. 15.6%)[15]. Avoiding tension during placement as well as rolling or bunching of the mesh can decrease the potential for pain. It is important to perform a full-thickness dissection to decrease the risk of mesh erosion.

Inherent properties specific to the mesh may have also contributed to mesh complications including mesh stiffness, immune reaction, and mesh shrinkage. Increasing stiffness of the mesh can result in a process termed stress shielding whereby the stiffer material carries the load for the weaker material (i.e., tissue) leading to degradation and atrophy of the tissue. Pore size and shape in addition to stiffness also dictates the response to axial forces and can result in the increased folding or wrinkling [16]. Decreasing porosity under tension leads to an increased density of mesh which can heighten the foreign body response [17]. Similar to any other implanted synthetic material, mesh induces an inflammatory reaction within the tissue. This can be beneficial early in the healing process, but profound or chronic inflammation may increase the rate of complications. It has been shown that lower weight and higher porosity meshes cause less of an inflammatory response [18]. Macrophage response to mesh tends to be that of a proinflammatory phenotype with high concentration of inflammatory cytokines. This inflammatory response has been found to persist years following implantation [19]. Finally mesh shrinkage is also a potential factor in complications. Experimental surgeries in rats have shown that mesh can shrink by an average of 25%–30%. A study by Lo et al. found a 19.6% reduction in the length of mesh on ultrasound by 1 month postoperatively; however, another study found no evidence of mesh contraction [20]. The normal vagina is a compliant structure and can change its confirmation during normal urination, defecation, and intercourse. A contracted mesh can lead to stiffness and decreased compliance with resultant dysuria, dyschezia, and dyspareunia.

The correlation of implanted transvaginal mesh with the development of systemic autoimmune disorders has also been suggested by many patients. Anecdotal reports of patients who developed diseases such as lupus, rheumatoid arthritis, and fibromyalgia were commonly found online. A 2017 study found no correlation with the development of these conditions up to 6 years following exposure. A separate retrospective 2019 study evaluating the frequency of implanted hernia or transvaginal mesh in patients cared for in an autoimmunity clinic found 40 patients who developed autoimmune syndromes following implantation. Importantly it was noted that 75% of these patients had a preexisting allergic disease [21].

Mesh and Pain

Transvaginal mesh can cause pain through a variety of manners such as nerve injury or irritation, immunological, and musculoskeletal mechanisms. Nerve injury or irritation is one of the most immediate presentations. Depending on the type of mesh and anatomical placement, nerve injury to the pudendal and/or obturator nerves can occur. These patients will often awaken in recovery with an intense burning, neuropathic pain limited to a specific nerve distribution. One study has shown that 5% of patients will have leg pain following placement of TOT slings and nerve injury has been reported in 0.7–0.9/1,000 [22]. In these cases, it may be imperative to immediately return to the operating room for removal. Expectant management may be pursued but symptoms that persist beyond 2–4 weeks should prompt return to the operating room. During this early postoperative phase, the scarring process is incomplete, and the mesh can be completely removed. Muscle spasm is a common, perhaps the most common, etiology for pelvic pain following pelvic mesh placement. Women with muscle spasm will typically have a more remote and insidious onset of their pain, typically more than 4 weeks postoperatively. This can commonly present in a subtle fashion with progressively worsening pain over years. The orientation of mesh arms through muscles of varying orientation can lead to pain with movement and resultant spasm of a variety of muscles.

The timing of pain onset can correlate with the etiology of pain as mentioned earlier. Immediate, acute, severe pain can be due to hematoma or nerve injury. Visceral injury or abscess may present over the first few days postoperatively. In the absence of identifiable cause and any lack of improvement, removal of the mesh should occur within 2–4 weeks of placement. If removed during this time, the scarring process is incomplete, and the mesh can be more easily removed. Delayed onset of pain (>4 weeks postoperatively) can signify mesh contracture or muscle irritation. Examination may reveal tight bands or pain along the course of the mesh arms. In this instance the decision to incise the arms to loosen the bands or remove the mesh is based on a discussion with the patient. It is common for this group of patients to have continued pain following mesh explantation and require ongoing postoperative treatment such as physical therapy or botulinum toxin injections. For patients who develop pain remote from mesh placement, a thorough evaluation to determine what component of pain may be related to the mesh is necessary. Some patients may not have tenderness along the course of the mesh but muscle spasm in alternative areas potentially limited benefit from mesh removal. In this group, it is reasonable to start with conservative management with physical therapy. If the patient has no improvement in her pain or is having severe rebound spasm, it may be appropriate to proceed with botulinum toxin injections or mesh removal. Some patients suggest mesh migration as an etiology for their pain; however, this is unlikely beyond 4–6 weeks once the mesh scars into place. While erosion and contracture can occur, these do not represent migration.

Location of pain may be dependent on the type of mesh implanted. In those with a transobturator arms, patients often present with groin, thigh, and vaginal discomfort. Obturator nerve injury presents as a radicular pain to the medial thigh that is exacerbated with internal rotation and hip extension and localizes inferior to the anteromedial thigh and inguinal region. Nerve irritation is more commonly due to myofascial causes produced secondary to hypertonia induced by the passage of the mesh through the muscle. Mesh with a sacrospinous attachment is more likely to entrap or injure the pudendal nerve. Patients will present with pain in the distal vagina, labia, clitoris, perineum, and anorectal region. Patients may also develop pudendal neuralgia from functional nerve irritation secondary to surrounding muscle spasm.

Patients often describe their pain as ranging from sharp, lancinating, and burning to a dull, heavy ache. The characteristics of the patient's pain may aid in determining the likely etiology.

Patients often describe symptoms of dyspareunia, dysuria, and dyschezia. Dyspareunia may be due to a variety of etiologies such as muscle spasm, mesh exposure, and decreased compliance of the vaginal walls. Male partners may also experience hispareunia in the instance of mesh erosion and exposed mesh edges scratching the penis. Depending on the type of mesh and its attachments, dysuria and dyschezia may result. In patients with dysuria it is important to rule out mesh erosion into the bladder with cystoscopy. Dyschezia is likely more related to contracture or muscle spasm but rectal erosion can also be evaluated by digital rectal examination or proctosigmoidoscopy.

Management of Pain Related to Mesh Implantation

The majority of patients with pain following pelvic mesh surgery have a component of muscle spasm. Data are conflicting on the role of mesh removal for pelvic pain but we have observed our patients to report a change in the character of their pain postoperatively. Danford et al. reported a series of 233 patients who underwent mesh removal for pain, with the majority (73%) experiencing improvement. Of the remaining, 27% did not improve and another 8% reported worsening of their pain [23]. Other studies have shown improvement rates closer to 50%. Management of mesh-related pain includes both conservative and surgical therapies.

Conservative management of pain may consist of physical therapy, medications, nerve blocks, and botulinum toxin injections. Physical therapy is the gold standard for management of myofascial pelvic pain. It is important for treating therapists to understand the need to relax the pelvic muscles rather than strengthen them, as strengthening exercises will significantly worsen symptoms. The initial treatment course typically consists of 3–4 months of therapy. Patients who are improving continue therapy, while those who do not may pursue mesh explantation. For those who have already undergone explantation, additional management with botulinum toxin is often pursued. We also frequently use muscle relaxants for patients with secondary spasm. Our preference is to use compounded vaginal suppositories of diazepam/baclofen ± ketamine or belladonna/opium. The literature is limited regarding benefit and while not all patients respond, those who do can utilize these suppositories two or three times daily for symptom management. Oral muscle relaxers such as cyclobenzaprine, methocarbamol, baclofen, and tizanidine can

also be utilized; however, anecdotally we see less response to these agents for pelvic spasm. Other medications such as gabapentin, pregabalin, duloxetine, or amitriptyline may help with pain modulation, as much of this population may have components of central sensitization. Nerve blocks may also be a useful adjunct for pain. Typically, for those with pudendal nerve irritation we will perform three CT-guided pudendal blocks with steroids at intervals of every 6 weeks, which may provide adequate improvement. Less commonly patients present with obturator nerve irritation that may also respond to nerve blocks. Perhaps the most successful conservative option is botulinum toxin, which has been approved for various spastic conditions such as cervical dystonia, upper limb spasticity, and chronic migraine but unfortunately has not yet been approved for myofascial pelvic pain. Botulinum toxin has been studied with symptomatic improvement noted and at time of publication the NIH has an ongoing study with promising early results. Our clinical experience has been quite reassuring. It is important to combine botulinum toxin injections with physical therapy to achieve the most benefit.

For patients who have failed conservative management or based on exam are expected to benefit from explantation, surgical treatment may be warranted. Prior to proceeding with mesh explantation it is extremely important to obtain operative and pathology reports for both the initial mesh placement as well as any prior excisions. Frequently patients are unaware of the type or location of mesh and it is imperative to identify the mesh placed in order to know the compartment and location of mesh arms as well as the route best utilized for removal. Pathology reports can be utilized to determine the amount of mesh likely left from prior removals. Most radiological studies have unfortunately not proven extremely useful to identify mesh in situ. 3-D ultrasound has proven to be most helpful, as a polypropylene mesh produces a distinct echogenic signal on sonography. Noncontracted mesh appears as a thin echogenic wavy structure just adjacent to the vaginal wall and has minimal acoustic shadowing. Contracted mesh appears thicker with more acoustic shadowing [24].

Mesh removal can be challenging for many reasons. The improved anatomical support created by vaginal mesh can inhibit adequate exposure and visualization. Due to the incorporation of the mesh into tissues, it can also be quite difficult to find. While the earlier generation meshes are stiff and more easily palpable, the newer lightweight meshes require appreciation of subtle changes within the tissue. The use of a surgical headlight can aid in identification due to the reflection of light off of the mesh fibers.

In general, we prefer total mesh excision in patients with pelvic pain, particularly those with concomitant muscle spasm. It cannot be stressed enough that one has knowledge of the type of mesh placed if this can be obtained. Following vaginal preparation, a Foley catheter is placed. We utilize a vaginal Bookwalter as well as elastic stays for retraction and exposure. In patients with a midurethral sling, a midline incision is made underlying the urethra. The epithelium is dissected out laterally for exposure. Once the mesh is identified in the midline the surrounding tissue is dissected away with Metzenbaum scissors. The mesh is followed as far laterally or superiorly as possible. In the case of a transobturator mesh, a 4- to 5-centimeter vertical incision is made in the genitofemoral fold at the level of the clitoris where the mesh would be expected to exit. The skin and fascia lata of the thigh are incised. A cerebellar or Weitlaner retractor is then used to expose the underlying thigh adductors. In general, we attempt to spread these muscles but at times it may be necessary to incise them for exposure. The location of the mesh can be quite variable making it challenging to find in this location. By not transecting the vaginal portion, it can be manipulated to help guide one to the location within the groin. Once the mesh has been removed, hemostasis is achieved through a combination of cautery, suture, or hemostatic agents, which are especially useful along the deep path of the arms. Paravaginal defects are closed followed by a Kelly plication. One may consider placement of an autologous sling at this time; however, our preference is to allow the site to heal and evaluate the patient's response in regard to her pain. In the case of a retropubic mesh, the dissection proceeds similarly as previously discussed; however, once the mesh has been dissected as far behind the pubic ramus as possible a laparoscopic approach is then taken. We prefer to utilize robot-assisted laparoscopy in these cases for improved dexterity. The bladder is filled with 300–400 milliliters of saline and the space of Retzius is opened. The bladder is dissected off the anterior abdominal wall until the pubic ramus is exposed. The vaginal mesh can then be manipulated again to help localize the retropubic portion. Dissection of the mesh is carried down to the pelvic floor, where it can ideally be removed in one piece. Paravaginal defects are repaired and Burch retropubic colpopexy may be performed. Mesh explantation of the larger prolapse meshes proceeds in a similar manner. A midline incision the length of the vagina is created and the vaginal epithelium dissected laterally. Once the mesh is identified, the midline portion is freed up and dissected laterally. At this juncture the mesh can be transected in the midline, allowing easier manipulation to trace the path of mesh arms. Depending on the type of mesh this may require deep dissection toward the sacrospinous ligament. Typically, this dissection occurs digitally or with Metzenbaum scissors to separate the mesh from the surrounding tissue. It is important to attempt to remove the complete arm, as it is extremely difficult to find remaining mesh in this location should the patient remain symptomatic. Care should be taken not to be too aggressive posterior to the sacrospinous ligament, as this can result in hemorrhage and nerve injury. Groin arms are dissected similarly to the technique for transobturator slings described earlier. Anterior or posterior repair may be attempted if there is adequate connective tissue remaining in an attempt to decrease recurrent prolapse. It is important not to perform an aggressive repair, as this can further perpetuate pain. Unfortunately, many patients will frequently continue to have pain following mesh excision; however, we have observed that they often describe that their pain has altered in its character.

Site-specific removal of mesh can alleviate symptoms especially for patients who have pain limited to a specific location such as the unilateral groin or along a tight band of tissue. A study of 17 patients with mesh contracture who underwent intervention consisting of mesh mobilization, division of mesh arms from the central graft, and excision of the contracted mesh resulted in an 88% reduction in pain and 64% reduction in dyspareunia [25]. Partial excision is also preferred for patients with mesh erosion in the absence of pelvic pain. This allows the patient to continue to receive the intended benefits of the mesh and decreases the risk of recurrent incontinence or prolapse.

If the patient continues to have pain following explantation, it is typically myofascial in nature and we pursue or repeat the conservative treatments previously mentioned. Patients who have developed central sensitization will require multiple modalities to effectively manage their symptoms.

Conclusion

Stress incontinence and pelvic organ prolapse are common conditions, with one in five women undergoing surgery for these conditions. Pain following the placement of a pelvic mesh for correction of these conditions is not a rare occurrence and is life changing for the women affected. The approval process for pelvic mesh shows the perils of the 510(k) process and the importance of trials in medical device development. Mesh-related pelvic pain can affect patients through a variety of mechanisms, and unfortunately removal may not completely alleviate all symptoms. Regardless, mesh removal can be a key part of treating these patients, especially those with musculoskeletal mechanisms of pain.

Five Things You Need to Know

- Stress incontinence and pelvic organ prolapse are common conditions with a significant impact on a woman's quality of life.
- The evolution of midurethral slings and pelvic prolapse meshes shows the importance of safety studies in medical device development and how the function and safety of a product in one area of the body does not translate to how it will act in another area.
- Mesh-related pain can occur through a variety of ways including neuropathic, immunological, and musculoskeletal mechanisms.
- When planning to remove a mesh it is of the utmost importance to obtain prior operative reports to aid in the ability to locate the mesh.
- Multimodal therapy including physical therapy, muscle relaxants, nerve blocks, and botulinum toxin injections are often important in both the pre- and postoperative management of mesh-related pelvic pain.

References

1. Wu JM, Matthews CA, Conover MM, Pate V, Funk MJ. Lifetime risk of stress incontinence or pelvic organ prolapse surgery. *Obstet Gynecol.* 2014;**123**(6):1201–6.

2. Foundation for the Global Library of Women's Medicine. Global Library of Women's Medicine. 2020.

3. Petros P, Papadimitriou J. Evolution of midurethral and other mesh slings: a critical analysis. *Neurourol Urodynam.* 2013;**32**:1–7.

4. Petros P. Creating a gold standard surgical device: scientific discoveries leading to TVT and beyond: Ulf Ulmsten Memorial Lecture 2014. *Int Urogynecol J.* 2015; **26**(4):471–6.

5. Wu MP, Huang KH. Tension-free midurethral sling surgeries for stress incontinence. *Incont Pelvic Floor Dysfunct.* 2008;**2**(2):53–60.

6. Moore RD, Miklos JR. Vaginal mesh kits for pelvic organ prolapse, friend or foe: a comprehensive review. *Sci World J.* 2009;**9**:163–89.

7. MAUDE Database. www.accessdata.fda.gov/scripts/cdrh/cfdocs/cfmaude/search.cfm

8. Shafaat S, Mangir N, Regureos SR, Chapple CR, MacNeil S. Demonstration of improved tissue integration and angiogenesis with an elastic, estradiol releasing polyurethane material designed for use in pelvic floor repair. *Neurourol Urodyn.* 2018;**37** (2):716–25.

9. Pelvic floor descent repair with modern mesh implants: the benefits outweigh the acceptable risks. Pfm Medical Ag, 2017.www.pfmmedical.com/en/press/press_releases/pelvic_floor_descent_repair_with_modern_mesh_implants_the_benefits_outweigh_the_acceptable_risks/index.html.

10. United States Judicial Panel on Multidistrict Litigation. 2017. www.jpml.uscourts.gov/sites/jpml/files/Pending_MDL_Dockets_By_District-November-15-2017.pdf.

11. Leone RMU, Finazzi AE, Soligo M, Li Marzi V, Digesu A, Serati M. Long-term outcomes of TOT and TVT procedures for the treatment of female stress urinary incontinence: a systematic review and meta-analysis. *Int Urogynecol J.* 2017;**28**(8):1119–30.

12. Barski D, Otto T, Gerullis H. Systematic review and classification of complications after anterior, posterior, apical, and total vaginal mesh implantation for prolapse repair. *Surg Technol Int.* 2014;**24**:214–24.

13. Welk B, AL-Hothi H, Winick-Ng J. Removal or revision of vaginal mesh used for the treatment of stress urinary incontinence. *JAMA Surg.* 2015;**150** (12):1167–75.

14. Withagen MI, Vierhout ME, Hendriks JC, Kluivers KB, Milani AL. Risk factors for exposure, pain, and dyspareunia after tension-free vaginal mesh procedure. *Obstet Gynecol.* 2011;**118**(3):629–36.

15. Achtari C, Hiscock R, O'Reilly BA, Schierlitz L, Dwyer PL. Risk factors for mesh erosion after transvaginal surgery using polypropylene (Atrium) or composite prolypropylene/polyglactin 910 (Vypro II) mesh. *Int Urogynecol J.* 2005;**16**(5): 389–94.

16. Feola A, Abramowitch S, Jallah Z, Stein S, Barone W, Palcsey S, Moalli P. Deterioration in biomechanical properties of the vagina following implantation of a

high-stiffness prolapse mesh. *BJOG*. 2013;**120**(2):224–32.

17. Brown BN, Mani D, Nolfi AL, Liang R, Abramowitch SD, Moalli PA. Characterization of the host inflammatory response following implantation of prolapse mesh in rhesus macaque. *Am J Obstet Gynecol*. 2015;**213**(5):668.e1–10.

18. Nolfi AL, Brown BN, Liang R, Palcsey SL, Bonidie MJ, Abramowitch SD, Moalli PA. Host response to synthetic mesh in women with mesh complications. *Am J Obstet Gynecol*. 2016;**215**(2):206.e1–8.

19. Chughtai B, Sedrakyan A, Mao J, et al. Is vaginal mesh a stimulus of autoimmune disease? *Am J Obstet Gynecol*. 2017;**216**: 495.e1–7.

20. Lo TS. One-year outcome of concurrent anterior and posterior transvaginal mesh surgery for treatment of advanced urogenital prolapse: case series. *J Minim Invasive Gynecol*. 2010;**17**(4):473–9.

21. Tervaert J. Autoinflammatory/autoimmunity syndrome induced by adjuvants (Shoenfeld's syndrome) in patients after a polypropylene mesh implantation. *Best Pract Res Clin Rheumatol*. 2018;**32**(4):511–20.

22. Kuuva N, Nillson CG. A nationwide analysis of complications associated with the tension-free vaginal tape (TVT) procedure. *Acta Obstet Gynecol Scand*. 2002; **81**(1):72–7.

23. Danford J, Osborn DJ, Reynolds WS, Biller DH, Dmochowski RR. Postoperative pain outcomes after transvaginal mesh revision. *Int Urogynecol J*. 2015;**26**(1):65–9.

24. Denson L, Shobeiri SA. Three-dimensional endovaginal sonography of synthetic implanted materials in the female pelvic floor. *J Ultrasound Med*. 2014;**33**:521–9.

25. Hokenstad EK, El-Nashar SA, Blandon RE, et al. Health-related quality of life and outcomes after surgical treatment of complications from vaginally placed mesh. *Female Pelvic Med Reconstr Surg*. 2015;**21**(3):176–80.

Chapter 19

Treatment of Sexual Dysfunction Arising from Chronic Pelvic Pain

Debra S. Wickman

Editor's Introduction

Sexual dysfunction is present in almost every patient with chronic pelvic pain, and often is the most significant problem that patients experience. This, in addition to a significant decrease of quality of life from pain, further negatively affects patients. Those who are unable to be intimate, may be abandoned by their partner, and not able to form new relationships. Sexual dysfunction therefore has to be taken very seriously, and it should be addressed with both the patient and her partner. Couples should be told that cure is possible and alternatives to vaginal intercourse should be discussed. Pelvic floor muscle spasm is often responsible for pain with intercourse. Treatment of this condition is discussed in Chapter 20.

Introduction

Women experience optimal sexual health through psychosomatic connection to their own bodies, synchronicity with their intimate partner(s), and through rewarding experiences with life overall. Sexual intimacy is a primary vehicle for that connection. Initially, with self-exploration, a woman discovers unique pathways to pleasure that later become reliable and reproducible, with a partner. Then, as partnered sexual activity becomes routine, she learns how her body functions when synchronized with another. Finally, as she actualizes in life, maturing through life goals – as a partner, perhaps as a mother, and/or in a career role, she develops the confidence, inner happiness, and serenity that play into satisfaction with the sovereignty derived from expressing her sexuality on her own terms, by her own definition.

The holistic, or biopsychosocial approach to sexual function is well established in medical diagnosis and treatment – especially with regard to interventions for sexual concerns [1]. Tenets of this view include physical

health, with appropriate neuroendocrine function; psychological wellness, with freedom from mood disrupters such as anxiety and depression; social/cultural acceptance within one's group(s); and the importance of relationship satisfaction, interpersonal competence, financial adequacy, and freedom from life stressors [2].

Blocks and barriers to sexual wellness are common in society, and as a result, sexual dysfunction is also prevalent, estimated to affect up to 43% of women worldwide – peaking at midlife, ages 45–64 [3, 4]. Similarly, chronic pelvic pain is common, striking one in seven women [5], and up to 26% of women worldwide [6], also increasing with age [7]. Overall health is an important predictor of satisfaction with sex – and multiple chronic health conditions exert a toll on sexual function more strongly than age alone [8].

Sexual concerns that persist for at least 6 months and cause personal distress are classified as "dysfunctions." However, in the true sense of holistic sexuality, wellness is more than absence of dysfunction – and must evoke elements of fulfillment in the physical, intellectual, emotional, and relational aspects of sexual being.

Classification of Sexual Dysfunctions

The most recent edition of the *Diagnostic and Statistical Manual of Mental Disorders* (DSM 5), the gold standard reference of psychiatric and behavioral disorders, refers to sexual dysfunction as a "heterogeneous group of disorders that are typically characterized by a clinically significant disturbance in a person's ability to respond sexually or to experience sexual pleasure" [9]. The term female sexual dysfunction encompasses gender-specific disorders outlined in the DSM-5, and an individual may have more than one sexual dysfunction simultaneously:

1. Female sexual interest/arousal disorder (FSIAD): – Formerly termed hypoactive sexual desire disorder and female sexual arousal disorder – two separate entities in the DSM-4

2. Female orgasmic disorder
3. Genito-pelvic pain/penetration disorder: Formerly dyspareunia and vaginismus in DSM-4

Sexual dysfunctions are subtyped according to "life-long versus acquired" and "generalized versus situational." The disorder must be experienced at least 75% of the time, cause significant distress, and be present for at least 6 months in order to qualify for the diagnosis.

A group of criteria called "associated features" provides five additional categories:

1. Partner factors (partner sexual problem; partner health status)
2. Relationship factors (poor communication, discrepancies in desire for sexual activity)
3. Individual vulnerability factors (poor body image; history of sexual or emotional abuse), psychiatric comorbidity (depression; anxiety), or stressors (job loss; bereavement)
4. Cultural or religious factors (inhibitions related to prohibitions against sexual activity or pleasure; attitudes toward sexuality)
5. Medical factors relevant to prognosis, course, or treatment [10]

Healthcare providers must be familiar with these classifications in order to recognize and intervene in the evolution of overlapping dysfunction in mood, behavior, and sexuality as one responds to life experience in the context of chronic pain.

The Female Sexual Response Cycle

The female response cycle has undergone revisions through the decades, as more information is gleaned about the ways women experience the pathway from desire and arousal to orgasm and beyond. A contemporary model, developed by Rosemary Basson, is a circular-type pathway, which takes into accounts the mind–body relationship of sexual function (Figure 19.1) [11]. It is crucial to understand this model, in order to make sense of the effects of chronic pain on sexuality. Mindset affects physiological function, and chronic pain alters the psyche.

This nonlinear model of sexual response incorporates the importance of intimacy/attachment, or the relationship aspect of motivation. It also explains that desire can be responsive or spontaneous, and that arousal can occur before, or after desire. Orgasm contributes to the reward component and reinforces motivation for more desire and arousal. This model normalizes the variability within desire and arousal, making it clear that the interplay between motivation, interest, arousal, desire, and orgasm is far from simple or straightforward. When chronic pelvic pain enters the situation, it affects many points along the sexual response model – shutting down arousal, preventing desire, and preempting intimacy, with emotions like resentment, disappointment, and shame. All points within the circular algorithm must be restored as much as possible in order to provide "flow" once again to sexual satisfaction.

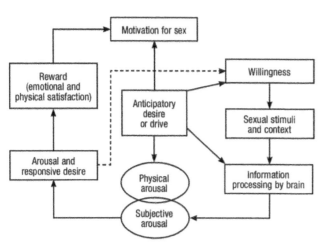

Figure 19.1 Circular sexual response cycle. Circular sexual response cycle shows overlapping phases of variable order. Reasons or motivations for sex are numerous, and sexual desire or drive may or may not be present at the outset but reached after the brain has processed sexual signals as sexual arousal, which conflates with sexual desire. The latter creates an urge for increased arousal, allowing acceptance of increasingly intense sexual stimulation. Reprinted with permission from Basson R. Sexuality and sexual disorders. *Clin Update Womens Health Care* 2014; XIII(2):1–81.

Effects of Chronic Pelvic Pain on Sexual Well-Being

Chronic gynecological pain has more far-reaching and all-encompassing effects on a woman than chronic pain arising from most other body regions because of the secondary effects it creates on the psychosocial factors related to sexual intimacy and intimate relationships. Optimal sexuality is derived from interrelated aspects of physical condition, intellectual beliefs, emotional responses, and relational connections in equal and profound ways. Until blocks and barriers in all these areas can be identified and resolved, true well-being and sexual health cannot be fully achieved.

Considering the sexual response cycle once again (Figure 19.1), one sees that impediments at any entry area, such as willingness, anticipatory desire, or subjective arousal can alter the flow of response, even stopping it. Physical pain is an obvious impediment; however, less apparent, more subjective, negative facets such as poor body image or low self-esteem, along with depression or anxiety, are just as destructive for the sexual response cycle.

Effects of Chronic Pelvic Pain on Mood

Chronic pelvic pain is correlated with significant levels of psychological distress and functional impairment; with more than half of women experiencing moderate-to-severe anxiety, and more than one-quarter with moderate-to-severe depression [12]. There is significant overlap between sexual dysfunction and depression, as seen in many prior studies. It follows, therefore, that chronic pelvic pain closely impacts the two related spheres of depressed or anxious mood and sexual dysfunction by being a stimulus for either or both. The medications used for the treatment of depression typically have a negative impact on the sexual function of women, though some have found the dopaminergic action of bupropion beneficial, and others advocate the possibility of using more traditional antidepressant medications – either at a lower dose, or providing occasional drug holidays to alleviate side effects.

Effects of Chronic Pain on Body Image

Chronic pelvic pain has a negative effect on female body image, and when body image is compromised, it impacts sexual function and satisfaction. Women may either develop a hypervigilant, obsessive focus on the painful part of the body, or complete dissociation and reduced awareness of the area. Women with chronic gynecological pain may have increased body exposure anxiety during sexual activities, especially if the pain is primary rather than developed secondarily [13]. A woman with primary chronic pelvic pain has not had a chance to develop a positive appreciation for her body, and its ability to function sexually in a pleasurable way. When the pelvic structures have always been a source of pain and distress, it is extremely difficult to experience normal sexual development, and unimpaired experiences of desire, arousal, or orgasm. Conversely, with chronic pelvic pain developed secondarily, a woman has had a span of healthy sexual function to provide a frame of reference – and a concrete cognitive goal to work back toward, as she takes steps to resolve the pain and return to prior levels of optimal function. It is important to establish whether chronic pelvic pain is primary or secondary, in order to evaluate and treat it effectively, as the two have different therapeutic trajectories. It is also helpful to address a woman's feelings about her body, and beliefs about her genital function, as these views are integral in planning holistic treatment [14].

Effects of Chronic Pain on Relationship/Intimacy

It is indisputable that chronic pelvic pain negatively affects relationship dynamics of the couple involved. It also follows that the quality of the relationship then likely influences the degree and intensity of the pain. This dynamic can have various presentations, from the virginal couple that marries, and then discovers that the female has pelvic floor tension and spastic pain, to the long-married couple that deals with pelvic pain from adhesive disease following multiple surgeries. It is crucial to enquire about how each partner has adjusted to pain within the relationship, and how he or she has navigated the ensuing difficulties with intimacy. It has been reported that male partner behavior has a modulatory effect on female sexual satisfaction. Increased facilitative, and decreased negative responses relate to higher sexual and relationship satisfaction, whereas more solicitous behavior on the part of the male creates less sexual satisfaction for both [15]. It is important to help the couple acknowledge these behavior patterns and provide a framework by which to rework them in order to circumvent continued negativity and reinforce positive relational satisfaction. The suggestion that partners' cognitive responses may influence the experience of chronic pelvic pain for women points toward the importance of considering and including the partner when treating this sexual health problem.

Tools to Evaluate Biopsychosocial Aspects of Female Pain

It is important to have efficient tools at hand in the clinical setting, to quickly identify all patients at risk for sexual dysfunction, in order to either deal with the problem(s) or provide appropriate referral for them.

Female Sexual Function Index

One comprehensive tool is the Female Sexual Function Index (FSFI) [16]. It is a 19-item measure of female sexual function yielding a total score, as well as individual scores relating to the six domains of desire, arousal, lubrication, orgasm, satisfaction, and pain. The FSFI questions are coded from 0.0 to 5.0, with the maximum score for each domain being 6.0. Summing item responses and multiplying by a correction factor derives the final score. The total composite sexual function score ranges from 2.0 (reflecting no sexual activity/no desire) to a high score of 36. An FSFI score of 19 or lower correlates to sexual dysfunction, with the specifics being identified by analyzing each of the domains. This comprehensive tool is useful in the research setting, but one drawback is that it requires considerable time for a woman to respond to the entire questionnaire. The provider must then take time to score the questionnaire, making it unwieldy in the busy clinical setting.

Female Sexual Dysfunction Index

One adaptation for the clinical setting is the Female Sexual Dysfunction Index (FSDI) (Figure 19.2), which is based on a shortened version of the FSFI, but features an additional item related to personal interest in having a satisfying sex life. The item rating sexual arousal was removed. The total score can range from 2 to 30, with a pathological sum considered ≥16 [17]. This tool is especially suited to nonspecialist settings, to quickly detect potential female sexual dysfunction (FSD), which could otherwise remain underrecognized.

Effects of Chronic Pain on Desire

The psychological implications of chronic pelvic pain exert a consistent effect on sexual function for women – especially with regard to desire for sexual activity. When chronic pain conditions comorbid circumstances in the pelvic floor and vagina to trigger more intense pain through pelvic floor tension, or vaginal spasm, it becomes very unlikely for a woman to experience either spontaneous or responsive-type sexual desire. Further, the high levels of anxiety and depression seen in women with chronic pelvic pain reduce the potential for sexual desire and arousal, both from central "shut-down" mechanisms resulting from alterations in brain neurochemistry, as well as local dryness, pain, and lack of lubrication from the disease process directly, or as consequences of treatment interventions. It is important to recognize the stepwise nature that must be undertaken in treating sexual dysfunction, as it is unrealistic to expect improvement in desire/arousal before resolving or improving the root cause(s) of chronic pelvic pain as much as possible. Sexual desire becomes more elusive if pain as a barrier is not reduced. Prescriptions or interventions aimed at improving desire are futile in the setting of chronic pain.

Sexual Anatomy: Implications for Genital Structures

Female genital form and function continues to be clarified and classified even in contemporary times. Structures such as the Skene's (paraurethral) glands, the clitoris, and the distal vagina are the focus of novel research further defining anatomical structure and physiological function in recent years. The concept of vaginal orgasm and the supporting role of anatomical structures in the anterior vaginal wall have garnered much interest of late, as consensus has shifted toward the clitoris, through its deeply rooted extensions underlying the labia, and diving deeply along the anterior vaginal wall, participating as more of a collaborative unit with the aroused anterior vaginal wall, rather than as a distinct entity. The "so-called" G spot is actually formed by an interactive, clitoral–urethral–vaginal complex, which is variable between women, due to diversity in relational measurements and routes of innervation [19]. These structures share some common vasculature and innervation and move in unison during sexual activity, especially when brought into even closer proximity during arousal through engorgement of genital tissues.

1. **How would you rate your interest in having an active sexual life?**
   (1) Extremely important
   (2) Very important
   (3) Important
   (4) Not important
   (5) Not very important

2. **Over the past 4 weeks, how would you rate your level (degree) of sexual interest/desire?**
   (1) Very high
   (2) High
   (3) Moderate
   (4) Low
   (5) Very low to none at all

3. **Over the past 4 weeks, how often did you become lubricated ("wet") during sexual activity or intercourse?**
   (0) Always or almost always
   (1) Most times
   (2) Sometimes
   (3) A few times
   (4) Almost never or never
   (5) No sexual activity

4. **Over the past 4 weeks, when you had sexual stimulation or intercourse, how often did you reach orgasm?**
   (0) Always or almost always
   (1) Most times
   (2) Sometimes
   (3) A few times
   (4) Almost never or never
   (5) No sexual activity

5. **Over the past 4 weeks, how often did you experience discomfort or pain during vaginal penetration?**
   (0) Always or almost always
   (1) Most times
   (2) Sometimes
   (3) A few times
   (4) Almost never or never
   (5) Did not attempt penetration

6. **Over the past 4 weeks, how satisfied have you been with your overall sexual life?**
   (0) Very satisfied
   (1) Moderately satisfied
   (2) Equally satisfied and dissatisfied
   (3) Moderately dissatisfied
   (4) Very dissatisfied

Figure 19.2 Female Sexual Dysfunction Index (FSDI). The score for each of the six items is added and total derived. A pathological sum is considered ≥16. Derived from Maseroli E, Fanni E, Fambrini M, Ragghianti B, Limoncin E. Bringing the body of the iceberg to the surface: The Female Sexual Dysfunction Index-6 (FSDI-6) in the screening of female sexual dysfunction. *J Endocrin Invest.* 2016;39:401.

The Skene's (paraurethral) gland is analogous to the prostate, and women display a wide range of variability regarding the number and location of Skene's gland ostia, opening both into the distal urethra internally, as well as lateral to the urethral meatus externally, in the vulvar vestibule. It remains unclear whether fluid emission from the Skene's gland ostia occurs as female ejaculate related to orgasm, or merely as lubrication in response to arousal. Examination of these ostia support the notion that the female body demonstrates plasticity in the genital tissues, much like in other areas of the

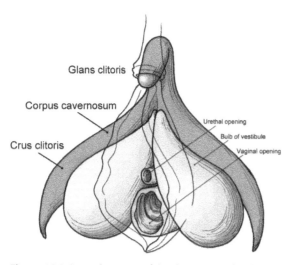

Figure 19.3 Internal structure of the clitoris. A graphic showing the internal anatomy of the vulva, with focus on the anatomy and location of the entire structure of the clitoris. External structures – the clitoral hood and labia minora – are depicted as transparent. Source: https://commons.wikimedia.org/w/index.php?title=File:Clit oris_anatomy_labeled-en.jpg&oldid=244771559" https://commons .wikimedia.org/w/index.php?title=File:Clitoris_anatomy_labeled-en.jpg&oldid=244771559.

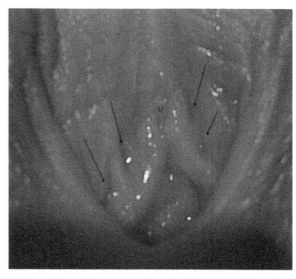

Figure 19.4 Skene's gland ostia in a subject *without* ejaculation history. Vaginal introitus displaying the external ostia of the Skene's gland in a woman who does not report ejaculation of fluid with orgasm. There are two ostia on each paraurethral location. Photo courtesy of Debra Wickman, MD, FACOG

body, in response to physiological challenges. There are differences in number of Skene's gland ostia between women who report ability to orgasm with expulsion of ejaculatory fluid (female ejaculation) as compared to those who do not expel fluid with orgasm (Figures 19.4 and 19.5). Women who report ability to ejaculate fluid have been found to have significantly more ostia than women who do not, possibly due to the body's ability to accommodate increased pressure or volume of fluid emitted [20].

Knowledge of these anatomical concepts is important for several reasons. First, there are obvious implications regarding the need for careful navigation among and around these important structures in performing surgery, to avoid creating or worsening pain or sexual dysfunction. Second, however, a less straightforward benefit is that physicians can utilize this information to educate women about their bodies, and encourage connection of intellectual facts with physical function, while separating myths from truth. When women understand the source(s) of their chronic pain, and its relationship to their body processes, they are likely to be more compliant in treatment, and successful as collaborators in healing.

Brain–Body Connections: Chronic Pelvic Pain and the Limbic Brain

The limbic portion of the brain is the center for neurochemical production related to sexual response and sexual function. It is made up of subcortical regions, which include important structures like the hippocampus, amygdala, hypothalamus, septal nuclei, cingulate cortex, and parahippocampal gyrus, among others. The brain receives messages about pain through the thalamus – which then directs signals to either the cerebral cortex, which mediates thought and analysis, or the limbic system, which links emotional responses to the stimuli. The cerebral cortex locates the source of pain, determines a course of action to alleviate it, and triggers pain-suppressive chemicals such as endorphins to modulate the pain message. The limbic system produces emotions that often accompany pain – fear, anxiety, or frustration, which can lessen or intensify the pain response felt. When pain is soothed, it is the limbic system that mediates the emotional response of security and reassurance, which lessens the experience of pain.

The limbic brain also mediates the euphoric and pleasurable experience of sex, with the interplay of dopamine and oxytocin among others. It reinforces the

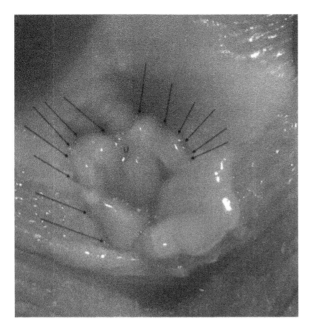

Figure 19.5 Skene's gland ostia in a subject *with* ejaculation history. Vaginal introitus displaying the external ostia of the Skene's gland in a woman who reports ejaculation of fluid with orgasm. There are seven ostia on the right, and six ostia on the left paraurethral location. Photo courtesy of Debra Wickman, MD, FACOG

repetition of pleasurable experiences. However, limbic dysfunction occurs in the setting of chronic pelvic pain. It is thought that allodynia results in increased sensitivity to pain afferents (hyperalgesia) from pelvic organs, with resulting abnormal efferent innervation of pelvic musculature (spasm)– both visceral and somatic. The pelvic musculature is triggered to undergo tonic contraction and generates more pain sensations. The pain afferents from these pelvic organs then follow the pain pathway back to the sensitized, hypervigilant limbic system, and the cycle repeats [21]. This mechanism is hypothesized to be responsible for communication between organ systems affected by chronic pain, or multiple close-by organ systems involved in pain syndromes. This type of influence on the limbic system is likely to alter normal liberation of dopamine and oxytocin pathways, blocking or muting the emotional benefits related to sex. Treatment should address this underlying limbic hypersensitivity, which can be treated with psychiatric medications or cognitive therapy. Targeted therapies to interrupt the loop anywhere along the mechanism is likely to be helpful as well, which speaks to the benefits of pelvic floor physical therapy, trigger point injections

or medications such as gabapentin or pregabalin, to normalize overactive pain pathways. Chronic pain should be addressed primarily, in order to mitigate its negative effect on the sexual response. Only after measures are taken to reduce or resolve pain, can appropriate limbic system responses be restored.

Implications of Suppressed or Absent Sex Hormones

Chronic pelvic pain due to menstrual abnormalities, such as dysmenorrhea or endometriosis is often primarily treated with suppressive agents such as an oral contraceptive or a gonadotropin-releasing hormone (GnRH) agonist. These medications are effective in suppressing the menstrual cycle and inhibiting pain but have a common secondary effect of causing hormonally mediated vulvar vestibulodynia. Serum free testosterone is reduced via suppressed production as well as binding to increased levels of serum sex hormone binding globulin. Female genital tissues, especially in the vulvar vestibule, require adequate local testosterone levels for health, in addition to estrogen. Without adequate local androgen levels, the Skene's and Bartholin gland ostia become erythematous and inflamed [22], creating a painful ring encircling the vaginal vestibule. Attempted penetration through this painful area triggers secondary spasm in the distal vagina and pelvic floor muscles, creating constriction of vaginal caliber, decreased oxygenation and increased lactic acid buildup in the pelvic floor muscles. This creates aching and discomfort for hours or even days afterward.

Low testosterone levels are associated with a decline in sexual arousal, genital sensation, libido, and orgasm. Currently, there are not Food and Drug Administration (FDA) approved testosterone preparations for women – leaving only manually compounded preparations, or medication packaged for men, used at approximately one tenth the usual male dose when prescribed for women. Compounded testosterone cream, for example, may be locally applied to resolve inflammation in the vulvar vestibular gland ostia, and dosed adequately enough to provide absorption for systemic uptake. Clinical studies continue to assess the benefits of testosterone and various modes of delivery for the treatment of female sexual dysfunction, both locally and centrally, but consensus has not yet been reached.

Premature surgical menopause may also be part of the treatment plan for chronic pelvic pain, and this can contribute to negative sexual consequences, due to low systemic and local estrogen levels as well as low testosterone levels, since the ovaries produce most of the body's estrogen, and a significant amount of the testosterone. It is important to discuss the potential risks and benefits of hormone therapy with the patient prior to surgery, so that she can make an informed decision ahead of time, and avoid the potentially dramatic symptoms from drops in hormone levels if she wants to supplement her sex hormones.

If she decides against systemic hormone therapy, she should be encouraged to consider local vaginal therapy – with intravaginal dehydroepiandrosterone (DHEA) or an estradiol product. Intravaginal DHEA, now in an FDA-approved form, provides local intracellular androgenic and estrogenic effects, which are very beneficial to vulvar vestibular gland health and local genital sexual response – supporting epithelial integrity, arousal, lubrication, and orgasm – free from the effects of local atrophy and inflammation.

The Integrative Pelvic Exam Protocol

Negative emotional memories intensify the experience of physical symptoms, and chronic pelvic pain is modulated by ongoing emotional responses, with input from significant relationship figures in a woman's life. Sexual activity, occurring in the setting of chronic pelvic pain, is layered with trauma, not only from the direct pain it causes, but also by indirectly fueling conflict or neglect in relationship intimacy. Further, traumatic memories are more vividly, consistently and completely remembered, along with any accompanying sensory component(s) over a longer span of time compared to positive, happy memories [23]. As a result, negative aspects influencing chronic pelvic pain are reinforced over time, and the woman experiencing it continues to react with compensatory emotional mechanisms that do not promote physical recovery or restoration of relationship health. Women become avoidant toward sexual intimacy in an effort to avert physical pain, as well as to elude relationship strain. This tendency toward disconnection can be seen as noncompliance with treatment recommendations or observed as perpetual helplessness in demeanor. The starting point to change this pattern is to facilitate an alliance and innate understanding between the woman's mind and her body, the end organ of perceived pathology. Although "talk therapy" is extremely helpful and necessary in most cases, it is not enough to offer counseling alone. To successfully

impact the course of treatment, it is necessary to shift cellular patterning/focus at the physical site of the trauma or chronic pain, in an intentional way.

This is accomplished through the pelvic examination, enhanced with digital technology, in order to engage, educate, and then empower the patient to understand and transcend her pain. The integrative pelvic exam protocol (IPEP) involves a detailed gynecological pelvic examination, using a digital colposcope, coupled with a digital tablet, via an app that provides a closed loop WiFi transmission of the colposcopic images to the tablet in real time.

The process is divided into a verbal preparatory phase, where a woman recounts the experience of her vulva/genitals using her own terms, along with how and where the pain is experienced. This is followed by a visual examination, allowing her to simultaneously engage with these structures, using the digital tablet, and guided by the examiner. This process is typically done in serial sessions, at a woman's individual pace, in a gynecological approach to sexuality counseling, and provides unifying, healing steps toward resolution of the traumatic aspects of the pain. Physical comfort and emotional calm are essential in order to allow full participation in the examination process. Women are given information and encouraged to ask questions throughout.

4-D Wheel of Sexual Experience

The 4-Dimensional (4-D) Wheel of Sexual Experience is based on work by Gina Ogden, PhD, who developed this therapeutic approach following her nationwide survey, which established that sexual experience for women is multidimensional, with the components of thoughts, emotions, meanings, and physical sensations evenly factored into the framework, in the form of quadrants, equally dividing a sphere. The 4-D process is an interactive creative structure through which patient/client explores her core sexual issues in the context of sexuality therapy, guided by a counselor/therapist who is versed in the 4-D process [24]. The IPEP takes the basic therapeutic premise of the 4-D Wheel and shifts the focus of the experience to the woman's vulva/genitals, allowing the story to be told from that unique perspective (Figure 19.6). The narrative unfolds while incorporating equal elements of body, mind, emotion, and relationship history in the recounting of pain/trauma and its consequences [25].

The physical dimension of the 4-D Wheel is the domain in which a woman explores a full range of sensory experiences, choosing both positive and negative descriptors that characterize her experience of chronic pain in her pelvis/genitals. Positive focus involves "wished for" characteristics such as pleasurable sensations or arousal, versus negative/shadow aspects, such as "burning" or "numbness."

The emotional dimension of the 4-D Wheel is the arena for exploring the full range of emotional feelings – relating to emotions such as happiness, trust, and passion versus anger, fear, sadness, or disappointment.

The mental dimension of the 4-D Wheel is the place where a patient exposes limiting beliefs and messages about why she has pain, or what meaning she ascribes to it.

Finally, the spirit dimension of the 4-D Wheel is the exploration of what sex and intimacy mean in the context of relationships and how they are molded and affected by the chronicity of pain and its effects. The guided assessment starts with one's relationship within herself and works outward to include her intimate relationship(s), other significant relationships, and finally life and all it encompasses.

These four dimensions vary from woman to woman, and the telling of each unique story is

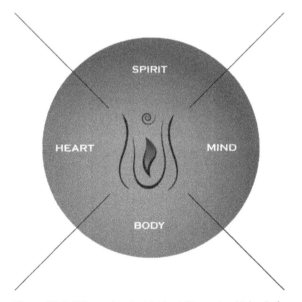

Figure 19.6 This graphic depicts the 4-Dimensional Wheel of Sexual Experience, a tool that provides the organizing framework in guiding a subject through the Integrative Pelvic Exam Protocol (IPEP), with the vulva/genitals leading the narrative through equal aspects of body/mind/heart/spirit, in recounting all facets of chronic pain and trauma. Artwork courtesy of Debra Wickman, MD, FACOG

therapeutic in confronting the multiple facets of chronic pain and integrating the layers of trauma affecting the nature of pain, and the ease with which it can lessen, resolve, and heal.

Integrative Pelvic Exam Protocol: Procedure in Detail

The woman is positioned in dorsal lithotomy position, with the upper body comfortably raised enough to allow her to hold the digital tablet in front and watch the examination in its entirety on the screen.

For the examination itself, a transparent, disposable plastic speculum is lubricated and inserted fully into the vagina, to the cervix. The cervix is located and pointed out on the tablet screen as a landmark starting point. If the cervix is surgically absent, then the vaginal cuff is used as the landmark.

While visualizing the cervix or vaginal cuff and all subsequent structures, the woman and examiner discuss the appearance of each of these structures, and the woman's reactions to seeing them, in the context of what she has already revealed during the preceding counseling session(s). She is encouraged to connect with the structures she sees on the tablet, as she perceives the examiner's touch, either with a gloved finger or a swab. The conversation between woman and examiner is organized around the 4-D Wheel quadrants, to evoke her physical, emotional, intellectual, and spiritual responses as she interacts with each body part.

The pelvic examination proceeds with a guided "tour" of the anterior and posterior vaginal fornices, the anterior vaginal wall (G spot), and the vaginal introitus – including the urethral meatus, the Skene's/paraurethral gland ostia, the hymenal remnants, and Bartholin gland ostia. Any unique aspects, that is, surgical/traumatic scars, prolapse/vaginal wall defects, atrophic changes, and so forth, are identified and discussed to the comfort level of the woman. The goal is to encourage discussion to expand beyond physical pain, or judgment about appearance, to include all of the 4-D Wheel quadrants: physical, emotional, mental, and spiritual.

The speculum is removed, and the examination continues externally to provide a digital view of the vulva, starting anteriorly with the mons, clitoral hood and clitoral glans, labia minora and majora, posterior fourchette, perineum, and anus. Each structure is discussed in terms of its contribution to sexual function and sensation – again using the 4-D Wheel quadrants as an organizing principle. Time spent on each anatomic structure varies depending on the individual need and circumstance. Opportunity for questions and answers flows freely during the process, and the examiner provides direct education regarding specific diagnoses and pertinent treatment options as the exam progresses.

Utilization of IPEP during the pelvic examination provides an integrative experience that links the examiner and woman in an active partnership as they interact and respond to each genital structure in view of all quadrants – body, mind, heart, and spirit. This process affords the women more control during the exam, as an active participant, able to document what she chooses with "screenshot" still photos, and to verbalize her thoughts and feelings about her body in her own timeframe, in a dialogue with the examiner. The process flows in a self-perpetuating fashion, as the woman becomes more comfortable and intrigued, opens up, shares more, and becomes engaged with it.

The IPEP process creates a body–mind connection to restore the loss created when a woman "shuts off" the feelings/sensations to her genitals in order to suppress current physical pain or the undesirable discomfort created by past traumatic experiences, long-term chronic pain, or self-neglect. By actively engaging in the physical exam, and seeing/feeling/discussing/reacting to her genital structures, she is invited to acknowledge their existence and deal with each part as a real entity.

The 4-D Wheel approach provides an organizing principle for this procedure, as the woman is guided to deal with each of her genital structures, issues, and concerns within the context of the whole being. The pelvic examination becomes a form of cognitive behavioral therapy, as a dynamic interventional process. One cannot successfully isolate an issue in the physical sense without also dealing with its related origins and consequences in the emotional, intellectual, and spiritual contexts as well.

Alternative Methods to Treat Sexual Dysfunction and Chronic Pelvic Pain

Acupuncture is associated with significant improvement in sexual function in all domains, but especially desire. This modality has also been practiced as part of traditional Chinese medicine for centuries in terms of treating both acute and chronic pain syndromes [26]. Similarly, hypnotherapy has also been shown to work

well in treating anxiety related to chronic pelvic pain and would therefore address related sexual deficits seen in the setting of pain.

Mindfulness is another long-practiced modality, brought from Eastern traditions, that provides focused awareness on the present moment, on the part of both clinician and patient, to relieve chronic pain, anxiety, and sexual dysfunction in most of its forms [27]. The patient focuses on newly emerging physical sensations and arousal, rather than on pain perception itself. The practice must be frequent, that is, daily, and consistent in order to provide maximum benefit. In turn, focus can also be turned toward all domains of the Female Sexual Function Index (FSFI), to improve desire through intention. It is beneficial, if not essential, that the clinician personally embody a mindfulness practice before he or she can successfully teach a patient the principles.

Summary

Management of sexual dysfunction arising from chronic pelvic pain is a long-term venture, involving all dimensions of sexuality in order to restore well-being and satisfaction. There is not a unifying algorithm to guide therapy, and treatment must be able to vary from one woman to the next, according to her unique situation and need. The clinician should work to resolve each component of pain as possible, in a stepwise fashion, in order to restore downstream sexual function, such as desire, arousal and orgasm. For ultimate success, a woman must be assisted in connecting her cognitive awareness with anatomical and physiological structure and function in order to surpass all roadblocks to sexual wellness.

Five Things You Need to Know

- Sexual dysfunction in women is multifactorial and complex, especially when arising from a setting of chronic pain. Do not delay inquiry about impaired sexual function – it is a significant quality of life indicator. It should be addressed from the onset of treatment for chronic pelvic pain so that appropriate intervention is planned in sync with the other treatment goals.
- Sexual dysfunction occurs in women of all ages and backgrounds. All women, from college-age to postmenopausal to elderly, should be asked about sexual satisfaction and concerns. The sexual problems may arise from different causes, but distress can occur at any age, and measures should be taken to address/alleviate them.

- Treatment of sexual dysfunction is biopsychosocial, and ideally involves a multidisciplinary team, including a sex therapist/psychologist to address needs related to psychological/cultural/relational factors; and a physical therapist trained in pelvic floor physical therapy, to manage pelvic floor disorders. Other resource personnel are enlisted as needed, such as acupuncturist, nutritionist, and compound pharmacist.

- Timing is critical. Work to resolve factors like atrophy or vulvar vestibulitis prior to referring for pelvic floor physical therapy. A stepwise treatment approach will maximize patient comfort as well as compliance. She will participate more in her care if the associated discomfort is minimized.

- Encouraging a woman to connect with her anatomy – both normal and abnormal, is key to optimizing patient participation in her treatment plan. Healthcare providers can promote this connection with education, illustration, and feedback. Women can learn by looking at a picture or model, or by viewing their own anatomical structures via a mirror or digital technology.

References

1. McCabe M, Althof SE, Assalian P, et al. Psychological and interpersonal dimensions of sexual function and dysfunction. *J Sex Med.* 2010;**7**(1 pt 2):327–36.

2. Naeinian MR, Shaeiri MR, Hosseini FS. General health and quality of life in patients with sexual dysfunctions. *Urol J.* 2011;**8**(2): 127–31.

3. Shifren JL, Monz BU, Russo PA, et al. Sexual problems and distress in United States women: prevalence and correlates. *Obstet Gynecol.* 2008;**112**(5):970–8.

4. Laumann EO, Nicolosi A, Glasser DB, et al. Sexual problems among women and men aged 40–80y: prevalence and correlates identified in the Global Study of Sexual Attitudes and Behaviors. *Int J Impot Res.* 2005; **17**(1):39–57.

5. Mathias SD, Kuppermann M, Liberman RF, et al. Chronic pelvic pain: prevalence, health-related quality of life, and economic correlates. *Obstet Gynecol.* 1996; **87**(3):321–7.

6. Ahangari A. Prevalence of chronic pelvic pain among women. *Pain Phys J.* 2014;**17**: E141–7.

7. Zondervan KT, Yudkin PL, Vessey MP, et al. Prevalence and incidence of chronic pelvic pain in primary care: evidence from a national general practice database. *Br J Obstet Gynaecol.* 1999;**106**(11):1149–55.

8. Appa AA, Creasman J, Brown JS, et al. The impact of multimorbidity on sexual function in middle-aged and older women: beyond the single disease perspective. *J Sex Med.* 2014;**11**(11):2744–55.

9. American Psychiatric Association. *Diagnostic and Statistical Manual of Mental Disorders: DSM-5.* Washington, DC: American Psychiatric Association DSM-5 Task Force;2013.

10. IsHak WW, Tobia G. DSM-5 Changes in diagnostic criteria of sexual dysfunctions. *Reprod Sys Sexual Disorders.* 2013;**2**:122.

11. Basson R. Sexuality and sexual disorders. *Clin Updates Womens Health Care.* 2014;**13**(2):11–15.

12. Bryant C, Cockburn R, Plante AF, et al. The psychological profile of women presenting to a multidisciplinary clinic for chronic pelvic pain: High levels of psychological dysfunction and implications for practice. *J Pain Res.* 2016; **9**:1049–56.

13. Maillé DL, Bergeron S, Lambert B. Body image in women with primary and secondary provoked vestibulodynia: a controlled study. *J Sex Med.* 2015; **12**(2):505–15.

14. Pazmany E, Bergeron S, Van Oudenhove L, et al. Aspects of sexual self-schema in premenopausal women with dyspareunia: associations with pain, sexual function, and sexual distress. *J Sex Med.* 2013;**10**(9):2255–64.

15. Rosen NO, Muise A, Bergeron S, Delisle I, Baxter ML. Daily associations between partner responses and sexual and relationship satisfaction in couples coping with provoked vestibulodynia. *J Sex Med.* 2015;**12**(4):1028–39.

16. Rosen R, Brown C, Heiman J, et al. The Female Sexual Function Index (FSFI): a multidimensional self-report instrument for the assessment of female sexual function. *J Sex Marital Ther.* 2000;**26**:191–208.

17. Maseroli E, Fanni E, Fambrini M, Ragghianti B, Limoncin E. Bringing the body of the iceberg to the surface: the Female Sexual Dysfunction Index-6 (FSDI-6) in the screening of female sexual dysfunction. *J Endocrin Invest.* 2016;**39**: 401.

18. File: Clitoris anatomy labeled-en.jpg. 2017, May 20. https://commons.wikimedia.org/w/index.php?title=File:Clitoris_anatomy_labeled-en.jpg&oldid=244771559

19. Graziottin A, Gambini D. Anatomy and physiology of genital organs – women. In Vodusek B, Boller F (eds), *Handbook of Clinical Neurology, Neurology of Sexual and Bladder Disorders.* 3rd series; Vol. **130**. Oxford: Elsevier BV Press; 2015.

20. Wickman DS. Plasticity of the Skene's gland in women who report ejaculation of fluid with orgasm (abstract). *J Sex Med.* 2016;**11**: 147.

21. Fenton BW. Limbic associated pelvic pain: a hypothesis to explain the diagnostic relationships and features of patients with chronic pelvic pain. *Med Hypotheses*. 2007;**69** (2):282–6.

22. Traish AM, Kim N, Min K, Munarriz R, Goldstein I. Role of androgens in female genital sexual arousal: receptor expression, structure and function. *Fertil Steril*. 2002;**77**(Suppl 4):11–18.

23. Porter S, Peace KA. The scars of memory: a prospective, longitudinal investigation of the consistency of traumatic and negative emotional memories in adulthood. *Psychol Sci*. 2007;**18** (5):435–41.

24. Ogden G. *Expanding the Practice of Sex Therapy: An Integrative Model for Exploring Desire and Intimacy*, 1st ed. New York: Routledge; 2013.

25. Ogden G. *Exploring Desire & Intimacy: A Workbook for Creative Clinicians*,1st ed. New York: Routledge; 2017.

26. Oakley SH, Walther-Liu J, Crisp CC, Pauls RN. Acupuncture in premenopausal women with hypoactive sexual desire disorder: a prospective cohort pilot study. *Sex Med*. 2016;4:e176–81.

27. Brotto LA, Goldmeier D. Mindfulness interventions for treating sexual dysfunctions: the gentle science of finding focus in a multitask world. *J Sex Med*. 2015;**12**:1687–9.

Chapter 20

Physical Therapy Interventions for Musculoskeletal Impairments in Pelvic Pain

Lauren Hill

Editor's Introduction

Pelvic floor muscle spasm is one of the most common reasons for pelvic pain, and it often coexists with other pelvic pain conditions. Oral muscle relaxants do not seem to be helpful in these patients and vaginal suppositories seem to relax muscles much better. A combination of diazepam 5 milligrams placed vaginally, baclofen 4 milligrams, and ketamine 15 milligrams used before bedtime works well on pelvic muscle spasm. The mainstay of treatment of pelvic floor muscle spasm is pelvic floor physical therapy. It is best done by Women's Health physical therapists who are specifically trained in pelvic floor dysfunction. Patients who fail physical therapy may be candidates for injections of botulinum toxin into pelvic floor muscles.

Treatment Planning and Goal Setting

The treatment of pelvic pain has notoriously been difficult due to the likelihood for multisystem involvement; interconnected symptoms; and lack of evidence demonstrating a clear benefit of one treatment, intervention, or technique over another. As discussed in Chapter 5, it is clear that often a patient's pain can be reproduced or aggravated by testing intrapelvic and extrapelvic structures. Deciding how to prioritize the multiple impairments and patient complaints can be challenging; however, it is necessary for successful treatment. The clinician must be able to tease apart the primary drivers causing the patient's symptoms: an organ or organ system, biomechanical deficiency, or pathological process.

There are various interventions including procedures, medications, and manual techniques that can be implemented to help address the patient's pain with specificity once the primary driver of the pain is identified. This chapter focuses on conservative treatments that can be utilized including referral to pelvic health physical therapy and education/techniques the primary clinician can provide if referral to physical therapy is difficult because of the location of the patient and lack of available referral sources.

To guide clinicians in their treatment and plan of care development, it is helpful to apply the definition of evidence-based medicine proposed by Sackett and Haynes, which is the "conscientious, explicit, and judicious use of current best evidence in making decisions about the care of individual patients" [1]. This involves integrating the best available current evidence, which in the case of pelvic pain is still evolving, with clinical expertise. As of now, there are no clear conservative techniques or treatment approaches that have been found to be superior therefore the clinician's proficiency and judgment they have acquired through clinical practice is heavily relied upon. Increased expertise in a clinical area is reflected in more effective and efficient diagnosis and in the integration of the individual patient's values and preferences that shape how the patient experiences and conceptualizes her pain symptoms. Within the context that the patient creates, it is important for the clinician to provide options to allow the patient to choose her preferred treatment that will help her progress toward her stated goals [2].

Utilizing this definition helps to not only identify the driver of the pain but also assists in the treatment planning process. When reflective critical thinking and expertise are integrated with a thorough assessment, the primary impairment, or driver, is often identified and an initial treatment plan can develop [2]. It is important to note that the primary driver of the pain may not always be a painful tissue and focusing treatment solely on the painful tissue may not yield successful results. Other systems, structures, or biomechanical habits may be dysfunctional and impaired but pain free and could be the underlying driver(s) that is/are causing pain in other systems or tissues due to excessive stress or overuse. To create a holistic picture of the patient's pain as well as develop a successful treatment plan, it may be these nonpainful structures or systems that need to be addressed in addition to the painful sources.

Identifying what tissue or structure hurts does not explain why it is hurting or why the patient is in pain. Often the question of why a structure is painful can and should be answered through a collaborative effort. It is often not possible for a clinician consulting in a medical setting to be able to take the time required to glean the necessary information from subjective interviewing; objective assessment of all integrated components to the patient's pain; as well as deciphering and discussing the patient's individual pain experience, goals, psychological status, and impacts to her functional abilities and daily life. Referral to collaborative and complementary providers is often necessary and recommended to help create a whole picture of the patient and her pain symptoms. This next section will specifically focus on what the pelvic health physical therapist is able to provide as a referral source to the clinician including an overview of treatment techniques often utilized in the pelvic pain population.

Faubion et al. suggest that referral to physical therapy early on in the patient's treatment planning should be a "cornerstone of management" for patients with pelvic pain [3]. Physical therapy is a profession grounded in a theoretical and scientific base with the goal to help individuals restore, maintain, and develop optimal physical functioning to allow for enhanced quality of life [4]. The focus in not just on the physical impairments of the body structures and functions but also on how those impairments impact a person's ability to participate in her activities of daily living and in her community and environment at large. This whole person approach is based on the concept developed by the International Classification of Functioning, Disability and Health (ICF), which is a World Health Organization approved system designed to classify heath and health-related states. The ICF is a biopsychosocial model of disability that conceptualizes a patient's level of functioning as a dynamic interaction between their health conditions, how that impacts her ability to function at the individual and society level, and how environmental factors affect her experience [4].

Physical therapists are experts in the assessment of the musculoskeletal system and how dysfunctions and impairments within this system can impact or be impacted by other bodily systems, pathologies, and injuries. Pelvic health physical therapists have additional knowledge and specific skill sets to be able to assess and treat musculoskeletal impairments of the pelvic floor and integrate how that relates to and impacts the larger body system and person. The role of the pelvic health physical therapist in the treatment of pelvic floor dysfunction is to work in concert with other medical professions such as urologists, urogynecologists, colorectal specialists, as well as psychologists, nutritionists, and integrative medicine doctors to help develop and implement an overarching individualized treatment plan. As discussed in Chapter 5, pelvic health physical therapists evaluate the structure and function of the pelvic girdle and address conditions or impairments noted through numerous hands-on and other modality techniques that will be described further in the next section. The development of goals and treatment planning is a collaborative process between the therapist and the patient, integrating the patient's conceptualization of their symptoms as described earlier to allow for the most optimal outcomes possible [4].

Through detailed evaluation and assessment of the patient with pelvic pain, the therapist is able to determine the primary driver(s) of the symptoms and treatment planning is then based on this information within the context of the patient's specific goals. It is typically difficult, if not impossible, to determine at times which dysfunction may have appeared first. The pain could be originating from pelvic floor muscle dysfunction in the form of overactivity that over time has led to dysfunctional voiding and painful bladder symptoms. Alternatively, visceral dysfunctions, although not directly related to muscular involvement, may over time cause guarding within the pelvic floor and eventually pain due to chronic holding patterns. The viscera and pelvic floor muscles may both be considered the drivers of the continued pain and both must be treated simultaneously to reach optimal interventional success. One can see how pelvic pain can begin as a singular issue or complaint that, if not addressed properly or due to chronicity of symptoms, can spread out to include other systems. The patient with an initial visceral issue such as irritable bowel syndrome (IBS), due to episodic and chronic pain the abdomen, may develop pelvic floor tension and overactivity from increased frequency of bowel movements eventually leading to pain during bowel movements and increased tissue tension in the extrapelvic muscles including within the abdomen and lower extremities. The patient may develop postural deviations and poor mechanics during activity, causing shortening in the hip flexors, abdominals, and diaphragm, which further limits trunk movement and perpetuates further cranial movement of the pain into the shoulders, jaw, and neck, causing headaches and further impaired function and activity participation [5]. Decreased participation and withdrawal from activity can impact the patient's mental status, leading to depression and further social isolation. At this point, the pain becomes a cycle with each system and area setting off the other, impacting the patient's ability to cope and the clinician's ability to effectively treat the pain. This type of patient presentation is not uncommon in the chronic pelvic pain world, and deciding where to start in terms of treatment is challenging; however, it is important to focus on what the potential initial drivers to the pain may have been including the visceral dysfunction of IBS and pelvic floor tension in this example. Working our way from the "central" pain driver can help to impact the more "peripheral" issues that are likely due to compensatory strategies the patient has developed in response to the pain.

In the process of establishing a treatment plan, the clinician must determine patient-identified goals and how to show incremental progress toward the desired outcomes. Patients are encouraged to describe their lifestyle and activities that they wish to resume and the therapist can work on creating measurable goals for each of the impairments and domains that are affected by the patients current conditions.

It is important to describe to the patients that the progress expected may be slow and may have some challenges as the body responds to the demands placed on the system to encourage adaptation and recovery. This means they may experience flare ups from overuse or fatigue as they try to establish how much they can do an activity or an exercise before they have maxed out the resources for their current tolerance.

The clinician should include goal setting, which involves not only increases in activity tolerance but recovery from activities as well. For a woman who may experience postcoital pain, her goal may include reducing the soreness and discomfort from 12 hours to 1 hour after sexual activity.

Keeping daily pain intensity journals is not usually recommended except to establish a pattern of the nature of the pain experience. It is the clinician's role to maintain records of activity-specific limitations and pain levels so that when reassessing a patient, it can be referenced to demonstrate progress or persistent disability.

Physical Impairment–Based Interventions

Interventions discussed in this section are considered conservative in nature and are targeted mainly at pelvic floor, abdominal wall, and hip musculature dysfunctions. These interventions are not used in isolation. One area of the musculoskeletal system may require a reduction of activation; another may require increased stability and strength. Patients with pelvic pain may be found to have overactivity at the puborectalis leading to dyspareunia symptoms, particularly during initial penetration; however, they also demonstrate true pelvic floor weakness and a lack of tenderness to palpation within deeper pelvic floor muscles as is sometimes the case with women who are postpartum reporting incontinence, low back pain, and dyspareunia. As there are overlapping symptoms, overlapping treatments are commonly implemented. In fact, a patient may need to begin with strategies to relax and lengthen the pelvic floor and then progressing to strengthening the intra- and extrapelvic muscles within the context of training the postural, respiratory, and biomechanical systems through facilitation techniques and education.

As discussed previously, pelvic floor overactivity can be the primary driver or a response to the patient's pain symptoms. Pelvic floor muscles that are overactive can be functionally short, meaning there is no length change to the muscles; however, the patient may consciously or subconsciously be clenching. Functionally short pelvic floor muscles will demonstrate elevated resting tone when assessed using surface electromyographic (SEMG) biofeedback. Alternatively, patients with pelvic floor overactivity may also demonstrate structurally short muscles. In this scenario, there is a length change of the muscles and therefore no elevated muscle activity is required to maintain the muscles in this shortened position, as they have become "fixed" into this position. During SEMG biofeedback, there would be no elevation in resting tone; however, on palpation trigger points reproducing pain would likely be present and the tissue quality of the muscles would appear taut. In addition to the intervention described earlier, these patients likely benefit from an increased frequency of manual stretching and use of dilators or other internal release devices depending on what areas of the pelvic floor are demonstrating this dysfunction. Interventions to address overactivity may include manual techniques, therapeutic exercise, dilators, modalities, relaxation training, and patient education. These various techniques will be further discussed in the following sections.

> The goal with patients with overactive pelvic floor muscles is to relax the pelvic floor muscles through bringing awareness to the clenching pattern, optimizing breath and postural patterns that could contribute to the holding of the pelvic floor muscles and relaxation techniques introduced to the intrapelvic as well as extrapelvic girdle muscles. Another goal with these patients is to lengthen the muscle to an appropriate resting state – ready for its tasks.

Interventions for Overactive Pelvic Floor Muscles

Manual Therapies

Manual therapy can encompass a multitude of techniques that are typically employed by the pelvic health physical therapist when focusing on pelvic floor overactivity. Indications for manual treatment may include pain with pelvic floor contraction, taut bands or trigger points identified within the pelvic floor, and presence of restricted movement of the fascia overlying the muscle fibers.

It was found in one study that myofascial trigger point release led to resolution or significant [6] improvement in symptoms in 83% of cases, lessening the overactivity of the pelvic floor musculature, and in turn decreasing bladder inflammation and central sensitization [7]. Manual release techniques provided by pelvic health physical therapy have shown success in the treatment of bowel and bladder dysfunction, pelvic pain, and sexual dysfunction [7–10]. It is important to consider that although release of the trigger point can be beneficial, the presence of trigger points is likely perpetuated by other factors that could

include postural malalignments, biomechanical dysfunctions, and asymmetries or poor movement patterns and habits. Addressing these factors is necessary to be able to resolve completely the symptoms caused by the trigger points. Thiele's massage is a classic manual intervention for relieving pain and trigger points in the levator ani and coccygeus muscle groups. This technique emphasizes a stroking motion along the overactive pelvic floor muscle from origin to insertion with periodic sustained holds when active trigger points are identified [11].

The prevalence of myofascial dysfunction in women with interstitial cystitis/bladder pain syndrome (IC/BPS) reported has varied from 14% to 23% to as high as 78% [12]. Restrictions in the fascia can be due to trauma, posture, musculoskeletal conditions, or inflammation. Myofascial release is a manual therapeutic approach developed by John Barnes that targets the fascia [13]. Myofascial release has been found to significantly improve pelvic pain related to urological dysfunctions compared to global therapeutic massage [9]. Release to the myofascial system involves a gentle, hands-on approach that can be applied throughout the entire body, helping to improve posture, range of motion, and pain reduction [14]. Once the therapist determines where the fascial restrictions lie, gentle pressure is applied in in the direction of the restriction focusing first on the elastic component of the fascia progressing to the collagenous barrier. This may involve maintenance of pressure for up to 120 seconds. As the barrier is released, the therapist follows the motion of the tissue until all barriers are released [13].

Visceral mobilization was developed in the 1970s by Jean-Pierre Barral, a French osteopath and physical therapist. This technique assists in aligning and balancing various functional and structural imbalances throughout bodily systems including the musculoskeletal, nervous, urogenital, digestive, lymphatic, and vascular. Within a healthy system working optimally, all of these interrelated components move with fluidity. Impairments or adhesions restricting the motion dynamics between internal organs, fascia, and ligaments can lead to chronic pain and irritation. Adhesions and strains in this connective tissue can be due to surgery, illness, injury, or habitual postures. The approach aims to evaluate and treat structural relationships between the viscera and their fascial or ligamentous attachments to the musculoskeletal system through a hands-on, gentle technique. The target system are the organs that are suspected to be causing or contributing to the dysfunction and pain based on patient report. Once dysfunction is identified, specific placement of the hands is meant to encourage optimal mobility of the viscera and its connective tissue. The goal is to improve the functioning of the individual organ, the system, and environment within which the organ is situated by facilitating the return of the organ to its appropriate position, thereby stimulating blood flow and optimal functioning and alignment to the area. The state and ability of the visceral organs to move freely can affect the musculoskeletal system in turn, such as in the example of recurrent infections within the urogenital viscera or injury contributing to symptoms such as pelvic floor muscle dysfunction due to sustained holding patterns and tension. The reverse can also be true: the pelvic floor muscles can create enough tension chronically leading to irritation and decreased mobility within the surrounding viscera. Both scenarios may, and likely will, produce similar patient reported symptoms such as urinary frequency, hesitancy, and dysuria leading the clinician to think this could be precipitated by a urinary tract infection when it fact it could also be pelvic floor tension that is creating or mimicking an infectious process [15].

Connective tissue manipulation is considered distinct from massage therapy in its technique as well as effects it has on the body. It is characterized by the movement and distortion of the connective and subcutaneous tissues with the goal being to release tension in the tissue and improve range of motion of the adjacent joints and neurodynamics. It is based on the principles that dysfunction of an internal organ is revealed in the increased tone of superficial muscles and disruption in the subcutaneous tissues. Typically the dysfunction is distributed in the dermatomes corresponding to the innervation of the affected organ, signaling where treatment should be targeted. Altered blood flow within the deep tissues or pain suppression is seen as the therapeutic benefit. In comparison to myofascial and visceral release techniques, the pressure exerted during connective tissue manipulation is firm, such as in the example of skin rolling creating a sensation felt as an uncomfortable scratching or cutting. Local effects include release of histamine, local swelling, and arterial dilatation increasing blood flow to the region and facilitating resolution of subacute or chronic inflammation, thereby reducing pain by removing noxigenic chemicals from the tissues. The more general effects are also thought to be

due to increased blood flow and stimulation to distance sites from the treatment area through stimulation of the autonomic nervous system, and more specifically, the parasympathetic nervous system [16].

Other manual therapy techniques can be utilized in this patient population to target overactivity in the pelvic floor in the form of neuromuscular reeducation activities to lengthen and coordinate the muscles of the pelvic floor. These techniques include contract–relax to promote relaxation at a point of limited range of motion with isometric contractions of the tensed muscle for 5–8 seconds followed by voluntary relaxation and movement into the newly acquired range of motion. Strain–counterstrain is a form of passive positional release that involves moving the dysfunctional tissue into a shortened position to allow for a reduction of tone [17].

Therapeutic Modalities/Devices

Vaginal dilators can be used a source of treatment to help address myofascial trigger points and to further elongate the shortened pelvic floor as well as a mechanism to allow for the patient to perform self-release as part of a home exercise program. Vaginal dilators are available in a variety of materials including silicone and plastic with and without handles to allow for improved ergonomics of the hand and wrist during release. The vaginal dilators provide a stretch to the vaginal muscles and tissue either at the vaginal entrance or for deeper release into the pelvic floor muscles if angled in that direction. Graded sizes are provided if the target tissue is at the vaginal introitus or second layer of the pelvic floor. The patient is encouraged to assume a comfortable, relaxed position when using the dilators to allow for optimal effect with the use of lubricants for improved ease of insertion and comfort [18]. Benefits of dilator use include restoration of soft tissue elasticity, improved relaxation and awareness of the pelvic floor muscles, desensitization of the vaginal tissue, and improved mobility of scars in the introital and perineal area [19]. Patients may benefit from concurrent use of topical creams to improve comfort and aid relaxation during release. Although vaginal dilators can be used to perform patient self-release into deeper pelvic floor muscles, internal release devices are also available that have curved shapes more conducive for releasing soft tissue into the vaginal side walls. The use of vaginal dilators and release devices has been noted to be successful in the treatment of pelvic pain syndromes including dyspareunia, however, in conjunction with physical therapy treatments to allow for education in proper use, graded progression, and relaxation techniques [20].

The use of SEMG biofeedback devices can be particularly useful in improving the patient's awareness of the pelvic floor muscles. SEMG biofeedback can be facilitated through internal vaginal or rectal probes or external electrode sensors placed on either side of the anal opening. SEMG biofeedback is not a measure of muscle strength; instead it records the voltage sum of muscle action potentials, giving feedback on muscle events. The use of biofeedback to improve overactive pelvic floor muscles is to facilitate "downtraining" or relaxation of the muscles. Patients may be overrecruiting pelvic floor muscles at rest, when experiencing stressors, or when performing basic mobility tasks such as transitioning from sit to stand. Using the SEMG biofeedback during functional activities, whether actual or simulated, can be a beneficial tool to allow patients to understand and become aware of how their pelvic floor muscles are responding to numerous activities. Various relaxation positions or techniques can be taught and practiced during the use of SEMG biofeedback and this will help the patient and therapist to determine what the pelvic floor muscles respond optimally to, thus developing a more individualized home program [5]. Relaxation of the pelvic floor muscles is an important skill not only in a relaxed supine position but also in various positions and during various activities, as this better corresponds with real life for the patient and allows the training to be more adaptable and pertinent. SEMG biofeedback should not be considered a treatment on its own but rather used in conjunction with other therapeutic techniques such as manual therapies [21].

Other modalities that have various levels of research as treatment for patients with pelvic pain due to overactivity in the pelvic floor muscles include ultrasound and transcutaneous electrical nerve stimulation (TENS). Ultrasound utilizes high-frequency sound waves applied through a wand or probe to the skin to penetrate deep tissue and produce deep warmth, decreased tension, and increased blood flow. Nonthermal settings aim to help promote healing and reduce inflammation within the target muscle [5]. Ultrasound has been used on perineal episiotomy scars as well as extrapelvic muscles that may be contributing to increased pelvic floor tension. Studies have shown women receiving therapeutic ultrasound versus placebo for treatment of acute and persistent perineal pain are more likely to report improvement in symptoms; however, no statistically significant differences have been shown and further research is warranted [22]. TENS is a frequently used modality in the management of musculoskeletal pain and is gaining evidence for its use in the pelvic pain population. This noninvasive and nonpharmacological method of pain relief has also been successful in the treatment of dysmenorrhea, labor pain, and overactive pelvic floor disorders with various placements of electrodes including bracketing the lumbar and sacral spine, along pudendal nerve dermatomes, and in suprapubic areas [5, 23, 24].

Mind–Body Techniques

Many patients with pelvic pain resulting from pelvic floor muscle overactivity will note an increase in symptoms related to increasing stress levels. Women with chronic pelvic pain have been found to have higher levels of hypervigilance, catastrophizing, and anxiety [25]. A large aspect of pelvic floor muscle overactivity retraining is devoted to education about this connection to allow patients to become aware of how their mental states are affecting their physical states as well as teaching the patients tools and methods they can utilize to help manage this connection.

Relaxation techniques have been found to be beneficial in this patient population. Peters et al. report in a clinical cohort of 87 women with IC/BPS that 25% reported relief with the use of relaxation techniques alone [26]. There are various techniques that can be utilized in the therapeutic setting to assist in relaxation. Autogenic training focuses on the physical sensation the patient experiences including her breathing and heartbeat with other psychosomatic cues such a describing a feeling of warmth throughout the patient's body or into the painful area. Guided imagery is the use of storytelling or descriptions that may be calming or have a positive connotation for the patient to replace negative associations or images. Progressive relaxation has the patient focus on contracting and relaxing each muscle group, working in a pattern throughout the body and typically combined with guided imagery and breathing. The benefits of relaxation training in chronic pain include a decrease in pain intensity, anxiety, depression, and fatigue; an increase in balance, mobility, and coordination;

improved coping strategies; and a decrease in medication usage and healthcare costs [27, 28]. These techniques are often beneficial to utilize in conjunction with physical and hands-on techniques that are traditionally employed by physical therapists. It is important to note that collaboration and referral to trained psychologists and counselors is beneficial and often necessary to continue to help the patient develop various stress management strategies that will impact their pain.

Modifications to a patient's breathing mechanics are another crucial aspect to relaxation training with benefits not only for the nervous system but also on the biomechanical movement of the pelvic floor. Deep breathing has been shown to have a calming effect on the central nervous system, with various recommendations for specifics of inhale and exhale timing employed [29]. The respiratory diaphragm is also known to synchronize with the pelvic floor, and optimal diaphragm descent during inhale helps the pelvic floor to descend properly as well. This synchronization can be used to the patient's advantage throughout the day or during activities when increased pelvic floor tension is noted, as she can be taught to perform an optimal inhalation that includes diaphragmatic descent, lateral lower rib excursion, minimal movement into the upper chest, and excursion of the abdomen and, in turn, relaxation of the pelvic floor muscles [30, 31].

Interventions for Underactive Pelvic Floor Muscles

Although not typically the most common finding in patients with pelvic pain, there are instances in which pelvic floor muscle hypoactivity or weakness may be present and contributing to the dysfunction and impairments a patient is describing. As discussed in Chapter 5, pelvic floor muscles that are weak do not typically produce pain on palpation, have increased extensibility, and may be present with concurrent patient complaints or issues such as prolapse, pelvic girdle pain, and incontinence. Patients may also demonstrate a combination of pelvic floor overactivity as well as hypoactivity; for example, a postpartum patient may report pain with intercourse on initial penetration and urinary leakage that on assessment demonstrates pain and taut muscle tissue at the vaginal entrance and on deeper palpation increased extensibility without pain reproduction. A patient

presenting with these symptoms may be provided verbal instruction to perform Kegel or pelvic floor contraction exercises for a prescribed number of repetitions per day. On return to the clinic, this same patient, having been diligent about performing upwards of 50 pelvic floor contractions per day, will likely report increased pain in the pelvic floor and during intercourse. Patients such as in this example require an individualized treatment plan, likely involving first a decrease in the pelvic floor tension and a "downtraining" approach that can be progressed to pelvic floor strengthening once demonstration of improved pelvic floor awareness and ability to relax the pelvic floor has been shown.

As with any other musculoskeletal dysfunction or impairment throughout the rest of the body, muscular tone first needs to be normalized to then progress into stability and strengthening exercises so as not to exacerbate and flare symptoms. This is not different in the pelvic floor. Patients with pelvic floor overactivity will also require pelvic floor strengthening to create optimal stability through the pelvic girdle, synchronization and support during functional movements, and improvement or maintenance of pelvic floor function; however, it has to be timed appropriately within the rehabilitation journey once the patient is able to demonstrate proper awareness and controlled relaxation of her pelvic floor.

> The goal of rehabilitation of underactive floor muscles is to restore the activation capacity and build dynamic muscular ability by focusing not just on the strength of a single contraction but also the endurance, coordination, and quick response of the muscle in various positions and during various challenges.

Therapeutic Modalities/Devices

In opposition to downtraining of the pelvic floor muscles, uptraining is the focus when wanting to retrain or strengthen into the pelvic floor. This involves pelvic floor muscle contraction, commonly known as Kegels. Verbal instruction in the performance of a pelvic floor contraction is often not sufficient, with research showing more than 50% of women performing contractions incorrectly after verbal instruction alone and 25% actually straining when asked to contract, therefore likely worsening their symptoms [32]. Repeated verbal instruction in conjunction with internal palpation and SEMG biofeedback can help to assess the accuracy of movement within the pelvic floor to ensure the patient is performing the correct maneuver. Depending on the significance of weakness present or inability of the patient to contract the pelvic floor, training into synergistic muscles including the hip adductors, gluteals, and low abdominals may be warranted in the initial phases of training to help produce pelvic floor muscle movement. Voluntary activity of the abdominal muscles has been shown to result in increased pelvic floor muscle activity, and this can be used to the patient and therapist's advantage when starting an exercise program [33]. As the patient continues to progress with her strength, accessory use of the synergistic pelvic girdle muscles will be encouraged to decrease with the goal for the patient to be able to produce an isolated pelvic floor muscle contraction.

Pelvic floor muscle training has been shown to be more effective than training with vaginal weighted cones alone when focusing on increased pelvic floor muscle strength as well as reduced urinary leakage. Treatment with weighted cones typically consists of holding the cone for 15–20 minutes, which may result in decreased blood flow to the area and therefore decreased O_2 consumption, muscle fatigue, and pain, promoting possible recruitment of compensatory muscles such as the abdominals and gluteals instead of a true pelvic floor contraction. Using the vaginal weighted cones in conjunction with pelvic floor muscle training may be more beneficial if the patient is advised to contract the pelvic floor around the cones in various positions for a number of repetitions at intervals throughout the day [34].

Similar to promoting relaxation of the overactive pelvic floor in various positions and situations, it is important as part of the individualized treatment program developed between the patient and therapist to progress strengthening exercises within a functional context. Patients are not static; therefore static training of muscles is not functional and will not produce the intended benefits. After initial training of how to accurately contract the pelvic floor, the therapist will guide patients through a graded program taking into consideration the effects of gravity, postures, body mechanics, and movements required for performance and participation in patient-desired activities.

The addition of SEMG biofeedback to a pelvic floor training program has not been found to be overwhelmingly beneficial. A review by Herderschee et al. of 24 randomized controlled trials comparing pelvic floor muscle training with and without biofeedback concluded the use of SEMG biofeedback may provide additional benefit however most available studies currently have small sample sizes and the largest two randomized controlled trials showed no additional benefit [35]. Studies that demonstrate the most improvement related to short-term cure rates of symptoms in patient with pelvic floor muscle weakness report thorough individual instruction by a physical therapist, training with SEMG biofeedback or electrical stimulation and close follow-up every 1–2 weeks [36]. In women with stress urinary incontinence or mixed incontinence, most randomized controlled trials have failed to show an additional effect or benefit of SEMG biofeedback to the training protocol for stress incontinence [4]. However, the use of SEMG biofeedback may be a helpful adjunct to other therapeutic techniques to increase patient awareness of her pelvic floor during various assessment and strengthening activities.

Electrical stimulation is another modality that is traditionally used to supplement a typical musculoskeletal strengthening program; however, there have not been robust studies to demonstrate the efficacy of electrical stimulation for pelvic floor muscle strengthening, as many studies have small numbers and poor methodological quality. Electrical stimulation can be applied to the pelvic floor through external electrodes or internal devices with the goal to stimulate the motor fibers of the pudendal nerve and a contraction of the pelvic floor muscles. When comparing electrical stimulation to pelvic floor muscle training, voluntary pelvic floor muscle contraction increases urethral pressure significantly more than electrical stimulation[37]. Conclusive evidence is lacking; however, pelvic floor muscle training seems to be more effective than electrical stimulation in women with stress urinary incontinence and there does not seem to be an extra benefit with the addition of electrical stimulation to pelvic floor muscle training.

Interventions for Pelvic Floor Incoordination/Dyssynergia

Muscles within the pelvic floor can be found to have appropriate contraction and relaxation capacity; however, their coordination in relation to functional activities may be disrupted. This inability to contract or relax the pelvic floor muscles when this is required and desired is termed pelvic floor dyssynergia. The result of pelvic floor dyssynergia can be difficulty emptying bowel and bladder, constipation, incontinence, straining, and even back and pelvic girdle pain due to lack of synchronization.

> The goal in retraining the pelvic floor muscle incoordination/dyssynergia is to improve the timing and sequencing of reflexive and dynamic contraction and/or relaxation in conjunction with functional activities.

The pelvic floor has an anticipatory function that is responsive to initiation of movement and increased intraabdominal pressure. In the case of stress urinary incontinence, the issue can be that the pelvic floor is found to bulge or descend in response to the increased intraabdominal pressure that accompanies coughing and sneezing, allowing urine to leak versus the optimal and correct movement of elevation during these involuntary activities [38]. Studies have shown that teaching patients with stress incontinence when they are found to have weakness and/or incoordination of movement to perform a pelvic floor contraction prior to coughing resulted in an 82% reduction in the amount of urine lost. This movement of the pelvic floor inward in response to an anticipated sneeze or cough is termed the "knack" [5].

Education and training on proper motor control and coordination are essential when trying to increase the awareness of the pelvic floor for a patient. Focusing on the coordination requires teaching the patient the difference between contraction and relaxation through verbal and tactile cues as well as SEMG biofeedback if indicated. Use of SEMG biofeedback may again be a helpful tool as well as internal palpation to assess the movement of the pelvic floor during activities. With internal palpation, the therapist is able to have the patient perform a simulated cough and assess the movement of the pelvic floor. External SEMG biofeedback sensors can be used during simulated voiding as well to assess if positioning on the toilet or breathing mechanics can be helpful in relaxing the pelvic floor [6].

Patients with dyssynergia may report symptoms of urinary urgency and frequency due to an uncoordinated biofeedback loop between the pelvic floor and the bladder. Pelvic floor muscles may be hyperactive, causing increased pressure around the bladder at lower bladder volumes and signaling the need to urinate even without substantial filling to bladder capacity. Bladder urge suppression techniques such as pelvic floor muscle contraction have been found to be effective if the main cause is likely incoordination of these muscles due to a concomitant short-term reflex inhibition of the detrusor muscle [5].

Constipation may also be a common complaint of patients with incoordination of the pelvic floor and impaired feedback loop to the brain for proper initiation and emptying of the bowels. There can be numerous factors contributing to constipation including visceral and autoimmune dysfunctions such as in the case of IBS or Crohn's, changes or deficiencies in food or fluid intake, or faulty voiding habits. We will focus here on the contribution of the pelvic floor and bowel habits to promoting and/or maintaining constipation. Coordination of abdominal and pelvic floor muscles as well as control of the intraabdominal forces are paramount to successful defecation. Dyssernergic dysfunction can also be associated with impaired anorectal sensation [5]. If holding or guarding patterns within the pelvic floor have become habitual either due to a history of impaired defecation techniques even as early as childhood or due to pain with defecation, the process of complete defecation can be disrupted. Education on toileting posture, decreased straining, and breathing mechanics during elimination can be beneficial and provided by the clinician during a clinic visit and/or through referral to pelvic health physical therapy. The therapist can then also focus on the important aspect of pelvic floor relaxation to allow for proper elimination and decreased associated pain if this is present through training relaxation techniques during defecation, use of SEMG biofeedback during simulated elimination, and manual release techniques into the abdomen and/or pelvic floor vaginally or rectally.

Other Pelvic and Abdominal Myofascial Dysfunctions

Painful or Restricted Scar Tissue

Along with abdominal and pelvic pain due to muscular or skeletal dysfunctions, scar tissue restrictions need to also be evaluated and addressed to create a larger picture of the contributing factors to a patient's pain. Scar mobilization can be applied to visible scars such as after cesarean section or episiotomy. This technique involves application of moderate pressure to and around the area of the scar while encouraging mobility various directions through repetitive motions and sustained holds. The goal of scar mobilization is to address the haphazard organization of the tissue by stimulating the body's healing process to realign the scar tissue in directions that are more in line with the angles of tissue pull and stretch in and around the scar area. It is recommended to perform scar mobilization during physical therapy treatments until optimal fluidity returns without signs of adherence to underlying tissues [8]. Patients can also be taught to perform their own scar mobilization as part of a home exercise program. Ultrasound therapy targeted at perineal and episiotomy scars resulting in dyspareunia after vaginal delivery has also been noted to be successful [22].

Impaired Pelvic Girdle Form/Force Closure

As discussed in Chapter 5 previously, the focus during evaluation of patients with pelvic pain cannot be limited to a small scope of only the pelvic viscera or pelvic floor muscles. The pelvic girdle is a highly interconnected system that includes muscles, bones, ligaments, vessels, and viscera that can all contribute in various ways to the production, exacerbation, and continuation of a patient's pelvic pain. We discussed in Chapter 5, the importance of alignment and posture in the evaluation of pelvic pain, and although a detailed musculoskeletal evaluation and treatment plan of the lumbopelvic complex is outside of the scope of this book, we will discuss here the necessity and benefit to focusing treatment on pelvic girdle alignment in this patient population. The pelvic girdle provides stability through form and force closure mechanisms. Form closure is how a joint's structure and orientation contribute to its mobility and ability to resist movement or translation when loaded [2]. Force closure is defined as the extra forces that increase articular compression and thus friction between the joint surfaces and also the joint's stiffness. These "extra forces" can be applied to the joint through resting tone and co-contraction of muscles that cross the joint or through muscles that do not cross the joint by way of increased tension placed through the fascia that does cross the joint [39]. All joints have a variable amount of form closure and the joint's anatomy and capsular/ligamentous compliance will dictate how much additional compression or support (force closure) is needed to ensure that integrity of the system is maintained when loads are increased. Therefore, translation, or shear, of the joints of the lumbo–pelvic–hip complex are prevented by a combination of the structure of the joint (form closure) and the compression created by ligaments, muscles, and fascia (force closure) [2].

Pelvic health physical therapists must address impaired flexibility and strength asymmetries of extrapelvic girdle muscles (including all hip prime movers) attaching to and crossing the pelvis to improve the mechanical robustness of the system during daily demands. A treatment plan that includes an active stretching home program should be initiated when restriction in these muscles is found. Return of the pelvic girdle muscles to an optimal length–tension relationship is important to promote a more optimal alignment, with the most significant restrictions to proper length and tension found in the iliopsoas, straight abdominal muscles, and femoral adductors in women with chronic pelvic pain [40]. Therapeutic exercise including strengthening activities that are progressed through functional movement patterns should be targeted at pelvic girdle muscles that are found to be weak and contributing to faulty posturing and habits. These could include gluteals and hip muscles as well as abdominal and back muscles although initiation of strengthening should not be performed in muscles containing trigger points, myofascial restrictions, or hyperactivity. The focus should then be to first downtrain or improve extensibility of these tissues prior to proceeding to strengthening activities. Excessive or inappropriate activation of abdominals, low back, hip, and gluteal muscles would be assessed during functional movements, as this can impact the movement of the pelvic floor muscles. A postural assessment, testing for leg length discrepancy, as well as functional movement assessment during load transfer tests in various positions and during patient goal-oriented movements, would also be performed.

Abdominal Wall Muscle Dysfunction

Abdominal muscle strength, flexibility, coordination, and function are of supreme importance in the treatment of pelvic pain, as it is often impacted or contributing to continued pelvic pain symptoms. According to Sapsford et al., "pelvic floor rehabilitation does not reach its optimum level until the muscles of the abdominal wall are rehabilitated as well" [41].

Common abdominal dysfunctions seen in patients with pelvic pain include poor breathing patterns, myofascial restrictions and trigger points within the abdomen, nerve entrapments or dysfunctions, and diastasis recti abdominus.

Breathing mechanics are of particular consideration because of the interconnectedness between the pelvic floor and respiratory diaphragm. Respiratory dysfunctions have frequently been noted to occur in conjunction with pelvic floor and low back dysfunctions because of this interconnectedness [40]. During inhalation, there is an eccentric relaxation of the diaphragm and pelvic floor and during exhalation a concentric shortening of the diaphragm and pelvic floor muscles, with exhalation being largely passive. Optimally, movement should occur into the abdomen and rib cage during inhalation including anterior/posterior as well as lateral expansion; however, in patients with pelvic pain there has been found to be increased vertical movement of the rib cage and increased movement in general into the chest versus abdomen [40]. Rehabilitation of breathing mechanics would include decreased overuse of the abdominal obliques and rectus abdominis; activation and uptraining of the transversus abdominis to optimize efficiency and control of breath; and education and facilitation of proper rib cage, chest, and abdominal movement assessing for dysfunctions or connective tissue restrictions that may be impeding expansion and full recoil, as well as postural education and retraining to allow for optimal lung excursion.

Myofascial release can be utilized in treatment of the abdominal area. Depending on the patient's ability to tolerate treatment to this area, the therapist may decide to alter treatment strategies by opting for an indirect vs direct approach to facilitate and improve movement. Direct techniques consist of applying the manual technique into the direction of the restriction, taking the tissue being manipulated into a maximal stretch or end range of motion position, whereas indirect techniques reduce the stretch on the tissue initially. Indirect techniques are typically seen as less painful or exacerbating for the patient and may be more appropriate for patients experiencing acute flares of pain or during initial stages of treatment with the goal being to progress and improve tolerance for direct techniques.

Entrapment or irritation of nerves as they course through the abdomen and innervate the abdominal wall can also lead to pain in the abdomen as well as into the pelvic girdle. Myofascial release as described earlier can be an aspect of treatment to help address any restrictions associated with the nerve irritation. Nerve mobilizations are also a targeted treatment to address the gliding and movement of the nerve as it travels through an area, thus improving axonal transportation and nerve conduction velocity. Neural mobilization is performed through manual techniques with the goal to restore dysfunctional neurodynamics through improving the mobility of the nerve as it travels through or near various structures, decreasing the pressure and irritation on the nerve. Treatment targeted at nerve mobility is indicated if there are signs of increased resistance of tissues surrounding the nerve and/or reproduction of symptoms with nerve mobility [6]. Improved mobility of the nerve is then reinforced through concomitant assessment and promotion of optimal postural and movement patterns to prevent habitual shortening and constriction.

Diastasis rectus abdominis (DRA) is another abdominal muscle and fascial dysfunction that can be seen in the pelvic pain population and is characterized by an abdominal wall separation at the linea alba between the rectus abdominus muscle bellies. Although not typically associated with overactive patients with pelvic floor pain, diastasis can be noted in conjunction with a wide variety of pelvic complaints including incontinence, dyspareunia, pelvic girdle pain, and incoordination and/or overactivity of the pelvic floor.

Upon palpation of the linea alba on a curl up/crunch, if DRA is suspected, a referral to physical therapy would be appropriate to further determine the impact the DRA is having on overall patient function and symptoms as well as to initiate a rehabilitation program. Physical therapy has been demonstrated to be an effective management approach for patients with DRA that may include manual release to myofascial trigger points if restriction is noted to movement, electrical stimulation, therapeutic exercise, breathing and postural retraining, and use of abdominal binders with the goal to wean off of these as strength and control develops all within the context of functional and patient goal-oriented movements and tasks. Some research is finding training of the transversus abdominis and movement patterns in prenatal patient's shows decreased incidence of DRA postnatal [42]. However, there are not studies to show the best rehabilitation approach to

DRA. The goal of DRA rehabilitation has shifted due to literature supporting the space between the rectus muscle bellies is less important than the ability to generate tension through the fascia connecting the muscles, which can provide stability in the spine and pelvis despite a continued DRA or actual separation [43].

Patient Education and Lifestyle Changes in Pelvic Health Physical Therapy

The foregoing information and description of treatments for pelvic pain and dysfunction are meant primarily to help the clinician understand the various evidence-based options to help this patient population, understanding that is it likely not within the scope of practice, nor is it possible within the limited timeframe provided, for clinicians to perform or progress the various conservative treatment modalities. The foregoing information can be helpful knowledge to the clinician when the decision is made to refer the patient for treatment with another clinician such as a pelvic health physical therapist, as the patient will likely want information regarding what to expect from such a referral. The largest aspect in the initiation of treatment that the clinician does participate in, other than surgical and intervention techniques obviously, is education. There are numerous education topics that the clinician can provide regarding anatomy of the pelvic floor and pelvic girdle, diagnosis, and interrelated symptoms as well as modifiable lifestyle choices and habits that can impact the success of the clinician-driven treatment plan.

There are many lifestyle modifications that the patient may be educated about because of their impact and relationship to pelvic floor dysfunction. Obesity has been shown to have a multitude of impacts on the patient's health and well-being, and in regard to pelvic floor dysfunction, has been shown to have an impact on urinary incontinence. A systematic review performed by Hunskaar found evidence to support waist–hip ratio and thus abdominal obesity may be independent risk factors for incontinence and that moderate weight loss should be seen as an adequate first-line therapy for urinary incontinence in women [44]. Women may be hesitant to initiate physical activity in the form of exercise if recommended to do so for fear that it may impact or worsen their incontinence. Studies have also found that in terms

of modifiable risk factors, exercise in the form of physical activity is negatively correlated with dysmenorrhea [45].

Smoking cessation is another common educational topic discussed with patients in relation to their pain as well as other symptoms. A systematic review found no studies to demonstrate that smoking cessation resolves or reduces urinary incontinence although urinary urgency and frequency have been shown to be up to three times more common among current than never smokers and this association seems to be a dose–response relationship. Current data suggest that smoking increases the risk of more severe urinary incontinence [46].

Dietary factors have shown to play a role in pelvic floor symptoms through their impact on the bladder and/or bowel. Avoiding bladder irritants has been a typical recommendation to patients, particularly those reporting symptoms consistent with IC/BPS or functional complaints of urinary frequency and urgency. Studies on counseling to reduce caffeine are more impactful in conditions with urge, not stress, primary incontinence symptoms. Fluid intake has not been supported by research as a method to help improve urinary incontinence due to the minor impact decreased fluid intake would have compared to the risk of limited intake including dehydration, urinary tract infections and constipation [4, 47]. Dietary changes have also been found to impact the incidence of stress urinary incontinence (SUI), with studies demonstrating the incidence of SUI is increased in women who consumed more total fat, saturated fatty acids, and monosaturated fatty acids as well as increased carbonated beverages, zinc, or B12. This was compared to the reduced incidence of SUI in women who ate more vegetables and chicken at baseline. A high intake of vitamin D, protein, and potassium has also been associated with decreased onset of overactive bladder in women [4, 47].

Education on bowel and bladder habits can also be initiated during clinic visits and can be invaluable information to patients with constipation and/or voiding difficulties associated with their chronic pain symptoms. Associations have been shown between constipation and urinary incontinence likely due to the chronic straining required for evacuation and associated pelvic floor dysfunction. Medical relief of constipation has been shown to significantly reduce lower urinary tract symptoms in the elderly although there has been no evidence to show that interventions targeted as reducing constipation in incontinent patients decreases urinary incontinence [48]. Education about bowel care including positioning with the knees elevated while on the toilet to decrease the anorectal angle, avoidance of straining, slight bulging of the pelvic floor on inhalation to encourage emptying, and consistency in meal amounts and times and other dietary changes can be beneficial information to this patient population.

In patients with chronic pelvic pain, instructions in pacing themselves to learn how to operate in the "safe zone" helps them to gain confidence in their body again, and not overdo their capability until they have built up the capacity with aerobic endurance, strength, neuromotor resilience, and reduced fear of movement.

Education provided by the clinician can help to initiate the treatment process for the patient; however, simply telling the patient about her condition and contributing behaviors is likely insufficient to motivate patients toward changing these behaviors. Various behavior modification theories and strategies have been studied and some consistencies are present. It is important when educating patients to individualize and personalize the information, focusing on how the change could impact the goals and activities they feel they are not currently able to tolerate or perform. Asking the patient about her belief in her ability to make the changes being asked and the feasibility of implementing the changes is also important. The clinician must understand what the patient perceives as "normal" in terms of her behaviors which will be influenced by her social group, with clinicians helping to modify misperceptions through evidence-based information. The clinician must stay aware that a patient's progress toward change will not be linear and she will move forward and backward along a continuum that will likely be affected by changes in her beliefs, perceptions of the impact of the changes, and input from her social circles and environment.

A patient's readiness and decision to change will shift forward and backward with time, and this is one of the main reasons advice-giving has limited effectiveness. Patients will accept advice and act upon it only when they are ready. The ambivalence toward behavioral changes can be met with motivational interviewing techniques that allow for reflective listening and open-ended questioning. This style offers the opportunity to build rapport with the patient, understanding her perceived importance of the behavior change, providing information if necessary, and exploring her level of perceived self-efficacy to make a change [49].

Concurrent Medical Interventions with Musculoskeletal Impairments

Patients may present with muscle dysfunction or joint or connective tissue conditions and even with appropriate physical therapy their current state may warrant additional supportive medical treatments.

Often patients who have long history of pelvic pain from muscle spasm may trial oral or local antispasmodics to reduce the muscle tension generated at rest that may also be too great to start to reduce with the correct physical therapy interventions. This pharmacological option may create a break in the spasm cycle that allows for progress to normalization of muscle tone and balance to be gained. In addition, if there is progress made but it is temporary, it may be beneficial to do a local trigger point injection (TPI) with analgesics to evaluate the effect on the local muscle immediately after to see if it was helpful to reset the muscle bias and continue to improve the muscle group relaxation with physical therapy techniques. For longer lasting effects, some physicians use steroid in the TPI, or they can opt to use Botox injections and send the patient back to pelvic health physical therapist to keep working on balancing the muscular system centrally and locally.

Another common pharmacological aid is the use of topical analgesic ointment, cream, or gel. This can improve the tolerance for palpation, release, and stretch and progressive desensitization of the vaginal introitus. At times it is valuable for initiating the mobility and flexibility back in an area that has been hypersensitive and presents with reactive muscle spasm and guarding.

Pelvic health physical therapists also count on their medical counterparts to adequately assess and manage the patient's hormonal status, as imbalance of estrogen or testosterone can set up painful mucosal conditions that impact function of the perineal and pelvic floor.

All pharmacological adjuncts must be screened for allergy, interaction, and appropriateness through the patients referring provider. Pelvic health physical therapists can report response or adverse reactions if noted on their visits.

Conclusion

Pelvic health physical therapists have a wide range of interventions that have been demonstrated as highly effective and low risk in addressing the primary muscle, joint, and soft tissue dysfunctions associated with pelvic pain conditions.

Encouraging patients to seek treatment early and establish goals and a treatment plan with a trained pelvic health physical therapist is valuable in their recovery and rehabilitation to help restore their function and minimize their disability.

Five Things You Need to Know

- To help effectively treat a patient's pelvic pain complaints, it is imperative to identify the primary driver of the painful condition whenever possible, recognizing it may not be a painful tissue or organ system but in fact dysfunctional or maladaptive biomechanics that over time lead to somatic manifestations.
- Referral and collaboration with various providers can be beneficial and often necessary to successfully treat multifaceted pain syndromes, including chronic pelvic pain. One such provider group that is integral in the plan of care development and treatment of chronic pelvic pain are pelvic health physical therapists who are experts in the evaluation of the musculoskeletal system and how it relates to other bodily systems and ultimately causes or perpetuates pelvic pain.
- Pelvic health physical therapy techniques can be applied to treat various pelvic floor issues. This includes manual treatments to target painful or dysfunctional tissues contributing to overactive pelvic floor muscles and pelvic floor muscle training for patients with underactive pelvic floor muscles. Neuromuscular reeducation and training should be provided for patients with pelvic floor dyssynergies, as well as optimization of breathing mechanics to benefit abdominal dysfunctions and pelvic girdle instabilities that might contribute or occur in conjunction with pelvic floor issues.
- Clinicians can intervene in a number of ways other than through their surgical techniques, and this includes thorough education about modifiable risk factors and optimal bowel/bladder habits that could be contributing to the patient's pelvic floor dysfunction.
- Adjunctive medical interventions can be valuable to help the patient with pelvic pain tolerate pelvic floor physical therapy in very acute stages or

hypersensitive situations and/or help continue progress the patient has made. This is often a two-way street, with medical interventions and pelvic health physical therapy helping to potentiate the effects of the other.

References

1. Haynes RB, Sackett DL, Gray JM, Cook DJ, Guyatt GH. Transferring evidence from research into practice: 1. The role of clinical care research evidence in clinical decisions. *ACP J Club*. 1996;**125**(3):A14–16.
2. Lee D, Lee, L-J. *The Pelvic Girdle*. Edinburgh: Elsevier; 2011.
3. Faubion SS, Shuster LT, Bharucha AE. Recognition and management of nonrelaxing pelvic floor dysfunction. Paper presented at Mayo Clinic Proceedings2012.
4. Bo K, Berghmans B, Morkved S, Van Kampen M. *Evidence-Based Physical Therapy for the Pelvic Floor: Bridging Science and Clinical Practice*. Philadelphia: Elsevier Health Sciences; 2014.
5. Irion JM, Irion G. *Women's Health in Physical Therapy*. Philadelphia: Lippincott Williams & Wilkins; 2010.
6. Padoa A, Rosenbaum TY. *The Overactive Pelvic Floor*. Cham, Switzerland: Springer; 2016.
7. Weiss JM. Pelvic floor myofascial trigger points: manual therapy for interstitial cystitis and the urgency-frequency syndrome. *J Urol*. 2001;**166**(6):2226–31.
8. FitzGerald MP, Kotarinos R. Rehabilitation of the short pelvic floor. II: Treatment of the patient with the short pelvic floor. *Int Urogynecol J Pelvic Floor Dysfunct*. 2003;**14**(4):269–75; discussion 275.
9. FitzGerald MP, Anderson RU, Potts J, et al. Randomized multicenter feasibility trial of myofascial physical therapy for the treatment of urological chronic pelvic pain syndromes. *J Urol*. 2009;**182**:570–80.
10. FitzGerald MP, Payne CK, Lukacz ES, et al. Randomized multicenter clinical trial of myofascial physical therapy in women with interstitial cystitis/painful bladder syndrome and pelvic floor tenderness. *J Urol*. 2012;**187**(6):2113–18.
11. Oyama IA, Rejba A, Lukban JC, et al. Modified Thiele massage as therapeutic intervention for female patients with interstitial cystitis and high-tone pelvic floor dysfunction. *Urology*. 2004;**64**(5):862–5.
12. Pastore EA, Katzman WB. Recognizing myofascial pelvic pain in the female patient with chronic pelvic pain. *J Obstet Gynecol Neonatal Nurs*. 2012;**41**(5):680–91.

13. Barnes JF. *Myofascial Release: The "Missing Link" in Your Treatment*. Norfolk, VA: Rehabilitation Services; 1995.

14. Laan EvL RHW. Overactive pelvic floor: Sexual functioning. In Padoa A, Rosenbaum TY (eds), *The Overactive Pelvic Floor* (pp. 17–29). Cham, Switzerland: Springer; 2016.

15. Barral J-P, Mercier P. *Manipulations viscérales*, Vol. 1. Paris: Elsevier Masson; 2004.

16. Goats GC, Keir KA. Connective tissue massage. *Br J Sports Med*. 1991;**25**(3):131–133.

17. Jones LH, Kusunose R, Goering E. *Jones Strain-Counterstrain*. Boise, ID: Jones Strain Counterstrain Incorporated; 1995.

18. Huffman LB, Hartenbach EM, Carter J, Rash JK, Kushner DM. Maintaining sexual health throughout gynecologic cancer survivorship: a comprehensive review and clinical guide. *Gynecol Oncol*. 2016;**140**(2):359–68.

19. Murina F, Bernorio R, Palmiotto R. The use of Amielle vaginal trainers as adjuvant in the treatment of vestibulodynia: an observational multicentric study. *Medscape J Med*. 2008;**10**(1):23.

20. Sorensen J, Bautista KE, Lamvu G, Feranec J. Evaluation and treatment of female sexual pain: a clinical review. *Cureus*. 2018;**10**(3):e2379.

21. Glazer HI, Rodke G, Swencionis C, Hertz R, Young AW. Treatment of vulvar vestibulitis syndrome with electromyographic biofeedback of pelvic floor musculature. *Obstet Gynecol Surv*. 1995;**50**(9):658–9.

22. Hay-Smith J. Therapeutic ultrasound for postpartum perineal pain and dyspareunia. *Cochrane Database Syst Rev*. 1998;(**3**).

23. Murina F, Bianco V, Radici G, Felice R, Di Martino M, Nicolini U. Transcutaneous electrical nerve stimulation to treat vestibulodynia: a randomised controlled trial. *BJOG*. 2008;**115**(9):1165–70.

24. Waldinger MD, de Lint GJ, Venema PL, van Gils AP, Schweitzer DH. Successful transcutaneous electrical nerve stimulation in two women with restless genital syndrome: the role of adelta- and C-nerve fibers. *J Sex Med*. 2010;**7**(3):1190–9.

25. Alappattu MJ, Bishop MD. Psychological factors in chronic pelvic pain in women: relevance and application of the fear-avoidance model of pain. *Physical Therapy*. 2011;**91**(10):1542–50.

26. Peters KM, Carrico DJ, Diokno AC. Characterization of a clinical cohort of 87 women with interstitial cystitis/painful bladder syndrome. *Urology*. 2008;**71**(4):634–40.

27. Persson AL, Veenhuizen H, Zachrison L, Gard G. Relaxation as treatment for chronic musculoskeletal pain: a systematic review of randomised controlled studies. *Phys Ther Rev*. 2008;**13**(5):355–65.

28. Bertisch SM, Wee CC, Phillips RS, McCarthy EP. Alternative mind–body therapies used by adults with medical conditions. *J Psychosom Research*. 2009;**66**(6):511–19.

29. Conrad A, Muller A, Doberenz S, et al. Psychophysiological effects of breathing instructions for stress management. *Appl Psychophysiol Biofeedback*. 2007;**32**(2):89–98.

30. Hodges PW, Sapsford R, Pengel LH. Postural and respiratory functions of the pelvic floor muscles. *Neurourol Urodyn*. 2007;**26**(3):362–71.

31. Talasz H, Kremser C, Kofler M, Kalchschmid E, Lechleitner M, Rudisch A. Phase-locked parallel movement of diaphragm and pelvic floor during breathing and coughing: a dynamic MRI investigation in healthy females. *Int Urogynecol J*. 2011;**22**(1):61–8.

32. Bump RC, Hurt WG, Fantl JA, Wyman JF. Assessment of Kegel pelvic muscle exercise performance after brief verbal instruction. *Am J Obstet Gynecol*. 1991;**165**(2):322–7; discussion 327–9.

33. Neumann P, Gill V. Pelvic floor and abdominal muscle interaction: EMG activity and intra-abdominal pressure. *Int Urogynecol J Pelvic Floor Dysfunct*. 2002;**13**(2):125–32.

34. Bo K, Talseth T, Holme I. Single blind, randomised controlled trial of pelvic floor exercises, electrical stimulation, vaginal cones, and no treatment in management of genuine stress incontinence in women. *BMJ*. 1999;**318**(7182):487–93.

35. Herderschee R, Hay-Smith EJ, Herbison GP, Roovers JP, Heineman MJ. Feedback or biofeedback to augment pelvic floor muscle training for urinary incontinence in women. *Cochrane Database Syst Rev*. 2011(7):CD009252.

36. Dumoulin C, Lemieux MC, Bourbonnais D, Gravel D, Bravo G, Morin M. Physiotherapy for persistent postnatal stress urinary incontinence: a randomized controlled trial. *Obstet Gynecol*. 2004;**104**(3):504–10.

37. Bo K, Talseth T. Change in urethral pressure during voluntary pelvic floor muscle contraction and vaginal electrical stimulation. *Int Urogynecol J Pelvic Floor Dysfunct*. 1997;**8**(1):3–6; discussion 6–7.

38. Sapsford RR, Hodges PW. Contraction of the pelvic floor muscles during abdominal maneuvers. *Arch Phys Med Rehabil*. 2001;**82**(8):1081–8.

39. Vleeming A, Stoeckart R, Volkers A, Snijders C. Relation between form and function in the sacroiliac

221

joint. Part I: Clinical anatomical aspects. *Spine.* 1990;**15**(2):130.

40. Haugstad GK, Haugstad TS, Kirste UM, et al. Posture, movement patterns, and body awareness in women with chronic pelvic pain. *J Psychosom Res.* 2006;**61** (5):637–44.

41. Sapsford RR, Hodges PW, Richardson CA, Cooper DH, Markwell SJ, Jull GA. Co-activation of the abdominal and pelvic floor muscles during voluntary exercises. *Neurourol Urodyn.* 2001;**20** (1):31–42.

42. Collie M, Harris B. Physical therapy treatment for diastasis recti: a case report. *J Sect Women's Health.* 2004;**28**:11–15.

43. Spitznagle TM, Leong FC, Van Dillen LR. Prevalence of diastasis recti abdominis in a urogynecological patient population. *Int Urogynecol J.* 2007;**18** (3):321–8.

44. Hunskaar S. A systematic review of overweight and obesity as risk factors and targets for clinical intervention for urinary incontinence in women. *Neurourol Urodyn.*2008;**27**(8):749–57.

45. Latthe P, Mignini L, Gray R, Hills R, Khan K. Factors predisposing women to chronic pelvic pain: systematic review. *BMJ.* 2006;**332**(7544):749–55.

46. Maserejian NN, Kupelian V, Miyasato G, McVary KT, McKinlay JB. Are physical activity, smoking and alcohol consumption associated with lower urinary tract symptoms in men or women? Results from a population based observational study. *J Urol.* 2012;**188**(2):490–5.

47. Abrams P, Andersson K-E, Birder L, et al. Fourth International Consultation on Incontinence Recommendations of the International Scientific Committee: evaluation and treatment of urinary incontinence, pelvic organ prolapse, and fecal incontinence. *Neurourol Urodyn.* 2010;**29**(1):213–40.

48. Charach G, Greenstein A, Rabinovich P, Groskopf I, Weintraub M. Alleviating constipation in the elderly improves lower urinary tract symptoms. *Gerontology.* 2001;**47**(2):72–6.

49. Emmons KM, Rollnick S. Motivational interviewing in health care settings: opportunities and limitations. *Am J Prev Med.* 2001;**20**(1):68–74.

Chapter 21

If Everything Else Fails

Michael Hibner and Elizabeth Banks

Editor's Introduction

Pelvic pain is one of the most difficult human conditions to diagnose and treat. The pelvis is composed of a complicated network of somatic and visceral nerves; connective tissues; as well as reproductive, urinary, and gastrointestinal organs. Pain in the pelvis can thus be from any of these areas. In order to diagnose and treat patient correctly it is very important to have a knowledge of all nongynecologic and gynecologic conditions leading to pelvic pain. Despite this knowledge, diagnosis may still be very difficult. Very often reexamining history and medical records may be helpful. In many patients pelvic floor is a main contributing factor to the pelvic pain.

The pelvis has multiple functions such as providing support to the upper body, locomotion, evacuation of waste, childbirth, and sexual pleasure (from stimulation of both external and deep structures). The nerves innervating the pelvis and lower extremity often originate in the same segments of the spinal cord, such as in the case of pudendal and sciatic nerves; thus, by the mechanism of crosstalk, pain originating in one nerve may subsequently lead to pain in a neighboring nerve Additionally, muscles of the lower back and anterior and posterior thighs attach to the pelvis and often become affected themselves in patients with pelvic pain.

Coexistence and opposing functions (such as continence and evacuation) of the pelvic organs often make the diagnosis and treatment of pelvic pain difficult. For instance, patients often complain of pain related to their bladder; however, there is a big difference if pain is at the beginning of urination, during urination, or at the end. Each one of these is caused by a different condition.

Unlike in other parts of the body, coexistence of pain conditions in the pelvis is well described. In the mechanism of viscerosomatic convergence when a patient has a visceral source of pelvic pain, such as endometriosis implants on the pelvic organs, the surrounding muscles may become spastic and tender as the painful stimulus from the visceral organ travels. This is demonstrated by the high incidence of pelvic floor dysfunction and muscle spasm in women with endometriosis. In a similar vein, via the mechanism of viscerovisceral convergence, patients with one source of visceral pain may develop pain in another visceral organ, as seen in women with endometriosis and other coexisting pain syndromes such as interstitial cystitis/bladder pain syndrome (IC/BPS) or irritable bowel syndrome (IBS).

Another difficulty in treating pelvic pain is that there is no single medical specialty that routinely treats the condition. The majority of women with chronic pelvic pain see their primary gynecologist as the first provider for their complaint. Unfortunately, specialists in general obstetrics and gynecology receive minimal education in residency regarding pelvic pain. Thus, the majority of general gynecologists are most comfortable with medical management and simple surgery for endometriosis. Some may attempt to treat IC/BPS, but most rarely treat lesser known but common conditions such as pelvic floor dysfunction, intraabdominal adhesions, or pelvic congestion syndrome. Urologists are well trained to treat IC/BPS but very rarely address any other pain-causing conditions. Other physicians such as gastroenterologists, neurologists, general surgeons, and orthopedists rarely address pelvic pain at all. Physiatrists (physical medicine and rehabilitation physicians) and pelvic floor physical therapists with special training in the pelvic floor may in fact be the best equipped to address the needs of pelvic pain patients, as pelvic floor muscle spasm is the main cause of pain for the majority of these patients.

Despite best efforts, it has been shown that approximately 60% of women with chronic pelvic pain seen in a general Obstetrics and Gynecology practice do not receive a proper diagnosis and therefore cannot get proper treatment [1]. This percentage is possibly less for patients seen in a specialized pelvic pain practice or in a multidisciplinary practice; however, this number is unknown. Unfortunately, there are still some patients who will not receive the correct diagnosis even when seen at the most specialized practices. This chapter aims to provide guidance and suggestions on how to proceed when this occurs. In these cases, there is little scientific evidence on how to proceed and many statements in this chapter are from very extensive personal experience treating many patients with pelvic pain over several years.

Multiple Sources of Pain

Most patients with chronic pelvic pain have multiple sources of pain [2]. There are frequently coexisting conditions such as endometriosis with IC/BPS, IBS, and spastic pelvic floor syndrome or pudendal nerve injury with spastic pelvic floor syndrome. Ideally all sources of pain should be identified and treated in order to improve a patient's pain. If all coexisting conditions are not addressed the patient will not be helped.

Think Pelvic Floor

The majority of physicians who see women for pelvic pain (gynecologists, urologists, gastroenterologists) are not familiar with pelvic floor muscle spasm, which is often a source or a contributing factor to pelvic pain [3]. Often patients with chronic pelvic pain undergo multiple laparoscopies and even hysterectomy, but their pain persists. More often than not they have spasm of the levator ani, obturator internus, and superficial pelvic muscles that is unrecognized and thus has never been addressed. Unfortunately, physicians don't know what questions to ask, nor are

Table 21.1 Causes of pelvic floor muscle spasm

Causes of pelvic floor muscle spasm	Possible mechanism
Endometriosis	Viscerosomatic conversion. Visceral organs with implants of endometriosis are innervated through the same segment of the spinal cord as the pelvic muscles. If the viscera is irritated, the pelvic muscle may develop a spasm in response.
Pelvic trauma/surgery/ mesh implantation	Direct trauma and irritation of the muscles.
Sexual and psychological trauma	Protective mechanism against penetration/rape.

Table 21.1 (cont.)

Causes of pelvic floor muscle spasm	Possible mechanism
Laxity of pelvic ligaments/joints	Increased laxity of pelvic joints may lead to overactivity and spasm of pelvic muscles to stabilize the joint.
Physical activity	Certain physical activity (gymnastics, ballet) may lead to overgrowth and increased tone of pelvic floor muscles.
Nerve compression	Nerve compression leads to significant pain that then causes reflex muscle spasm in the area close to the injured nerve (somatosomatic reflex).
Unknown	Possible genetic or anatomical predisposition to muscle spasm

Table 21.2 Symptoms indicative of pelvic floor muscle spasm

Symptom	Comment
Urinary hesitancy	Possibly the most sensitive symptom. Women without muscle spasm should be able to urinate immediately after sitting down on the toilet. Any delay is abnormal. Pelvic floor muscle spasm puts pressure around the urethra, causing hesitancy. This also explains why some patients have difficulty emptying their bladder after pelvic surgery. In extreme cases patients may have to self-catheterize.
Constipation	In a mechanism similar to urinary hesitancy, patients with pelvic floor muscle spasm often develop constipation. Patients will often complain of thin pencil-shaped stool. In some cases patients may also complain of severe bloating. This may be due to difficulty in passing gas.
Pain after intercourse	The majority of patients with pelvic pain have pain with intercourse. Patients with pelvic floor muscle spasm also have pain after intercourse. Some patients will complain of pain after intercourse lasting for 1–2 days.
Pain with physical activity	Patients with pelvic floor muscle spasm often have more pain after physical activity.

Table 21.2 (cont.)

Symptom	Comment
Increased pain in the evening (at the end of the day)	Patients with pelvic floor muscle spasm usually have less pain when they wake up and pain increases as the day goes by.
Pain improved with heating pad	Pain improved with the application of heat is almost always indicative of pelvic floor muscle spasm.

they taught to properly examine for pelvic floor muscle spasm. If there is any doubt if the patient has pelvic floor muscle spasm she should be referred to a pelvic floor physical therapist.

Repeat History

The most important component of diagnosis and evaluation of chronic pelvic pain is the history (Figure 21.1).

Questions regarding the events that lead to the onset of pain are central to the diagnosis. Often, at the patient's initial visit, when the history is taken for the first time, she may not remember all the events leading up to the start of her pain (Figure 21.2). Thus, it may be very beneficial to retake the history from the very beginning. Patients who complain of pain since menarche are more likely to have endometriosis. On the other hand, if their pain started with pregnancy, delivery, surgery, athletic activity, or trauma they most likely have another etiology causing their pain. Many patients with complex pain conditions have several reasons to have pain, and it is very important to identify all the sources of pain. Often pain from different sources may begin at different chronological points; thus obtaining a detailed history with a precise timeline is crucial. For example, pain caused by endometriosis, which often starts with onset of menstrual periods, with time may become related to physical and sexual activity. This usually signifies involvement of pelvic floor muscles. As time progresses

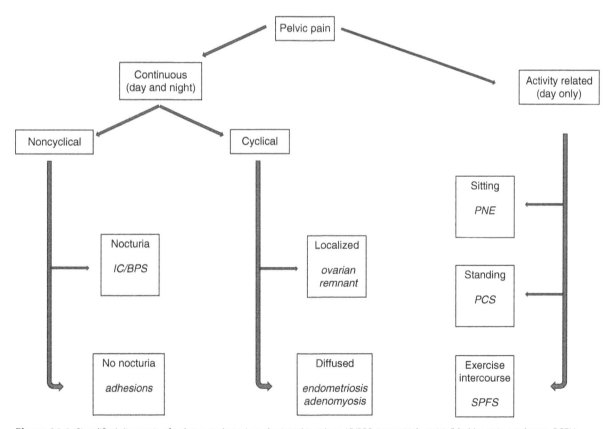

Figure 21.1 Simplified diagnosis of pelvic pain based on the initial incident. IC/BPS, interstitial cystitis/bladder pain syndrome; PCFN, posterior cutaneous femoral nerve; PCS, pelvic congestion syndrome; PFTM, pelvic floor tension myalgia; PNE, pudendal nerve entrapment.

Table 21.3 Review of patient's history

Onset of pain	Pain beginning with menarche – endometriosis Pain after pelvic trauma, surgery, vaginal delivery – musculoskeletal/nerve pain Pain after pregnancy – pelvic congestion Pain after abdominal/pelvic surgery – adhesions
Location	Localized pain – nerve pain, ovarian remnant Diffuse pain – muscular pain, visceral pain, endometriosis
Aggravating factors	Physical activity – musculoskeletal/nerve pain, adhesions Upright position – pelvic congestion syndrome Pain with sitting – pudendal neuralgia Pain with full bladder – IC/BPS Pain at the end of urination/bowel movement – pelvic floor muscle spasm Pain worse in the evening – musculoskeletal pain, pelvic congestion syndrome Pain at night when turning in bed – adhesions Pain with menstrual periods – endometriosis, adenomyosis Pain with ovulation – mittelschmerz, ovarian entrapment/remnant
Alleviating factors	Pain decreased with heating pad – musculoskeletal pain Pain decreased after urination – interstitial cystitis
Sexual symptoms	Pain during intercourse – any pelvic pain condition Pain lasting after intercourse – pelvic floor muscle spasm, pelvic congestion syndrome Pain with sexual arousal without penetration – pudendal neuralgia, pelvic congestion syndrome Persistent sexual arousal – pudendal neuralgia Pain with intercourse in quadripedic ("doggy") position – IC/BPS
Urinary symptoms	Urinary hesitancy – pelvic floor muscle spasm Nocturia – IC/BPS Pain with full bladder – IC/BPS Pain at the end of urination – pelvic floor muscle spasm

IC/BPS, interstitial cystitis/bladder pain syndrome.

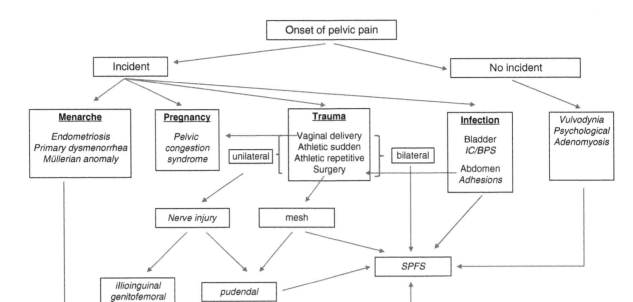

Figure 21.2 Simplified diagnosis of pelvic pain based on the nature of pain and additional symptoms. Abbreviations as for Figure 21.1.

the bladder may become affected and patients may begin complaining of nocturia and pain with a full bladder. In addition to taking a repeat history from the patient it is sometimes very helpful, with the patient's permission, to talk to family members, especially parents or partners. People close to the patient may notice patterns that the patient herself may be unaware of. Another good technique, especially if the patient is referred from another physician, is to "start clean." It may be more helpful to first obtain a full history directly from the patient before reviewing notes from another provider. This may allow the clinician a broader perspective and may prevent the clinician from coming to the same conclusion as prior providers.

Determine if Pain Is Somatic or Visceral

If the etiology of the pain cannot be determined, it may be helpful to determine if pain is somatic or visceral. This may help later on to narrow down the pain to a specific location.

Pelvic pain may be nociceptive somatic, nociceptive visceral, or peripheral neuropathic. Often if pain has persisted for a long period of time through previously described mechanisms of viscerosomatic and viscerovisceral convergence, patients may have a mix of all of the above.

Reexamine Medical Records

Pelvic pain patients are usually seen by many providers before being seen by a pelvic pain specialist.

In the process of working up their pain condition patients often undergo multiple tests, consultations, and procedures. Often, at the time of the first visit, patients will provide hundreds of pages of records from other providers and it is almost impossible to review those records in the allocated time for their visit. It is thus important to choose which records should be reviewed first, and those that may need to be reviewed at a later time.

Operative Reports

In patients in whom pain began after a surgical procedure the most important record to review is the report of that surgery or surgeries. It is crucial to determine what was the indication for the procedure, if there was any pain present prior to the procedure, and if the pain that patient has now is the same pain but worse or if this this a new onset of pain. Additionally, it is important to note how the patient was positioned for surgery and if there's any possibility of compression of the pelvic nerves from positioning. Location of the incision(s) should also be determined to assess the possibility of injury to the abdominal wall nerves secondary to the surgical incision(s). This may be especially important in laparoscopic surgery, since incisions are placed close to the anterior superior iliac spine and consequently may injure the iliohypogastric or ilioinguinal nerve. In open abdominal or vaginal surgery it is important to determine which retractors were used, where the

Table 21.4 Types of pain

	Nociceptive somatic	Nociceptive visceral	Peripheral neuropathic
Location	Localized	Diffuse	Radiating
Characteristics	Pinprick, stabbing, sharp	Ache, pressure or sharp	Burning, shooting, tingling, numb, electric shock-like, or lancing
Mechanism	A-delta fiber located in the periphery	C fiber	Dermatomal innervation
Examples of medical treatment	Opioids and NSAIDs	Opioids and NSAIDs	Antidepressants, anticonvulsants, local anesthetics
Examples of surgical treatment	Trigger point injections	Resection of endometriosis, adhesiolysis	Neurolysis neurectomy
Examples in the pelvis	Spastic pelvic floor syndrome	Endometriosis, IC/BPS, IBS, abdominal/pelvic adhesions	Pudendal nerve entrapment

IBS, irritable bowel syndrome; IC/BPS, interstitial cystitis/bladder pain syndrome; NSAIDs, nonsteroidal antiinflammatory drugs.

blades were positioned, and how deeply they were placed. Equally important is the physical exam. The purpose of the exam is to determine which structures may have possibly been affected by the surgical procedure. This is particularly important in surgeries where sutures or any other surgical material may have been placed deep into the muscles or close to the nerves. Permanent sutures or permanent surgical material such as mesh may cause irritation to the muscles or nerves. Direct nerve injury, although rare, also needs to be anticipated. Furthermore, it needs to be determined if this surgical material needs to be removed, and if yes what is the best route to remove it. The surgical report should also be scrutinized to identify if there are any descriptions of difficulties or complications encountered during the procedure.

Pathology Reports

Examining the pathology report may be especially important in cases of endometriosis. Too often patients have multiple surgeries for presumed endometriosis, but there are no pathology reports present that corroborate the diagnosis of endometriosis. Pathology reports are also very important in patients with pain caused by pelvic mesh placement who had mesh removal surgery. The pathology report will specify the size of the removed piece and therefore will allow the treating physician to determine whether the entire piece was removed or if there is any mesh left behind.

Radiology Reports

Other medical records that are important to review may include radiological reports. Pelvic MRI may be helpful in diagnosing conditions such as pelvic congestion, pelvic masses, deep infiltrating endometriosis, abdominal wall endometriosis, hernias, ovarian remnant, and nerve compression. Radiological imaging is not very accurate for determining the presence of permanent sutures and mesh. Pelvic and abdominal ultrasound may also be useful in ruling out conditions such as abdominal and pelvic masses, ovarian remnant, as well as pelvic congestion. Both MRI and ultrasound require experienced radiologists and sometimes it may be useful to have the existing study be reviewed by another radiologist with excellent knowledge of pelvic pain and pelvic pathology.

Other Specialty Consultations

One needs to be careful in reviewing the notes of other providers, as providers of other specialties may not be experts in pelvic pain; thus the results of these consultations should be interpreted with caution. On the other hand, reports from pelvic floor physical therapists are very important and often have invaluable insight to the patient's pain.

Laboratory Tests

Blood and urine test results are rarely helpful. One of the exceptions is in the case of ovarian remnant syndrome in a premenopausal patient who has had the contralateral ovary removed. In this case serum hormone levels (follicle-stimulating hormone, estradiol) may reveal premenopausal levels.

By far the most important case in which to review medical records, as previously mentioned, is in patients with pain that originated after placement of pelvic mesh. These patients often have more than one type of mesh kit placed either for prolapse or incontinence. Additionally, it is important to determine if these patients have already had parts of the mesh removed. One needs to be familiar with all types of meshes used in pelvic surgery, points of attachments, technique of placement, and anatomical correlations of mesh and pelvic nerves/muscles. As mesh is very difficult to identify on radiological tests, a surgeon who is planning to remove the patient's mesh must have a clear understanding of how much mesh is left in situ and where it is located.

Pelvic MRI

One of the most useful radiological tests in diagnosing causes of pelvic pain is pelvic MRI. It has the potential of demonstrating pelvic congestion, deep infiltrating endometriosis in the rectovaginal septum, endometriosis in the adnominal wall layers, pelvic and abdominal masses, spinal abnormalities, and nerve compression. Routine MRI on every patient with pelvic pain may not be warranted, but if the patient has no diagnosis despite workup this test should be ordered. It is important, though, to communicate with the radiologist regarding the presumed pathology before ordering the study, as multiple protocols exist for MRI and the correct test must be ordered.

From the author's experience there have been multiple cases where diagnosis was very difficult to establish. After discussing the case with a radiologist

Table 21.5 Medical records to review

Operative reports	Indications for surgery Positioning Location of incisions Retractors used Structures operated Surgical materials used Mesh type, location, and amount removed
Pathology reports	Confirm endometriosis Confirm amount of mesh removed Confirm removal of ovarian remnant
Radiology reports	MRI – pelvic congestion, deep infiltrating endometriosis, pelvic masses, nerve compression
Other specialty consultations	Need to be carefully interpreted since few providers have deep knowledge of pelvic pain Pelvic floor physical therapist reports may have important insight to the patient's pain
Laboratory tests	Rarely helpful with the exception of premenopausal patients with suspected ovarian remnant syndrome in whom the contralateral ovary has been removed

Table 21.6 MRI protocols for various pain causing conditions

Condition	Protocol	Comments
Pelvic congestion syndrome	Dedicated pelvic time resolving MRA angiogram w/wo contrast	Assessment of early arterial enhancement of dilated gonadal veins and parauterine, paravaginal venous plexus
Deep infiltrating endometriosis	Dedicated MRI female protocol w/wo, vaginal and rectal contrast enhancement	Evaluation of the uterus, adnexa, deep pelvic spaces, ligaments, rectovaginal septum, and colonic wall for endometriosis
Endometriosis of the abdominal wall	Dedicated MRI female protocol w/wo, + vaginal contrast to include abdominal wall in the FOV	Assessment of abdominal wall endometriosis
Pelvic/ abdominal masses	Dedicated MRI female protocol w/wo, + vaginal contrast	Assessment of uterine, cervical, ovarian, and vaginal pathology
Spinal abnormalities	Dedicated MRI of lumbosacral spine w/wo contrast	Evaluation of disk level, neural foramen
Nerve compression	Dedicated pudendal MRI w/wo contrast	High-resolution T2 andT1 WI in paraxial and paracoronal planes, dynamic axial contrast enhanced examination for evaluation of neurovascular bundle morphology, course, and pathology

well versed in pelvic pathology, specific protocol pelvic MRI helped establish the underlying etiology of the pelvic pain.

Selective Nerve Blocks

In some patients the diagnosis of pain has been narrowed to nerve injury. In these patients pain usually begins after some traumatic event such as sport trauma, accident, childbirth, or surgery. Pain is usually localized, burning, and tingling in nature. Patients often have allodynia, which is pain in response to a stimulus that is normally not painful. If the nerve also has a motor component there may be motor deficit noted as well. Unfortunately, with the significant overlap of innervation in the pelvis it is at times difficult to determine which nerve is responsible for the patient's pain. In these cases, selective pelvic nerve blocks may be very helpful. These blocks must be completed with radiological guidance to ensure that the proper nerve is being blocked. The majority of pelvic nerves can be blocked using ultrasound guidance, but some nerves are better blocked with CT guidance. Blocks done with local anesthetic and steroid serve mostly diagnostic purposes, but there may also be therapeutic benefit, as the steroid can decrease inflammation around the nerve.

Autonomic Nerve Blocks

When laparoscopic assessment and somatic nerve blocks have failed to provide the diagnosis for the patient's pain, it may be appropriate to offer patients autonomic nerve blocks. For pelvic pain they include the superior hypogastric plexus (SHP) block, inferior hypogastric plexus block, and the ganglion impar block. These blocks are usually performed by anesthesiologists specialized in the treatment of pain or interventional radiologists and are completed under fluoroscopic or CT guidance.

The superior hypogastric plexus is located anterior to the bifurcation of the aorta. It receives sympathetic contribution from L3–L4 lumbar splanchnic nerves and parasympathetic contribution from S2–S4 pelvic splanchnic nerves. Inferiorly the SHP forms the right and left hypogastric nerves, which continue into the pelvis to form right and left inferior hypogastric plexi. In patients with genitourinary cancer who receive SHP block, almost 80% have a positive response to a diagnostic block and more than 70% have significant reduction in pain following neurolytic block. This number remains almost unchanged at 6 months follow-up.

The inferior hypogastric plexus (IHP) is paired and located on either side of the rectum and vagina. It is a continuation of the hypogastric nerves. IHP block has been shown to help in patients with endometriosis, bladder pain, and rectal pain.

The ganglion impar is formed by the convergence of the right and left sympathetic trunks in front of the coccyx. It provides sympathetic innervation to the coccygeal, perineal, and rectal area. Ganglion impar block has been shown to help with pain in the rectum, anus, distal urethra, distal third of the vagina, and vulva. In one study patients with nonmalignant pelvic pain there was 50% reduction in pain lasting on average 2.2 months [4].

Sacral Nerve Stimulation

Sacral neuromodulation is a well-established treatment for patients with urinary dysfunction. The most commonly used device (InterStim) involves insertion of electrodes in the third and/or fourth sacral foramen next to the nerve root. Sacral nerve stimulation is currently not FDA approved for treatment of chronic pain; however, there are several studies that have shown promising results [11].

Spinal Cord Stimulation

The use of spinal cord stimulation (SCS) is well established in the treatment of neuropathic pain from various conditions such as complex regional pain syndrome, failed back surgery syndrome, and ischemic limb pain. SCS provides analgesia through electrical stimulation of the dorsal column of the spinal cord via electrode leads placed into the epidural space. It is currently FDA approved for the treatment of neuropathic pain of the trunk and lower limbs. Outcomes

have been favorable for the treatment of the aforementioned conditions. SCS may be beneficial for treatment of select patients with neuropathic pelvic pain [12].

Hysterectomy for Chronic Pelvic Pain

Preforming hysterectomy for chronic pelvic pain is one of the most controversial issues in gynecology. Different providers have different conflicting options on the outcomes of hysterectomy in patients with pelvic pain. Unfortunately, the research and literature are not helpful either, as published results are conflicting. One of the first studies was published by Stovall in 1990. He reported on long-term outcomes of hysterectomy preformed on 99 women for idiopathic chronic pelvic pain. This study found that 78% of women had significant improvement in pain 12–64 months after surgery [5]. Another study preformed 5 years later on 308 women by Hillis and colleagues found that 74% of women with pelvic pain a year after hysterectomy had complete resolution of pain, 21% of women had a decrease of pain, and in 5% pain was unchanged or worsened [6]. In certain subgroups – women who were younger than 30 years of age, who were uninsured or on Medicaid, who did not have identifiable pathology, and who had a history of pelvic inflammatory disease – 40% of patients continued to be in pain after hysterectomy. Both of those studies proved that hysterectomy is more effective when hysterectomy is done for identifiable disease that is causing pelvic pain.

A study of quality of life and sexual functioning in women with preoperative pain and depression was performed in 1,200 women who underwent hysterectomy [7]. They were monitored up to 24 months after surgery. It was found that 78%–86% of women with preoperative pain, depression, or both reported improvement in pain after surgery. Also 50%–52% of women reported improvement in mental, physical, and social function and 60% reported decrease in dyspareunia. It is also debated whether ovaries should be removed in patients with pelvic pain. This is discussed in chapter 7.

Centralized Pain and Complex Regional Pain Syndrome

Central pain may be one of the most difficult pain conditions to treat. In patients with central pain and central sensitization the central nervous system amplifies sensory inputs from many organ systems and treatment of peripheral organ only rarely leads to resolution of pain. In those cases in which patients continue to be in pain despite successful treatment of organic causes of pain the treating physician concludes that patient must be fabricating pain. Some patients with pelvic pain demonstrate many features of complex regional pain syndrome [8]. Those are pain in response to minor stimulus, pain exacerbated by movement, pain improved by sympathetic block. Minor stimuli in pelvic pain may be ovulation, minimal adhesions, and minimal endometriosis. Disruptions of sympathetic pathways that are helpful in patients with pelvic pain are presacral neurectomy, superior and interior hypogastric plexus block, and ganglion impar block.

Ketamine infusions have been shown to be helpful in patients with centralized pain and complex regional pain syndrome [9].

Psychosomatic Pain

Psychosomatic disorders are conditions in which physical diseases have mental component derived from stresses of everyday living. Chronic pain is certainly one of the best described conditions that may be caused by stressful and traumatic events of the past. It has been estimated that 40%–60% of women with chronic pain have a history of being abused during childhood or adulthood [10]. This is twice to four times higher than in the general population.

Use Discussion Boards

Sometimes despite multiple diagnostic procedures a diagnosis still cannot be reached. Fortunately, there are several chronic pelvic pain discussion boards for providers where information and ideas can be exchanged. One of the best discussion boards is managed by the International Pelvic Pain Society (pelvic pain.org). This society is composed of physicians from multiple medical fields as well as numerous pelvic floor physical therapists; thus discussion board questions are answered by specialists from numerous medical fields. Another frequently used discussion board is managed by AAGL (aagl.com). This society of minimally invasive gynecological surgeons is composed of several physicians who specialize in pelvic pain.

There are also numerous support groups and discussion boards for patients. These boards are usually not monitored by healthcare professionals. Often, information exchanged on these boards is inaccurate and should not be used by physicians; however, physicians should be aware that patients are reading them and may be receiving incorrect information.

Many patients arrive to their medical appointments already having researched their condition and their physician on the internet. Physicians themselves are often discussed and ranked on these patient-targeted discussion boards.

Refer the Patient Out

If despite all the tests and treatments the patient still has no relief of her pain, the best course of action might be to refer the patient out to the specialized pelvic pain center. There are several renowned practices in the United States and abroad who specifically see patients for chronic pelvic pain, and the knowledge and resources available to them allow for much better care of patients with chronic pelvic pain. One of the societies most involved in chronic pelvic pain is International Pelvic Pain Society (pel vicpain.org). Their website lists providers (physicians and physical therapists) who have an interest in seeing patients with pelvic pain. Another good resource is website of Women's Section of American Physical Therapy Association (women shealthapta.org).

When referring a patient for psychiatric treatment, it is important not to lead the patient to believe that the root cause of her pain is psychiatric. It very rarely is. A patient who is told that the pain is "in her head" makes her feel as though medical providers don't believe that her pain is real. Moreover, when a patient's family member learns that the patient is being referred to a psychiatrist the family may blame the patient for "making her pain up." A patient's partner, especially, may feel that the patient is using her pain to avoid sexual intimacy.

Offer Random Treatment

Sometimes even if the patient does not have a diagnosis it is better to offer random treatment rather than doing nothing. If the treatment helps it may lead to the correct diagnosis. This diagnosis by treatment is called *ex juvantibus* in Latin. One of the more commonly used treatments without diagnosis is gonadotropin-releasing hormone analogs for presumed endometriosis. Other treatments may include doing pelvic nerve blocks or botulinum toxin A injections to the pelvic floor. The data remain limited on these treatment modalities; however, our patients have had excellent success with both pelvic nerve blocks and botulinum toxin A injections into the pelvic floor. Please refer to Chapters 15, 16, and 20 for additional information.

Alternative medical treatments that may be beneficial include platelet rich plasma injections into the pelvic floor, cannabidiols, acupuncture and dry needling. The literature is very limited on the use of these therapies for pelvic pain; however, these are safe interventions that patients may explore and find beneficial.

Psychological Treatments

Nonpharmacological interventions such as exercise, mindfulness, and cognitive behavioral therapy (CBT) have been shown in several studies to improve pain, function, and quality of life in patients with chronic pain. These interventions target the experience as well as the psychosocial sequalae of pain [13]. CBT has traditionally been the first-line psychological intervention; however, in recent years mindfulness has been used increasingly for the treatment of chronic pain as well as other medical conditions. Preliminary studies have shown similar beneficial outcomes from both CBT and mindfulness treatments [14]. For patients who do not have access to a trained psychologist there are several smartphone apps on the market that provide guided mindfulness treatments. Psychological interventions may be especially useful adjuvants for patients with a history of trauma. Larger randomized control trials are needed to detail the efficacy of psychological interventions compared to first-line biomedical treatments for chronic pain.

Five Things You Need to Know
- If all else fails, consider starting fresh and reexamining all the evidence from the beginning.
- Pelvic pain is often myofascial and assessment by knowledgeable pelvic floor physical therapist or physiatrist may be invaluable.
- Most of the patients have more than one reason for pain and all the causes have to be identified. Treatments often fail because not all causes of pain are addressed.
- One of the most important questions to ask is how did the pain start – was it trauma related, menstrual cycle related, instant, or did it happen over time?
- Treat *ex juvantibus*. Sometimes when everything else fails institute the treatment you think may help and if it does establish the diagnosis based on that treatment.

References

1. Mathias SD, Kuppermann M, Liberman RF, Lipschutz RC, Steege JF. Chronic pelvic pain: prevalence, health-related quality of life, and economic correlates. *Obstet. Gynecol.* 1996;**87**:321–7.
2. Chung MK, Chung RP, Gordon D. Interstitial cystitis and endometriosis in patients with chronic pelvic pain: the 'Evil Twins' syndrome. *JSLS.* 2005;**9**:25–9.
3. Gyang A, Hartman M, Lamvu G. Musculoskeletal causes of chronic pelvic pain. *Obstet. Gynecol.* 2013;**121**:645–50.
4. Reig E, Abejón D, Del Pozo C, Insausti J, Contreras R. Thermocoagulation of the ganglion impar or ganglion of Walther: description of a modified approach. Preliminary results in chronic, nononcological pain. *Pain Pract.* 2005;**5**:103–10.
5. Stovall TG, Ling FW, Crawford DA. Hysterectomy for chronic pelvic pain of presumed uterine etiology. *Obstet. Gynecol.* 1990;**75**:676–9.
6. Hillis SD, Marchbanks PA, Peterson HB. The effectiveness of hysterectomy for chronic pelvic pain. *Obstet. Gynecol.* 1995;**86**:941–5.
7. Hartmann KE, Ma C, Lamvu GM, Langenberg PW, Steege JF, Kjerulff KH. Quality of life and sexual function after hysterectomy in women with preoperative pain and depression. *Obstet. Gynecol.* 2004;**104**:701–9.
8. Janicki TI. Chronic pelvic pain as a form of complex regional pain syndrome. *Clin Obstet Gynecol.* 2003;**46**:797–803.
9. Correll GE, Maleki J, Gracely EJ, Muir JJ, Harbut RE. Subanesthetic ketamine infusion therapy: a retrospective analysis of a novel therapeutic approach to complex regional pain syndrome. *Pain Med.* 2004;**5**:263–275. DOI: 10.1111/j.1526-4637.2004.04043.x.
10. Rubin JJ. Psychosomatic pain: new insights and management strategies. *South Med J.* 2005;**98**:1092–1099, 1138.
11. Mahran, A, Baaklini G, Hassani D, et al. Sacral neuromodulation treating chronic pelvic pain: a meta-analysis and systematic review of the literature. *Int Urogynecol J.* 2019;**30**:339–52.
12. Song JJ, Popescu A, Bell RL. Present and potential use of spinal cord stimulation to control chronic pain. *Pain Physician.* 2014;**3**:235–46.
13. Till SR, Wahl HN, As-Sanie S. The role of nonpharmacologic therapies in management of chronic pelvic pain: what to do when surgery fails. *Curr Opin Obstet Gynecol.* 2017;**4**:231–9.
14. Dunkley CR, Brotto LA. Psychological treatment for provoked vestibulodynia: integration of

Index